BEATING CANCER WITH NUTRITION

Optimal nutrition can improve outcome in
medically treated cancer patients

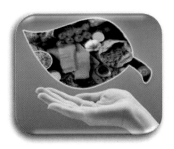

Patrick Quillin

Nutrition Times Press, Inc.
Copyright 2020

ISBN 978-1-7352347-0-0

Printed in the United States of America.

Bulk purchases of this book available through:
Bookmasters, 800-247-6553

Nutrition Times Press, Inc.
Box 130789
Carlsbad, CA 92013
Ph.760-804-5703
Email: support@gettinghealthier.com

IMPORTANT NOTICE
   This book is intended for educational purposes only and is not to be considered a substitute for appropriate medical treatment. Every effort has been made to insure accuracy of facts and details, but publisher and author assume no liability for errors in printing and changes in websites. Patient profiles are real people, most of whom, the author worked with. These profiles are not typical.   No results are guaranteed.
   Many books, organizations, products, websites, clinics, and people are mentioned in this book. No one paid to be listed here.

Table of Contents

Dedicated to

Claude Bernard "Doc" Pennington
(1900-1997)
For belief in my project to write
the first version of this book. Thank
you for your generosity.

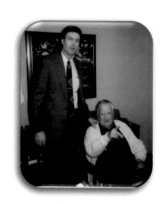

Thank You!

Camille Hughes, for your awesome computer talents in making this book a professional package.

Hugh Riordan, MD (1932-2005) for your trailblazing courage in moving the frontiers of the healing arts forward.

Adelle Davis (1904-1974), for your books that inspired me to enter the complex and rewarding field of nutrition.

T. Townsend Brown, for your support, gentle spirit, and giving me "shelter from the storm".

Jeffrey Bland, PhD, for your leadership in functional medicine.

Carol Rapson, for giving me an opportunity to start a new life.

Bill and Mary McNulty, for sending me out west.

Rob Fagot, for sending me in the right direction.

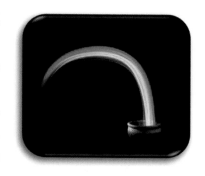

Ty and Charlene Bollinger, for your brilliant and relentless quest to bring The Truth About Cancer to the public.

Chapter 1

YOU HAVE ALREADY BEATEN CANCER
AND YOU CAN DO IT AGAIN

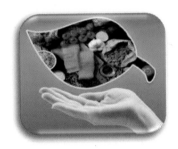

"The doctor of the future will give no medicine, but will interest his patient in the care of the human frame, in diet and in the cause and prevention of disease."
Thomas Edison, inventor the light bulb and over 1,000 patents, 1903

You have already beaten cancer. While millions of people have died from this dreaded disease and trillions of dollars spent on research and therapies, you have within you the ability to beat cancer. The purpose of this book is to awaken the healer within you.

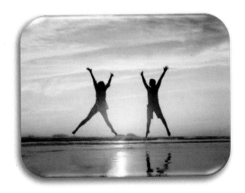

First proposed by Erhlich in 1909, the surveillance theory of cancer has been well accepted by scientists worldwide.[1] Your intact immune system recognizes and destroys the inevitable tumor cells that crop up daily. By one estimate, each of your 37 trillion cells experiences 5,000-10,000 DNA "hits" per day or potentially cancer-causing damage from free radicals. Yet, your body finds and repairs these DNA hits.

There is a mysterious yet irreplaceable force in all of life that "knows" how to heal itself. The broken bone, the scab on your arm, the baby being made in that woman's uterus, the ability of children to regenerate a severed fingertip--all tell us that Nature has an incredible plan for good health and long life. But only if those same natural forces within us have been given the raw building blocks of physical nutrients and meta-physical thoughts and feelings, plus relative freedom from toxic blockages.

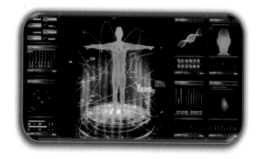

Pregnancy is not a 9-month illness to be cured by a doctor. Heart disease is not caused by a deficiency of statin drugs. Cancer is not caused by a deficiency of chemo drugs. Heart disease, cancer, wounds, infections, arthritis, and other conditions are abnormalities. Restore your body's ability to regulate itself, and these common ailments oftentimes will disappear. Reverse the obesity and the diabetes goes away. Eliminate the offending food and allergies clear up. Fix the underlying cause of cancer, and the cancer can clear up.

MIRACLES OF MODERN MEDICINE

If you are in a car accident, then head to the nearby big city emergency center for the best medical care the world has ever seen. If you have a bacterial infection that has a targeted antibiotic, then you are in luck with modern medicine. However, if you are among the 99% of medical patients who suffer from a degenerative disease (e.g. heart disease, cancer, diabetes, auto-immune, fatty liver, mental illness) then:

"Modern medicine is based on a lie."
Dale Bredesen, MD, UCLA, author THE END OF ALZHEIMER'S

Micro surgery, 3 D printing of spare body parts, DNA cloning, targeted gene therapy, telemedicine, computer simulated drug development, and more are all noteworthy accomplishments of modern medicine. Yet your body has innate mechanisms of self-regulation and self-repair that are poorly understood by the brightest minds on the planet earth. We cannot reproduce this wonder of healing. But we can encourage it. That is what this book is all about.

88% of Americans have some metabolic disorder. 2/3 of Americans are overweight. The incidence of diabetes has skyrocketed from the rare rich obese man to now 30 million Americans have it and another 60 million are prediabetic. Nearly 6 million Americans have Alzheimer's disease. In one generation autism incidence has grown from 1 in 5,000 to now 1 in 59. Cancer incidence has increased from 1% of deaths in 1900 to 24% of deaths in 2017. Technology and our modern lifestyle have come with a cost.

Genetics shows us that you look something like some of your ancestors. Hard wired information that is irreversible. Epigenetics shows us that much of our lifestyle plays a powerful role in modifying our genetic risk factors for disease. Soft programming, or epigenetics, says that we can literally change the way our body works.

CANCER OVERTAKES SICKER AND WEAKER CELLS.

In the Disney movie, "Never Cry Wolf", a biologist was assigned the task of observing wolves in the Arctic north to see if wolves were killing the elk, and whether the wolves must be killed. The biologist found that wolves primarily eat rodents, such as mice and rats. When the wolf pack ran down a herd of elk, the wolves caught and ate the slowest and sickest of the elk herd. The biologist ran out to the elk carcass that the wolves had finished feasting on, broke off a piece of ribbing, and found that the elk had been suffering from leukemia. In other words, the wolves pruned the sick and feeble in the elk herd. Similarly, cancer and infections attack a feeble and compromised host. Cancer cannot invade a healthy body. Make your body healthy, and the cancer simply

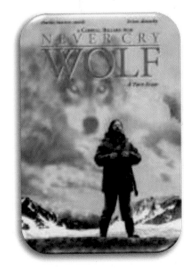

goes away. Improve the health of the elk herd, and the wolves cannot catch the healthy ones. Only the sick elk (or body cells) are vulnerable to the wolves (or cancer).

In the 2020 Covid virus global pandemic, it was found that the average age of death for Covid victims was 78. The average lifespan in America is 78. Over 90% of the victims were both old and had underlying medical conditions, such as diabetes, heart disease, etc. Over 50% of the deaths were in 1% of the counties in the US. 99% of those infected recovered. And the authorities shut down everything. Unprecedented in American history. Covid-19 was an opportunistic infection that attacked the frail. So does cancer. This book will show you how to get your body so healthy that cancer is unwelcome in your body.

CANCER IN A HOST AS A SEED IN THE SOIL

If you drop a watermelon seed on the concrete, then the seed will not grow, because the conditions required for growth (warm temperature, fertile soil and moisture) have not been met. For decades, American doctors have spent 100% of their time trying to kill the "seed", or the cancer cell. Yet Antoine Bechamp (1816-1908), a French biologist, was the first to notice that the "soil" or the environment on which the yeast or bacteria fell was crucial in germinating the disease.

Dr. Stephen Paget wrote in *Lancet* in 1889 "Cancer metastasis involves a complicated biochemical 'conversation' between the seed and the soil." Professor Bruce Ames at the University of California Berkeley has shown that cancer can be generated in animals simply by depriving the animal of certain nutrients, which results in "biochemical chaos" and cancer.

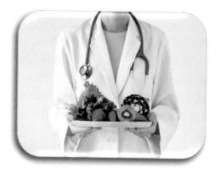

Oncologist Isaiah Fidler at the MD Anderson Cancer Center in Houston has recently added his endorsement of this "seed and soil" theory in cancer: "The time has come to put major emphasis on the soil." The "soil" is your body which is highly dependent on the nutrients in your diet.

WHAT IS YOUR VITALITY RATING?

Your body is composed of 37 trillion well-orchestrated cells that perform miracles each and every second. Your body is built from food that you have consumed over your lifetime, plus the inevitable toxins that come with living in 21st century developed nations. When you are young, well-nourished, rested, well-exercised, free of toxins and negative emotions, excited about life, trusting of your surroundings, with something to do, someone to love, and something to look forward to--then your vitality rating is high. It is unlikely that you will get cancer or any other disease. You can be around infected people and not get an infection. You can live in an invisible sea of allergenic substances (pollen, dust, mold) and not get an allergic sneezing attack.

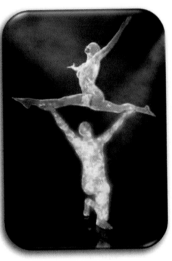

When we live on highly refined junk food that is full of toxins and does not provide our body with the necessary nutrients for optimal health, when we feel imprisoned, when we consume more toxins than our body can neutralize or eliminate, when we do not get the prerequisite of exercise--then our bodies lose that magical self-regenerating ability. Heart disease, diabetes, or cancer may be the result. If you have cancer, then your vitality rating is low. This book has information that will help you boost your vitality rating. You will at least become a healthier cancer patient. Ideally, you will become cancer-free.

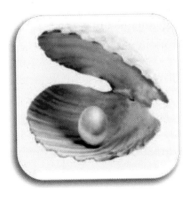

A clam has two pieces to its protective shell. Imagine if one piece of that shell is your physical protection: proper nutrient intake, exercise, avoidance of chemical toxins, and proper alignment of your body structure and energy meridians. The second half of that clam shell is represented by your metaphysical protection: love, connection to others, sense of purpose in life, fun things to do, pleasure, and relying on a Higher Power. Put the two shell halves together and the clam is well protected. If either side is missing, the fragile clam body becomes vulnerable to infections and predators. If either side of your "non-specific host defense mechanisms" (physical or metaphysical) is missing, then you become vulnerable to cancer and other ailments.

Through the information provided in this book, we are going to restore the protective and recuperative powers that are yours. To finish the clam metaphor, a pearl is a beautiful and valuable item that starts out as an irritation in the clam, which is covered by multiple layers of calcium that only the clam can make. My hope is that the irritation of cancer will be covered over by your miraculous healing abilities so that when the cancer is gone, all that is left is a "pearl" that improves your life.

The bad news about all of this "vitality rating" and personal involvement in cancer recovery is that we will never develop a magic bullet drug for all cancer patients. The good news is that you can become actively involved in your healing process.

CRISIS=DANGER + OPPORTUNITY

"Cancer is the best thing that ever happened to me." The words almost knocked me over. I was listening to the testimonials from several cancer survivors who had gathered in a class reunion to celebrate life. These people later went on to explain this strange statement. "My life wasn't working. I didn't take care of my body. I didn't eat right. I didn't get enough rest. I didn't like my job, or myself, or those around me. I didn't appreciate life. I rarely stopped to smell the roses along the way. I asked too much of myself. I was too busy. Cancer was a great big red light flashing on the dashboard of my car saying 'pull this vehicle over and fix it now.'"

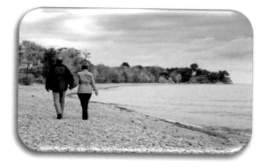

These cancer victors had shown the ultimate courage by turning adversity into a major victory. In Oriental language, "crisis" is written by two characters, one meaning "danger" and the other meaning "opportunity". Cancer is a crisis of unparalleled proportions, both for the individual and for humanity. For a minority of cancer patients, cancer has become an extraordinary opportunity to convert their lives into a masterpiece.

THE BIG CANCER PICTURE

Cancer is now the number one cause of death in America, surpassing heart disease as of January 2005. About 17 million Americans alive today have been treated or are still in treatment for cancer. By some estimates, about 8 million Americans are currently in the cancer "pipeline" or in treatment or watchful observation.

Each year, over 1.6 million more Americans are newly diagnosed with cancer with another 5 million skin cancers that are treated on an outpatient basis at the doctor's office. Half of all cancer patients in general are alive after five years. 42% of Americans living today can expect to develop cancer in his or her lifetime. Today, 24% of Americans die from cancer--a sharp contrast to the 1% who died from cancer in the year 1900. Europe has an even higher incidence of cancer. For the past four decades, both the incidence and age-adjusted death rate from cancer in America have been steadily climbing. Some people claim that the recent very modest improvements in cancer survival are explained by earlier diagnosis from more cancer screening procedures such as PSA, colonoscopy, breast exam, etc. Ironically, amidst the high-tech wizardry of modern medicine, at least 40% of cancer patients will die from malnutrition, not the cancer itself. This book highlights proven scientific methods that use nutrition to:

- ◆ Prevent or reverse the common malnutrition that plagues cancer patients.
- ◆ Make the medical therapies of chemotherapy and radiation more of a selective toxin to the cancer while protecting the patient from damage.
- ◆ Bolster the cancer patient's immune system to provide a microscopic army of warriors to fight the cancer throughout the body, because when the doctor says: "We think we got it all" that's when we are relying on a well-nourished immune system to locate, recognize, and destroy the inevitable remaining cancer cells.
- ◆ Help to selectively starve sugar-feeding tumor cells by altering intake of sugar, blood glucose levels, and circulating insulin.
- ◆ Slow down cancer with high doses of nutrients that make the body more resistant to invasion from tumor cells, aka using nutrition factors as biological response modifiers.

All of this good news means that cancer patients who use the comprehensive therapies described in this book may expect significant improvement in quality and quantity of life, and chances for a complete remission--by changing the underlying conditions that brought about the cancer. Cancer is an abnormal growth, not just a regionalized lump or bump. Chemo, radiation, and surgery will reduce tumor burden, but do nothing to change the underlying conditions that allowed this abnormal growth to thrive. In a nutshell, this book is designed to change the conditions in the body that favor tumor growth and return the cancer victor to a healthier status. More wellness in the body means less illness. We are going to take your body beyond surviving and into thriving.

Once Louis Pasteur discovered how to kill bacteria by heat processing (pasteurization), he embarked upon an energetic but ultimately frustrating career to eliminate all bacteria from the planet earth. Didn't work. And a century later, after the development of numerous "super drugs" to kill bacteria, Americans now have infections as the third leading cause of death, right after heart disease and cancer. Many bacteria are now drug resistant and virtually unstoppable. Similarly, after spending the last half century trying to poison the insects out of our fields with potent pesticides, we now have "super bugs" that are chemically resistant to all poisons and a net INCREASE in crop loss to insects. Same goes for cancer. We thought that we could poison the cancer out of the patient. But many

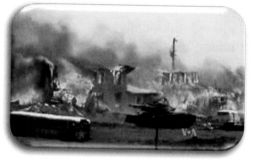

cancers develop drug resistance or hormone independence, while the toxic drugs compromise our immune systems and leave us "naked" in the battle with the cancer. Military refer to "carpet bombing" the enemy, which is to bombard repeatedly and excessively. We have tried that on cancer with more collateral damage (patient damage) than imaginable.

There is a new philosophy emerging in science and medicine. According to several articles in major cancer journals, oncologists are asking the question: "Must we kill to cure?" In the prestigious *Journal of Clinical Oncology* (April 1995, p.801), Drs. Schipper, Goh, and Wang provide a compelling argument that curing the cancer patient need not include killing the cancer cells with potent cytotoxic therapies. In many ways, from our fields to our bacterial infection patients to our cancer patients, we need to re-examine Dr. Pasteur's grand deathbed epiphany: "The terrain is everything." The terrain is your human body. Nourish it properly with nutrients, oxygen, good thoughts, and exercise, and it will perform miraculous feats of disease recovery. We don't fully understand these "non-specific host defense mechanisms", but we need to respect and utilize them. That is how we will win the "war on cancer."

HOW IS THIS BOOK DIFFERENT?

Attacking Cancer on Many Levels. A hammer, pliers, and screwdriver belong in any good tool box, just as chemo, radiation, and surgery have their place in cancer treatment. But that tool box is far from complete. There are many alternative cancer therapies that can be valuable assets in cancer treatment. This book offers other "tools" to support the basic, but incomplete, toolbox that we currently use against cancer.

This book offers a unique multi-disciplinary approach to treating cancer that is based on both scientific studies and actual clinical experience. My basic strategy is a three-pronged attack on cancer:

1) Change the cause of the cancer. Use nutrition, exercise, attitude, and detoxification to elevate the body's own internal healing abilities.

COMPREHENSIVE CANCER TREATMENT INCLUDES:

1	2	3
change underlying cause(s) of disease	restrained tumor debulking	symptom management
NUTRITION	CHEMO?	PAIN**
DETOXIFICATION	RADIATION?	NAUSEA
DYSBIOSIS	SURGERY?	ANOREXIA
HORMONE BAL.	IV Vit C	ANEMIA
HYPERGLYCEMIA	CURCUMIN	LEUKOPENIA
INFECTIONS	Oxygen/OZONE	DEPRESSION
STRESS	BURZYNSKI	CACHEXIA
EXERCISE	HYPERTHERM	HAIR LOSS
ENERGY PATHWAYS	ALKALINIZE	
ETC.	PEMF	
	HERBALS	

2) Restrained tumor debulking. Reduce cancer burden with chemo, radiation, hyperthermia, and other appropriate therapies.

3) Symptom management. Cancer can bring many symptoms that make life a purgatory. There are many allopathic and naturopathic therapies to manage the symptoms and make the disease and medical treatments more tolerable.

4) Avoid tunnel vision. It is important to avoid the mistake of the past, which is to focus on one aspect of cancer treatment and forget the other potentially valuable therapies. Avoid monomania, or obsession with one "magic bullet" idea. This book pays homage to the complexities of the human body and mind and draws on many fields to provide maximum firepower against cancer. We need all the weapons we can muster, for cancer is no simple beast to kill.

NUTRITION: THE MISSING PIECE OF THE CANCER TREATMENT PUZZLE

American health care is nearing a financial "meltdown". We spent $3.6 trillion in 2018 on disease maintenance, which works out to $11,000/person which is 18% of our gross national product--twice the expense per capita of any other health care system on earth. Notice that I said "disease maintenance", because we certainly do not support health care in America, and "health insurance" is neither related to health nor solid actuarial insurance.

The most expensive disease in America is cancer at $150 billion/yr. These opulent expenses would be easier to swallow if we were obtaining impressive results. But many experts argue that we have made limited progress in the costly and lengthy "war on cancer".

By 1971, cancer had become enough of a nuisance that President Richard Nixon launched the long-awaited "war on cancer", confidently proclaiming that we would have a cure within 5 years, before the Bicentennial celebration in 1976. With over $200 billion spent on research in the past 49 years, $2 trillion spent on therapy, 600,000 deaths per year and no relief in sight from traditional therapies--it is blindingly obvious that we must re-examine some options in cancer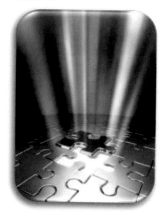

prevention and treatment. If 4 fully loaded 747 planes crashed every day, that would equal the death toll from cancer...and someone would do something to improve the situation.

Experts estimate that 45% of males and 39% of females living in America will develop cancer in their lifetime. Breast cancer has increased from one out of 20 women in the year 1950 to one out of eight women. With some cancers, notably liver, lung, pancreas, bone, and advanced breast cancer, our five-year survival rate from traditional therapy alone is virtually the same as it was 30 years ago.

This book is about options. If our current results from traditional cancer treatment were encouraging, then there would be no need for alternative therapies against cancer. Unfortunately, traditional cancer therapies have plateaued--some might say that they hit a dead-end brick wall. In many instances, the treatment is worse than the disease, with chronic nausea and vomiting, hair loss, painful mouth sores, extreme fatigue, and depression as common side effects of therapy and minimal improvements in lifespan.

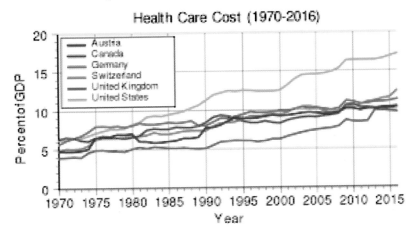

Health Care Cost (1970-2016)

Long-term complications include toxicity to the heart, kidneys, and bone marrow. While many children may recover from cancer, they are placed at much higher risk for getting cancer later in life from their cancer therapy. And if the cancer patient recovers from the disease, which is no small task, then recovering from the therapy may be even more challenging. Many patients come to me suffering from peripheral neuropathy (tingling numbness and pain in the hands and feet), after too much chemo with no nutrients to protect the delicate nerves.

Obviously, if what we are doing isn't working, then we need to look at some sensible, scientific, non-toxic, and cost-effective options that can amplify the tumor-killing abilities of traditional therapies. Nutrition is at the top of that list. Many experts call our health care crisis a "ticking time bomb". By using lifestyle medicine we can defuse that bomb.

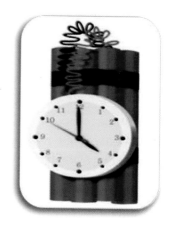

The recommendations provided in this book are scientifically-backed, time-tested, logical, and supported by my clinical observations in working with thousands of cancer patients over the course of 30 years. Follow the program outlined in this book and you, the cancer patient, can surpass the recovery predictions of your oncologist.

WHAT'S NEW IN THIS REVISED VERSION

This book was 14 years in the making and is the fifth major revision of the original 1994 version. This book is meant to be a companion to my 12 KEYS TO A HEALTHIER CANCER PATIENT, which provides an excellent overview of the epigenetic forces that can help the cancer patient with a better outcome; including attitude, nutrition, exercise, toxins, microbiome, and energy alignment. BEATING CANCER WITH NUTRITION focuses heavily on the subject of nutrition as a key component for cancer recovery.

This book is a consolidation of my 20 years of education, 40 years of professional experience, thousands of patients that I counselled, hundreds of textbooks that I have read, thousands of peer reviewed journal articles I have read, and over 600 hours of postgraduate training at seminars. Do not underestimate the power in this information.

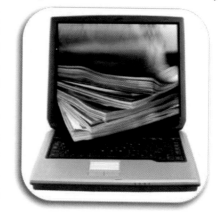

The feedback I received over the past years has helped to shape this book into its format. Plenty of color illustrations are used. "A picture is worth a thousand words." And a lot easier and more enjoyable to grasp. Large type is used since many cancer patients are older and may have compromised vision. No words are wasted in this book. Words are simply tools to bridge the gap between my mind and your mind. I am not trying to impress anyone with my vocabulary, but simply choosing the proper tool for the job.

Each of these chapters could have been a semester class in college rich in bombastic scientific language. I have spared you the trouble. This book is interactive. Those who are reading the e-book or Kindle version will be able to click on hyperlinks to visit the original study or website. This book is meant to provide you with a short, punchy, easy to read, colorful, bullet point guide to get your body back into prime healing mode. Without further ado, let's do this.

Our general axiom:

> "A well-nourished cancer patient can better manage and beat the disease."

For more information on how your body can fight cancer go to GettingHealthier.com.

PATIENT PROFILE:

L.M. was diagnosed in 1994 with late stage breast cancer. She read and followed the principles in BEATING CANCER WITH NUTRITION while using her doctor's selective tumor debulking therapies. While her prognosis had been poor, L.M. went into complete remission. L.M. attended a lecture by your author in Atlanta in November of 2018 and was delighted with her newfound health. 25 years after her death sentence, L.M. looks and feels fabulous.

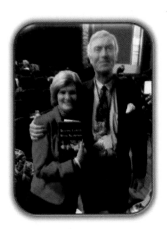

ENDNOTES

[1] https://www.jci.org/articles/view/32136

Chapter 2

SHORTCUT: EXECUTIVE SUMMARY

IF YOU ARE TOO SICK TO READ MUCH, THEN READ THIS SECTION

21 Days to a Healthier Cancer Patient

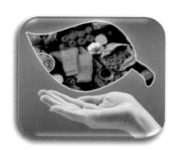

BEATING CANCER THROUGH:

DAY 1: HOPE, OPTIMISM, AND A FIGHTING SPIRIT

Focus on the parts of your body that are working properly, not on the cancer. Since you are alive enough to read this book, then something and perhaps quite a bit are working in your body. Give thanks for everything that you can think of. Thanksgiving is a healing balm on the body and soul.

What are your priorities in life? Have they changed since finding out about your cancer diagnosis? Have they changed for the better? Is it possible that cancer has become a life-threatening, yet valuable wakeup call for you?

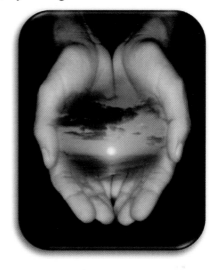

We are all going to die. The question is not "if", but rather "when". For cancer patients, sometimes this "when" becomes a more immediate issue. But our finite lives should be an issue for all of us, all of the time. Life is precious. Not to be wasted. Many of us cram our days with minutia, trivial details. We spend too much time worrying about insignificant events and lose sight of the real issues in life:

- ◆ be here now
- ◆ value your mission
- ◆ cherish your friends and family
- ◆ savor sunsets and sunrises
- ◆ soak up the beauty and music and laughter and play that is all around you, but drowned out by the cacophony of crass commercialism
- ◆ be at peace with your Creator, however you conceive that Higher Power

People beat cancer all the time. But fear of death is not a reason to live. What do you want them to say at your funeral? "Look, I think she's moving!!" Not going to happen. Begin today with a renewed sense of purpose and proper perspective for the truly memorable things in life. Build a fighting "can-do" spirit that will serve you well for the coming journey of treating your cancer. Find a "co-patient", a loved one, or family member who is so supportive that they will keep you motivated when you have run out of steam.

Be enthusiastic. The word "enthusiasm" comes from the Greek words meaning "God within". With joy, enthusiasm, appreciation, and altruism, we literally become a conduit for Divine healing power.

Chapter 2 – Executive Summary. If You Are Too Sick to Read Much...

20

DAY 2: KNOWLEDGE, OPTIONS, DATA GATHERING

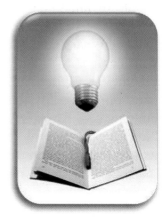

While your doctor who made the cancer diagnosis may have a plan for you, it is probably not the only therapy that is appropriate for your cancer and may not even be the best therapy. You need to explore your options. In today's society, getting information is easier than ever before. Get on the Internet and spend a few hours gathering data and phone numbers on who can help you with your particular cancer. The more knowledge that you have on the treatment and curing of your cancer, the more likely you are to make the right decision on which "wagon master" to choose for your vital treatment ahead.

Consider seeking a second and third opinion from a local doctor who has a firm grasp on nutrition, such as found in the directories on the web:

♦ The <u>Institute for Functional Medicine</u> has a website that helps you to locate a health care professional who can help you solve the mystery of etiology of disease.[1]

♦ The <u>American Association of Naturopathic Physicians</u> has a website to help you find a local talented doctor.[2]

♦ <u>Life Extension Foundation</u> has a listing of innovative practitioners.[3]

DAY 3:

THE POWER OF FULL SPECTRUM CANCER TREATMENT

White light is composed of the colors of the spectrum: red, orange, yellow, green, blue, indigo, violet...ROY G. BIV. Comprehensive cancer treatment, like the spectrum, requires all of the colors or modalities for enhanced chances of a successful outcome.

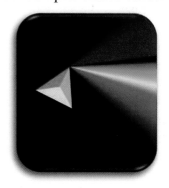

Synergism means that $1 + 1 = 3$ or 500, but a whole lot more than 2. Synergism tells us that the combined efforts of certain factors yield more than what would have been expected. Do not rely on any "magic bullet" nutrient to beat your cancer. There are no such things. Your body needs the 50 recognized essential nutrients plus a couple of hundred other valuable nutrients that can only be found in a wholesome diet that is supplemented with the right nutrients.

"What is the most important part of a car?" Some people answer: "The engine." Fine. Then I will give you an engine and let's see you drive it home. A car, like a healthy human body, is composed of many essential parts. The most important part of the car is the one that is not working. In building a house, all of the raw materials must arrive in the proper ratio at the proper time, otherwise you cannot build a sturdy home. Same thing with the human body. Nutritional synergism says that when you gather the right nutrients together at the right time in the right ratio, the body becomes a lean, mean, disease-fighting machine. Full spectrum cancer treatment employs a wide array of therapies to change the underlying causes of the disease, while using restrained tumor debulking, while managing symptoms to improve quality of life. Nothing less will do in your quest to beat cancer.

DAY 4: STARVE THE CANCER

Cancer is a sugar-feeder. The scientists call it an "obligate glucose metabolizer". You can slow cancer growth by lowering the amount of fuel available to the tumor cells. Americans have become like a moth to a flame, seeing the flame (junk food) as tasty, but failing to recognize that this junk food, especially sugar, can kill you. The resulting constant high blood 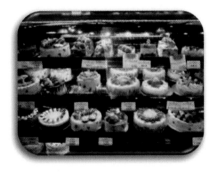 glucose levels yield many diseases, including cancer, diabetes, heart disease, hypertension, and yeast infections. Trying to beat cancer while eating a diet that constantly raises blood glucose is like trying to put out a forest fire while someone nearby is throwing gasoline on the trees.

Stop eating refined carbs, including white flour and sugar. Begin an exercise program to burn blood glucose down to a manageable level. Practice intermittent fasting, in which you narrow your feeding window to only 8 of the 24 hours in the day, then water fast for one day a week. You may develop sugar cravings worse than you currently have. Ignore them and push through the discomfort.

Chapter 2 – Executive Summary. If You Are Too Sick to Read Much...

22

Focus on a plant-based diet rich in whole fruits, vegetables, whole grains, legumes, nuts, seeds, seaweed, mushrooms. Add some yogurt, butter, grass fed meat, eggs, and wild caught fish. Use cinnamon liberally, since it helps to stabilize blood glucose. Take supplements of chromium and magnesium. To beat cancer, you must starve it of glucose.

DAY 5: AVOID MALNUTRITION

Cancer is a wasting disease. Over 40% of cancer patients actually die from malnutrition, not from the cancer. Cancer generates chemicals that lower appetite while increasing calorie needs. The net effect is that many cancer patients begin to lose weight. You cannot fight a life-threatening disease while malnourished. You need all the proper nutrition you can get to feed your immune system, which is your army assigned to killing the cancer cells. The backbone of the immune system is protein. If you cannot eat solid foods, then try the Dragon-slayer shake mentioned later in this book.

DAY 6:
NUTRITION + MEDICINE= IMPROVED RESULTS

While chemotherapy and radiation can kill cancer cells, these therapies are general toxins against your body cells also. A well-nourished cancer patient can protect healthy cells against the toxic effects of chemo and radiation, thus making the cancer cells more vulnerable to the medicine. Proper nutrition can make chemo and radiation more of a selective toxin against the cancer and less damaging to the patient.

DAY 7: TURBOCHARGE YOUR IMMUNE SYSTEM

Your immune system consists of 20 trillion cells that compose your police force and garbage collectors. The immune system is responsible for killing the bad guys, any cells that are not participating in the processes of your body, including cancer, yeast, bacteria, virus, and dead cells. "Kill the bad guys and take out the trash." That is what your immune system 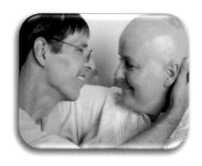 is supposed to do. But since you have cancer, something is wrong with your immune system: usually either stress, toxic burden, or malnutrition.

Eat well and take professionally designed nutrition supplements. Lower your stress levels. Use guided imagery to imagine your immune cells like sharks gobbling up the cancer cells. Detoxify your body. The average American body has 1,000 times more heavy toxic metals than our primitive ancestors before the dawning of the industrial age. Toxins shut down the ability of the immune system to mount a good battle against the cancer cells.

As your cells divide billions of times daily, mistake cells are the inevitable consequence. These mistake cells sometimes grow into cancer cells, which your immune system recognizes as being defective and then gobbles them up. The average adult gets 6 bouts of cancer in a lifetime, yet only 42% of Americans will end up in a cancer hospital. The other 58% had a competent immune system, which protected the person against defective cells rising up to become palpable life-threatening cancer. Get your immune system working and the end of your cancer is in sight. That is what this book is all about.

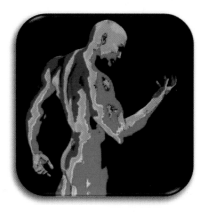

DAY 8: THE HEALING POWER OF WHOLE FOODS

It is amazing how simple the answer to cancer can be. Our brilliant researchers have spent almost a half century and $200 billion of your tax dollars at the NIH wrestling with the complex issue of curing cancer. Yet Nature has been solving the dilemma for thousands of years. All of us get cancer all of the time, yet magical ingredients in a whole food diet are there to help the body beat cancer. Ellagic acid from berries induces "suicide" in the cancer cells. Lycopenes from tomatoes help to suppress cancer growth. Genistein in soy, glutathione in green leafy vegetables, and S-allyl cysteine in garlic are examples of the new scientifically-validated cancer fighters of the 21st century.

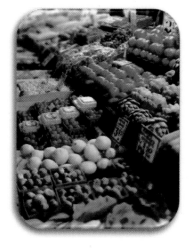

Chapter 2 – Executive Summary. If You Are Too Sick to Read Much...

24

You don't have to wait for 7 years while some drug company goes through the $800 million drug approval process, nor for FDA approval, nor for a doctor's prescription for some drug that has many toxic side effects and costs thousands of dollars each month. These miracle anti-cancer agents are waiting patiently at your nearby grocery store and health food store.

- ◆ Eat foods as close to their natural state as is possible.
- ◆ Eat as much colorful vegetables as your colon can tolerate.
- ◆ If a food will not rot or sprout, then throw it out.
- ◆ Shop the perimeter (outside aisles) of the grocery store.

DAY 9: NUTRITIOUS AND DELICIOUS RECIPES

Now that you understand the importance of eating wholesome foods to beat your cancer, you will need some tips on making this food palatable. You are trying to take simple food straight from Nature and use healthy seasonings to make a quick and tasty meal. Crock pot, pressure cooker, steaming, and grilling are all wonderful means of cooking nourishing foods. Some produce is most nutritious when eaten raw, such as many vegetables and all 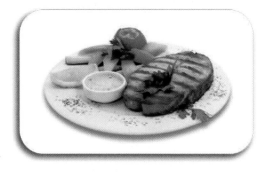 fruit. A high-speed blender can take any leftovers or foods that are not appealing and blend them in to a smoothie drink or a nice soup.

Your will be surprised at how delicious and nutritious the recipe section can be. You do not have to sacrifice flavor to get well. Food as medicine. Accept the concept that food can deliver all that you need: health and taste. Foods that are easy to prepare, and easy to find at your local grocery store. And it will help you to beat your cancer. See the chapter on Quick and Easy Recipes.

DAY 10: HERBAL MEDICINE

There are thousands of herbs that have been used for thousands of years to treat cancer. None are guaranteed cures for all cancers, but many are non-toxic boosters of immune function and detoxification pathways. Garlic--as a food, seasoning, and/or pill supplement has merit for cancer patients.

Many other herbs merit attention, as you will see in the chapter on herbs. Astragalus, turmeric, horseradish, echinacea, goldenseal, licorice, ginseng, ginkgo, ginger, Rhodiola rosea, and cat's claw are on the golden hit parade of herbs to help you toward recovery from cancer. Work with a professional who can help guide you toward which herb is best for your disease, your therapy, your wallet, and your stomach tolerances.

DAY 11: HEALTHY FATS

While too much fat and the wrong kind of fat have been killing millions of Americans for the past 50 years, we are now finding a new form of fat malnutrition: deficiencies of the essential fats. Fish oil (EPA), borage or primrose oil (GLA), conjugated linoleic acid (CLA from the meat and milk of ruminants like cows and sheep), and shark liver oil are all fats that can help you to beat your cancer. For a simple starter, begin taking a few capsules of fish oil daily, preferably basic cod liver oil or krill oil with all the good vitamin A and D still intact. You can also make a delicious, healthy Italian salad dressing by using olive oil, water, vinegar, and some seasonings.

The right fats in your diet will feed the precious pathways for beneficial prostaglandins, which are crucial to beating cancer. Healthy fats line the cell membranes and help to lower blood glucose by making insulin more effective. Healthy fats make the immune cells more likely to recognize and destroy cancer cells.

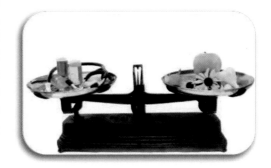

DAY 12: MINERALS

Before modern agriculture, farmers would use manure and compost to nourish the soil before planting the crops. Today, we use only nitrogen, phosphorus, and potassium (N:P:K) as the basic fertilizer. With each passing harvest, the American soils and our bodies become more deficient in essential minerals for health. For instance, scientists have found that a dust speck of selenium (200 micrograms daily) can lower cancer incidence by 60% and raise immune functions dramatically.[4] Deprive animals of magnesium and they spontaneously develop lymphoma. Some of our

Chapter 2 – Executive Summary. If You Are Too Sick to Read Much...

26

cancer epidemic in America is due to our serious and widespread deficiency in essential minerals.

Buy a basic mineral supplement, containing decent amounts of calcium, magnesium, chromium, and selenium. Add some kelp, which is rich in the trace minerals that are found both in the ocean and supposed to be found in your body fluid.

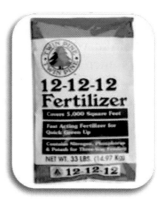

DAY 13: VITAMINS

Vitamins are the factory workers that get things done. Calories are the fuel for energy, and minerals are part of the structure or help vitamins to get things done. Most Americans are deficient in vitamins and minerals and plant phytochemicals, even on the basic survival Recommended Dietary Allowance level.

When you buy "supplemental" life or car insurance, you are still expected to make a decent effort to maintain your health, life, and car. When you take nutrition supplements, you are still expected to make a decent effort to maintain your diet and other lifestyle factors for health. Vitamin pills will not replace an optimal diet nor healthy lifestyle. See the chapter on supplements for more details.

DAY 14:
NOURISH YOUR MICROBIOME: HEALTHY GUT

Professor Elie Metchnikoff won a Nobel prize in 1908 for his work on the immune system. He later discovered the bacteria that makes yogurt (lactobacillus) and declared "Death begins in the colon." Indeed, it may. And the colon and gut of most Americans are under siege by unfriendly organisms and free radicals.

When we eat nourishing food, our well-established colony of friendly bacteria in the colon competes with yeast. Many Americans eat too much fat, too much sugar, not enough fiber, and very little probiotic food (like yogurt and tempeh); take antibiotics (which wipe out all bacteria in the body, including the friendly bacteria); and subject ourselves to stress-- all of which affects the balance of power between good and bad microorganisms in the gut. The net effect is an overgrowth of yeast, along with a deficiency of friendly bacteria that feed the immune system via the lining of the intestines. The yeast, which are there to degrade feces upon elimination, become hateful dictators in the gut. Many health problems result from what is called "dysbiosis" of the gut, or not having the right kind of microorganisms in charge.

Eat more fiber and no white sugar. Drink plenty of clean water. Eat yogurt daily or take a probiotic supplement. Make sure that you have a daily bowel movement. Use gentle herbal laxatives, like senna, if necessary. After 40 years of poor diet and chronic constipation, some people need colon flushing. Find a qualified expert to help on this issue.

About 70% of our immune system surrounds the gastro-intestinal tract. For better or for worse, the status of our gut will begin the healing or the deterioration of a cancer patient.

DAY 15: WATER

Only one substance is found in all forms of life from virus to plants to humans: water. Our bodies and the earth's surface are composed of 2/3 water. Water is the most amazing substance on earth, providing the fluid of life in your body and the bathing solution for all cells in your body. Yet, most Americans do not get enough water and are drinking contaminated water.

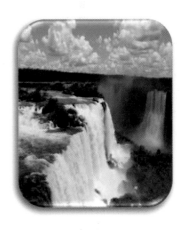

Our water pollution situation in this country has been called "a ticking time bomb." by the Environmental Protection Agency. We have used our rivers, lakes, and oceans as if they were sewers to dump unconscionable amounts of toxins. And we end up drinking that stuff. Pollution in our water supply is part of the reason for our growing cancer epidemic in this country.

Buy yourself a good water filter system and install it on your kitchen tap. Dual stage carbon filtration may cost $100-$200, with reverse osmosis costing two or three times that much. If need be, buy bottled water from a respectable vendor. Some bottled water is merely bottled city tap water with sugar added to make it taste better. Drink enough water to dilute your urine so that it is nearly clear in color and inoffensive in odor. Chronic dehydration first shows up in wrinkled skin, poor concentration, constipation, frequent infections, and eventually may appear as cancer. Water is your friend. Drink lots of clean water.

Chapter 2 – Executive Summary. If You Are Too Sick to Read Much...

28

DAY 16: BREATHING

In 1931 German scientist/physician Otto Warburg was awarded the Nobel prize in medicine for his work in explaining the <u>abnormalities of cancer cells</u>.[5] Some "shift" occurs from a normal cell that can metabolize amino acids, fats, and glucose to a cancer cell that favors glucose and emits lactic acid to subdue its host. The modern PET scan device found in the best hospitals in the world uses the Warburg principle to find the tumors in the patient.

Some experts postulate that a change in the pH of the cell leads to lower oxygen concentration leads to the cell suffocating leads to the cell switching to glucose for fuel. Cancer feeds on glucose like a primitive cell. Healthy cells in your body are aerobic, meaning that they need oxygen. Cancer hates well-oxygenated tissues of the body. Lung tissue, which is well oxygenated, develops cancer as the result of smoking carcinogens and excessive "rusting" of tissue in the absence of antioxidants to protect the lung tissue.

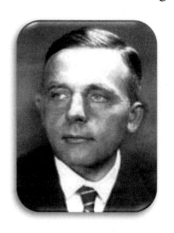

Of all nutrients required by the human body, oxygen is the most essential. We can go weeks and even months without food, days without water, but only a few minutes without oxygen. We are aerobic creatures by design. Cancer is the opposite. Unfortunately, many Americans breathe shallowly, thinking that sucking in our stomach is more important than diaphragm breathing to fully oxygenate our tissues.

Get some exercise. Do some yoga. Start breathing properly all the time. Lay on the floor with a book on your stomach. Begin breathing by pushing the book up and sucking in air to the bottom of your lungs. Continue breathing by filling the lungs fully and expanding your chest. Reverse the process on exhaling. This "belly breathing" will fully oxygenate your body to help make it less friendly to cancer cells, like shining sunlight on a vampire.

DAY 17: CHANGE THE UNDERLYING CAUSE

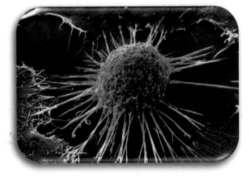

No one with a headache is suffering from a deficiency of aspirin. And no one with cancer has a deficiency of chemo or radiation. While these therapies might temporarily reduce tumor burden, they do not change the underlying cause of the disease.

Mrs. Jones might be suffering from metastatic breast cancer because, in her case, she is still hurting from a hateful divorce of 2 years ago, which drives her catecholamines into a stress mode and depresses her immune system; she goes to bed on a box of high sugar cookies each night; she has a deficiency of fish oil, zinc, and vitamin E; and she has an imbalance of estrogen and progesterone in her body. Her oncologist may remove the breasts, give her Tamoxifen to bind up estrogen, and administer chemo and radiation; but none of these therapies deals with the underlying causes of the disease. And it will come back unless these driving forces for the disease are reversed.

Find a nutritionally-oriented doctor and determine what got you into this condition, which will provide a detailed map on how to get you out of this situation.

DAY 18: IS CANCER AN INFECTION?

There is compelling evidence that some or many cancers are advanced infections. Medline literature shows us that stomach cancer is often from the bacteria Helicobacter pylori, liver cancer from the infection hepatitis, cervical cancer from the infection human papilloma virus, and more.

Hence, the need to address the infection is crucial in reversing the cancer. Yeast (fungi), virus, bacteria, mycoplasma, and parasites are among the critters that dwell within us and can create life-threatening

Chapter 2 – Executive Summary. If You Are Too Sick to Read Much...

30

diseases, like cancer. There are over 400,000 different strains of yeast, of which 400 can cause diseases in humans. Yeast is the "undertaker and the ecologist", decomposing all of life back to mother earth. Unfortunately, due to lowered vitality we are becoming premature victims of yeast and other infections. Just like wolves attack the weakest of the herd, opportunistic pathogens attack the weakest of cells within our body. Your mission is to make your body so full of wellness that there is no room for illness.

Take a simple urine test to see if you have a yeast overgrowth or blood test to see if you have other infections. Your doctor will then:

- ◆ kill the infectious organism with prescription medication and/or nutrition supplements
- ◆ starve the yeast, by eating a diet that lowers simple carbohydrate intake
- ◆ make the environment uncomfortable for the infectious agent, by bolstering your body's defense mechanisms

DAY 19: BEATING CANCER SYMPTOMS

"If the heat don't kill you then the humidity will." "And if the cancer don't kill you then the side effects will." Actually, both are worthy of your attention. Nausea, depression, insomnia, constipation, diarrhea, anemia, weakness, fatigue, pain, and more can be common side effects of cancer. Depending on how advanced your cancer is, your medical therapies being given, your general health, etc., you can reduce symptoms to a tolerable level. This is crucial because some cancer patients just give up, after suffering too much for too long. Much of this suffering can be reduced by allopathic and naturopathic treatments. Pain and discomfort induce stress, which lowers immune functions, which can be a real show-stopper for cancer patients. Pain management is crucial for many cancer patients. Get help.

DAY 20: SELECTIVELY REDUCE TUMOR BURDEN

It is very likely that your body needs some help in removing 10 or 20 trillion cancer cells, in order to reduce tumor burden enough to get your own anti-cancer defenses up and running. Working with the information that you gathered on day 2 (know your options of treatment), begin the process of debulking your tumor. Surgery, chemo, radiation, immune therapies, and hyperthermia are all common options. The key here is "restrained" tumor debulking. Anyone can kill all the cancer cells in your body.   A thimble full of arsenic will do the job.   No more cancer cells. No more you.

Surgeons used to take the aggressive cowboy approach and remove all surrounding tissue near the tumor.   Then they found that by removing too many lymph nodes, that lymphedema, or pooling of lymph fluid, could create such pain that amputation of limbs became necessary. "Remove the target organ" was

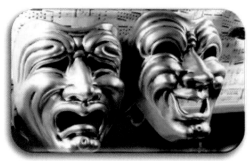

the battle cry of many an oncology surgeon.   The hemicorporectomy was the pinnacle of aggressive surgery, where the cancer patient with a sarcoma below the waist had the body removed from the waist down.   The survival statistics of these poor victims were no different than sarcoma patients who did nothing.   Pelvic exenteration, taking out all internal organs near the tumor, yielded no improvement in survival curves and a serious reduction in quality of life for the remaining months.   "Maximum sub-lethal chemo" has been the mantra of many oncologists.   Bring the patient to the therapeutic brink of death, and then salvage the patient if possible.

Find a doctor who will work with you on RESTRAINED tumor debulking. Just like the childhood fable of Goldilocks, you want a doctor to remove--not too much, not too little, but just the right amount of tumor mass.   Consider intravenous vitamin C, medical cannabis, hyperthermia, sodium bicarbonate, and intravenous turmeric therapies.

Choose   your   doctor "wagon master" wisely.   Just like the wagon master of the old west who was entrusted with getting the pioneers through the treacherous journey out west, you   are   entrusting   your physician to get you through the treacherous   journey   toward health.

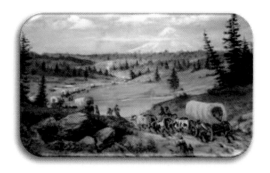

Chapter 2 – Executive Summary. If You Are Too Sick to Read Much...

32

DAY 21: ILLNESS AS A TEACHING TOOL

What have you learned since being diagnosed with cancer? How have your priorities changed? Do you see life differently? Do you appreciate sunsets and friends more? If so, then you are heading in the right direction toward healing. If not, then wake up.

In working with over 3,000 cancer patients individually and speaking to many thousands of cancer patients, there is a clear message in the appearance of a serious disease in anyone's life. Illness can be an unavoidable teaching tool. You can ignore advice from friends and loved ones. But you cannot ignore a terminal diagnosis.

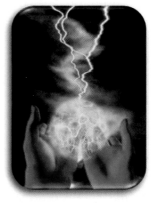

I have had my own health challenges and each has taught me much. We are here on this earth for a very limited amount of time. What are we doing with our precious time and talents? Are you a human being or a human doing? Do you hate more than you love? Take more than you give? See the glass as half empty rather than half full? Spend more time contemplating regrets than your dreams? Treat people with respect or victimize them? Understand your unique skills that the world needs?

Cancer is more than just a physical systemic disease. And it requires more than just good nutrition and medicine to cure. It is a wakeup call of the highest magnitude. Cancer patients who heed the call become better people having experienced this acid bath, this gauntlet, this baptism of fire. Many a cancer patient has stood in front of an audience and said: "Cancer is the best thing that ever happened to me." If you are nodding in agreement with this statement, then you are moving toward healing.

In Oriental language, "crisis" is written with two characters: one meaning "danger", the other character meaning "opportunity". For thousands of cancer patients, the disease has forced them into rearranging their priorities and lifestyle. Respect your body, your "temple of the Holy Spirit". Fill your mind and your hours so full of joy, passion, helpfulness, music, laughter, play, worship, thanksgiving, friends, family, and your work that there is no room left for cancer in your life. A diamond is nothing more than a piece of coal that was put under a lot of pressure. You can become a diamond through the healing of your cancer.

PATIENT PROFILE: BEAT ENDSTAGE TUBERCULOSIS

True story. The number one cause of death throughout most of the 19th century was tuberculosis. Galen Clark went to Yosemite Valley to die of end stage tuberculosis at age 42 in the fall of 1856. His doctor told him that coughing up chunks of his lungs meant he had up to 2-6 months to live. There was no cure for this disease. Clark reasoned that "If I'm going to die soon, then I'm going to die in Yosemite, the prettiest place I've ever seen." He got happy. Scientists now tell us that happiness brings on the flow of endorphins, which supercharge our immune system and may slow down cancer.

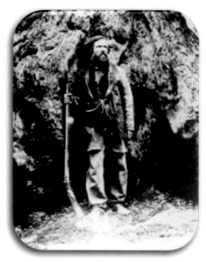

Next, Galen Clark carved his own tombstone, thus accepting his mortality, a ritual that would give us all a better appreciation of our finite time on earth. He then started eating what was available in Yosemite in those days; clean and lean wild game, mountain trout, nuts, berries, vegetables, and lots of clean water. No sugar and no dairy products. He then began doing what he wanted to do, hiking and creating trails, in the place he treasured the most, Yosemite Valley. He didn't die 6 months later, but rather 54 years later, just shy of his 96th birthday. He bolstered his "non-specific host defense mechanisms" with good thoughts and good nutrition.

Our bodies want to be well. There is an innate wisdom within all of life that knows how to fix disease. No one has to tell the scab on your hand how to heal properly. Your body knows what to do. We just have to give our body the proper physical and metaphysical resources to do its job right while purging our systems of toxins that inhibit healing.

Feed your mind the good thoughts of music, beauty, laughter, play, art, and friends; share a glass of wine or a cup of tea at sunset, and discuss the events of the day with a loved one. Feed your heart the good feelings

Chapter 2 – Executive Summary. If You Are Too Sick to Read Much...

34

of love, forgiveness, confidence in your abilities, a sense of purpose in your life, and a trusting relationship with your Creator. And feed your body good nutrients through diet and supplements, thus providing your body the raw materials that it needs to rebuild itself. You can recover from your cancer.

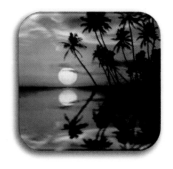

For more information on how your body can fight cancer go to GettingHealthier.com.

ENDNOTES

[1] https://www.ifm.org/find-a-practitioner/

[2] https://www.naturopathic.org/AF_MemberDirectory.asp?version=2

[3] http://health.lifeextension.com/InnovativeDoctors/

[4] https://iubmb.onlinelibrary.wiley.com/doi/abs/10.1002/biof.5520140120

[5] http://symposium.cshlp.org/content/70/363.short

Chapter 3

WHAT CAUSES CANCER

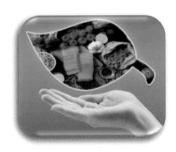

"Illnesses do not come upon us out of the blue. They are developed from small daily sins against Nature. When enough sins have accumulated, illnesses will suddenly appear."
Hippocrates, father of modern medicine, circa 400 BC

WHAT'S AHEAD?
A healthy human body has many built-in mechanisms to recognize and destroy invading cancer cells. It is a breakdown of these protective mechanisms that allows cancer to become a health risk. Restoring these protective mechanisms is crucial for long term cancer recovery.

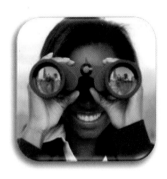

In the terrifying film, "The Predator", a chameleon-like beast from outer space descends upon the sweltering jungles of Central America to hunt humans, including Arnold Schwarzenegger. If you sweated through this film, then you have an idea of how hard it is to kill cancer. But fear not, we are going to turn your body into a lean, mean, cancer fighting machine.

The Predator wore a shield that allowed it to blend into the surrounding environment, making it almost invisible. Cancer mimics the chemistry of a fetus, and hence becomes invisible to the human immune system. Cancer also mutates by changing its DNA composition almost weekly, which is a major reason why many cancers develop a drug resistance that often limits the value of chemotherapy. Cancer also weakens its host by installing its own abnormal biochemistry, including:

- changes in the pH, or acid/base balance
- creation of anaerobic (oxygen-deprived) pockets of tissue that resist radiation therapy like someone hunkered into a bomb shelter
- blunting the immune system
- elevating metabolism and calorie needs, while simultaneously lowering appetite and food intake to slowly starve the host
- ejecting by-products that create weakness, apathy, pain, and depression in the host
- siphoning nutrients out of the bloodstream like a parasite.

With its invisible, predatory, and every-changing nature, cancer is truly a tough condition to treat. Cancer is essentially an abnormal cell growth. Its unchecked growth tends to overwhelm other functions in the body until death comes from:

1) organ failure, e.g., the kidneys shut down

2) infection, e.g., pneumonia, because the immune system has been blunted

3) malnutrition, because the parasitic cancer shifts the host's metabolism into high gear through inefficient use of fuel, while also inducing a loss of appetite.

SUBDUE SYMPTOMS OR DEAL WITH THE UNDERLYING CAUSE OF DISEASE?

There is a basic flaw in our thinking about health care in this country. We treat symptoms, not the underlying cause of the disease. Yet, the only way to provide long-lasting relief in any degenerative disease, like cancer, arthritis, and heart disease, is to reverse the basic cause of the disease. For example, let's say that you developed a headache because your neighbor's teenager is playing drums too loudly. You take an aspirin to subdue the headache, then your stomach starts churning. So, you take some antacids to ease the stomach nausea, then your blood pressure goes up. And on it goes. We shift symptoms with medication, as if in a bizarre "shell game", when we really need to deal with the fundamental cause of the disease.

Let me give you another example. What if I strike my thumb with a hammer. Boy, that hurt! Yet I keep doing the same masochistic act of striking my thumb with a hammer every morning for a week. And by then, my thumb is swollen, painful, discolored, and bleeding. So I go to Dr. A who recommends analgesics to better tolerate the pain. Dr. B suggests an injection of cortisone to reduce the swelling in my thumb. And Dr. C recommends surgery to cut off the finger because it looks defective. Of course, the real answer is to stop striking my thumb with a hammer.

Let's make this analogy relevant to modern healthcare. Let's look at the millions of Americans with rheumatoid arthritis, such as Mrs. Smith, whose condition is caused by eating too much sugar, plus an allergy to milk protein, and a deficiency of fish oil, vitamins C and D, 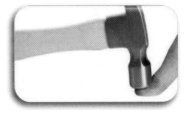 and the mineral zinc. Mrs. Smith goes to Dr. A, who recommends analgesics to better tolerate the pain. Dr. B suggests cortisone to reduce the swelling. And Dr. C recommends hip replacement surgery to cut off the defective parts. The real answer is to change the underlying cause of the disease, e.g. stop striking your thumb with a hammer.

A more common example is heart disease. There are over 60,000 miles of blood vessels in the average adult body. When a person develops blockage in the arteries near the heart, open-heart bypass surgery will probably be recommended. This procedure is done 200,000 times each year in the US to reestablish blood flow to vessels near the heart. But what has been done to improve the other 59,999 miles left that are probably equally obstructed?

A Harvard professor, Dr. E. Braunwald, investigated the records from thousands of bypass patients in the Veteran's Administration Hospitals and found no improvement in lifespan after this expensive and risky surgery.[1] Why? Because the underlying cause, which could be a complex array of diet, exercise, stress, and toxins, has not been resolved. Bypass surgery treats the symptoms of heart disease in the same way that chemo and radiation treat the symptoms of cancer. Each provide temporary relief, but no long-term cure.

Meanwhile, Dr. Dean Ornish was working as a physician doing bypass surgery in the early 1970s and watching some patients come back for their second bypass operation. Ornish reasoned: "Obviously, this procedure is not a cure for heart disease." At the time, there was convincing data that a low-fat diet, coupled with exercise and stress reduction, could lower the incidence of heart disease. Ornish wondered if we took that same program and cranked it up a notch or two, making it more therapeutic, might it reverse heart disease? And it did. The Ornish program is reimbursable through many insurance companies and <u>scientifically proven to reverse heart disease</u>.

Many of the nutritionally oriented medical doctors started their careers as cardiologists, no doubt hoping to make a difference in the lives of their patients. Eventually, these people hit a brick wall of futility with drugs and surgeries and turn to lifestyle, beginning with nutrition. The textbook <u>LIFESTYLE MEDICINE</u> from James Rippe, MD showcases a brilliant list of MDs and PhDs who endorse the notion of changing the underlying causes of disease. John Abramson, MD of Harvard authored his <u>OVERDOSED AMERICA</u> about the broken promise of American medicine and the need to use nutrition and lifestyle to reverse most degenerative diseases.[2]

While the American Cancer Society was violently opposed to Dr. Max Gerson's nutritional program to treat cancer patients in the 1950s, the ACS then released in the 1980s its dietary guidelines for the prevention of cancer, which was very similar to the Gerson program.

The crucial missing link in most cancer therapy is stimulating the patient's own healing abilities, because the best medical equipment cannot detect one billion cancer cells. Imagine leaving behind only one billion dandelion seeds on your lawn after you thought you got them all.

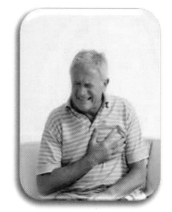

The "war on cancer" is an internal microscopic war that can only be won by working within the laws of nature: stimulating the patient's own abilities to fight cancer while changing the abnormal conditions that allow cancer to grow. All other therapies are doomed to disappointing results. Combined together, these treatments of restrained external medicine coupled with stimulating the cancer patient's internal healing abilities hold great promise for dramatically improving your chances of success against cancer.

WHAT CAUSES CANCER?

Most degenerative diseases, including cancer, do not have a readily identifiable enemy. In a bacterial infection, you can attack the "cause" of the disease with an antibiotic. Although, one could argue that a compromised host immune system is more at fault than a deficiency of antibiotics.

Cancer seems to be caused by a collection of lifestyle and environmental factors that accumulate over the years. Since success against any degenerative disease requires getting to the root of the problem, let's examine the accepted causes of cancer.

Toxic overload. The Environmental Protection Agency lists 85,000 chemicals in its registry of substances that fall under the Toxic Substances Control Act. At least 20,000 are known carcinogens. Each year, America alone sprays 1.2 billion pounds of pesticides on our food 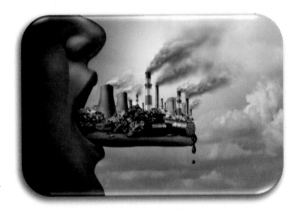 crops, feeds 30 million pounds of antibiotics to our farm animals to help them gain weight faster, and generally bombards the landscape with questionable amounts of electromagnetic radiation. Environmental activist Erin Brockovich has written a new book on the water pollution crisis facing America and the world with 300 million tons of plastic created annually, half as disposable one use items.

Bruce Ames, PhD, of the University of California at Berkeley, has estimated that each of the 37 trillion cells in your body undergoes from 1,000 to 10,000 DNA "hits" or potentially cancer-causing breaks every day. Newer studies examining the role of the immune system in protecting us against cancer show that the average adult has one cancer cell appear each day. Yet somehow, for most of us, our DNA repair mechanisms and immune system surveillance are able to keep this storm of genetic damage under control. Wallowing in our own high-tech waste products is a major cause of cancer in modern society, since carcinogens add to the fury of the continuous assault on the DNA.

Host Defenses: how do we heal?

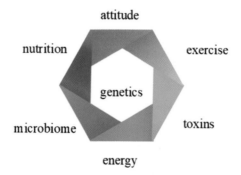

attitude

nutrition   exercise

genetics

microbiome   toxins

energy

Mother Nature's algorithm

Noted authority Samuel Epstein, MD, of the University of Illinois, says that a major thrust of cancer prevention must be detoxifying our earth. Toxins not only cause DNA breakage, which can trigger cancer, but also subdue the immune system, which then allows cancer to become the "fox in the chicken coop", with no controlling force.

Early research indicated that once cancer has been upregulated, or " the lion is out of the cage", then no amount of detoxification is going to matter. Newer evidence says otherwise. Cancer growth can be both slowed and even reversed, under the right conditions. According to the National Cancer Institute, there are 17 million American cancer survivors who have lived 5 or more years after their cancer diagnosis. Cancer is reversible. If toxins caused the problem, then detoxification is the solution. For more on detoxification, see the chapter on changing the underlying causes of cancer.

Distress. It was the Canadian physician and researcher, Hans Selye, MD, who coined the term "the stress of life", so he could document the physiological changes that took place in lab animals when exposed to noise, bright lights, confinement, and electric shocks. The thymus gland is a pivotal organ in immune system protection against infections and cancer. Dr. Selye noted that stress induces thymus gland shrinkage, increases fats in the blood (for the beginnings of heart disease), and erodes the stomach lining (ulcers).

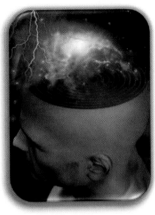

Candace Pert, PhD, a celebrated researcher at the National Institutes of Health, discovered endorphins in human brains and led the charge toward unravelling the chemical mysteries of the mind. Dr. Pert says that the mind is a pharmacy and is continuously producing potent substances that either improve or worsen health.

Since stress can create cancer, it should seem a logical leap that the mind can help to prevent and even subdue cancer. Noted physician and researcher at the University of California San Francisco, Kenneth Pelletier, MD, PhD, wrote his ground-breaking book, MIND AS HEALER, MIND AS SLAYER, to show that certain personalities are more prone to certain diseases. Many alternative therapists use a wide variety of psychological approaches to help rid the body of cancer.

ETIOLOGY FOR MOST DISEASES
pull out the weed by the root

primary etiology	→	secondary etiology	→	diagnosed diseases
NUTRITION		INFECTIONS		HEART DISEASE
INFECTIONS		INFLAMMATION		CANCER
EXERCISE		HYPERCOAGUL		DIABETES
ATTITUDE		DYSBIOSIS		STROKE
TOXINS		HYPOTHYROID		AUTO-IMMUNE
ENERGY ALIGN		MALDIGESTION		CHRONIC FATIG
GENETIC VULN		IMMUNE DYSFUN		MENTAL ILLNESS
		HYPERGLYCEMIA		ALZHEIMER'S
		ALLERGIES		PARKINSON'S
		HORMONE IMBAL		et al.
		OXIDATIVE STRES		
		ACIDOSIS		

Clearly, there is some mental link in the development of cancer for many patients.[3] I have worked with many cancer patients whose major hurdle was spiritual/emotional healing. While dietary changes are difficult for many people, it is far easier to change the diet or take some nutrient pills than change the way we think. Pulling emotional splinters is a painful but essential experience. Not only is there a metaphysical link to cancer, but the site of the cancer may provide clues regarding how to fix the problem. Many breast cancer patients have experienced a recent divorce, which results in the loss of a feminine organ. One patient of mine suffered from cancer of the larynx, which began one year after his wife left him with the thought "there's nothing you can say that will make me stay." Another patient was an attorney with stomach cancer who said "when I go to work, I get a pit in my stomach." If spiritual wounds started the cancer, then spiritual healing is an essential element for a cure.

Nutrition. The human body is built from, repaired by, and fueled by substances found in the diet. In the most literal sense, "we are what we eat...and think, and breathe, and do." Nutrition therapy merely tries to re-establish "metabolic balance" in the cancer patients. After decades of living outside the accepted realm of cancer therapies, nutrition therapy has found a new level of scientific acceptance with the 1990 report from the Office of Technology Assessment, an advisory branch of Congress, whose expert scientific panel wrote in UNCONVENTIONAL CANCER TREATMENTS:

"It is our collective professional judgment that nutritional interventions are going to follow psychosocial interventions up the ladder into clinical respectability as adjunctive and complementary approaches to the treatment of cancer."[4]

Exercise. While 40% of Americans will eventually develop cancer, only 14% of active Americans will get cancer. A half hour of exercise every other day cuts the risk for breast cancer by 75%. Exercise imparts many benefits, including oxygenation of the tissues to thwart the anaerobic needs of cancer cells. Exercise also helps to stabilize blood glucose levels, which can restrict the amount of fuel available for cancer cells to grow. Exercise improves immune function, lymph flow, and detoxification systems.

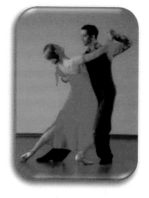

Exercise helps us better tolerate stressful situations. Exercise improves tolerance to chemotherapy. Some therapists use hydrogen peroxide or ozone to oxygenate the tissue. Humans evolved as active creatures. Inactivity is an abnormal, under-oxygenated metabolic state--so is cancer.

PATIENT PROFILE

I read your book and started on ImmunoPower. I was diagnosed with Stage 4 rectal cancer in February and I am now half way through my 12 chemo treatments. The progress CT scan I had last week has now been read and commented on by my doctor. All pelvic and retroperitineal nodes (para-aortics) where the original rectal tumor had spread to now appear anatomically normal on the scan. Even the rectal tumor itself cannot not presently be detected. We are going to get through the full 12 sessions, for the therapeutic dose.

I just wanted to thank you again for writing your book and providing insight on nutrition and other factors, such as my faith, which I know sits on top of all of this. I hope to wrap up all treatment requirements by the end of the calendar year and I plan on following the tips in your book for a lifetime after that. I know that I am not out of the woods yet, but I am going to think that way anyway and I am certainly grateful to God for this amazing news to date.

BZ

For more information on the epigenetic (lifestyle controlled) factors that can help your body recognize and destroy cancer, read <u>12 KEYS TO A HEALTHIER CANCER PATIENT</u> by Patrick Quillin.[5]

ENDNOTES

[1]. Braunwald, E., New England Journal Medicine, vol.309, p.1181, Nov.10, 1983

[2] https://www.amazon.com/Overdosed-America-Promise-American-Medicine/dp/0061344761/ref=sr_1_1?dchild=1&keywords=overdosed+america&qid=1590791226&sr=8-1

[3]. Newell, GR, Primary Care in Cancer, p.29, May 1991

[4]. Office of Technology Assessment, UNCONVENTIONAL CANCER TREATMENTS, p.14, IBID

[5] https://www.amazon.com/Keys-Healthier-Cancer-Patient-Incredible/dp/0578564297

Chapter 4

PROGRESS REPORT ON THE WAR ON CANCER

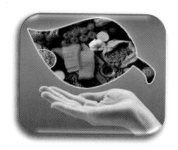

Insanity is doing the same thing over and over again, but expecting different results."
Albert Einstein, PhD, Nobel laureate

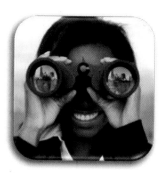

WHAT'S AHEAD?

If oncology was as effective as emergency room medicine, then there would be no need for "alternative cancer treatment". The risk-to-benefit ratio is heavily in favor of using nutrition as part of every cancer patient's comprehensive treatment program.

Cancer is not a new phenomenon. Archeologists have discovered tumors on dinosaur skeletons and Egyptian mummies. From 1600 B.C. on, historians find records of attempts to treat cancer. In the naturalist Disney film, "Never Cry Wolf", the biologist sent to the Arctic to observe the behavior of wolves found that the wolves would kill off the easiest prey, which were sometimes animals suffering from leukemia.

Cancer is an abnormal and rapidly growing tissue, which, if unchecked, will eventually smother the body's normal processes. Cancer may have been with us from the beginning of time, but the fervor with which it attacks modern civilization is unprecedented.

President Richard Nixon declared "war on cancer" on December 23, 1971. Nixon confidently proclaimed that we would have a cure for cancer within 5 years, by the 1976 Bicentennial. In 2005 Guy Faguet, MD, an oncologist who spent his career as a researcher at the National Cancer Institute wrote an expose <u>THE WAR ON CANCER: AN ANATOMY OF FAILURE</u>.[1] Dr. Faguet noted that "chemotherapy is curative in about 2% of cancers."

US CANCER INCIDENCE: EPIDEMIC PROPORTIONS
Projections of Cancer Cases between 2000 to 2050 by Age

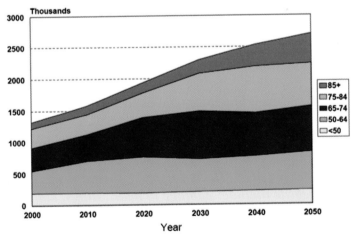

Source: SEER program, NCI and population projections from US Census Bureau

- Our ability to treat and cure most cancers has not materially improved."[2] The unsettling bad news is irrefutable:
- newly-diagnosed cancer incidence continues to escalate, from 1.1 million Americans in 1991 to 1.7 million in 2020
- deaths from cancer in 1992 were 547,000, with 609,000 in 2018
- since 1950, the overall cancer incidence has increased by 44%, with breast cancer and male colon cancer up by 60% and prostate cancer by 100%

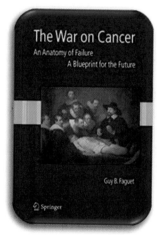

- for decades, the 5-year survival has remained constant, for non-localized breast cancer at 18% and lung cancer at 13%
- only 5% of the $6.5 billion annual budget for the National Cancer Institute is spent on prevention
- grouped together, the average cancer patient has a 50/50 chance of living another 5 years, which are the same odds he or she had in 1971
- claims for cancer drugs are generally based on tumor response rather than prolongation of life. Many tumors will initially shrink when chemo and radiation are applied, yet tumors often develop drug-resistance and are then unaffected by therapy.
- In <u>2005 cancer surpassed heart disease</u> as the leading cause of death for all but the elderly (over 85).[3] It is already the number one fear.
- 42% of Americans living today can expect to develop cancer.

IS CHEMO EFFECTIVE?

When examining risk to benefit to cost ratio of chemo for cancer patients, we find that the *side effects for most chemo drugs as listed on the Mayo Clinic website include: damage to heart, lungs, kidneys, nerves (causing painful neuropathy), inducing cancer, and the routine nausea, vomiting, hair loss, fever, loss of appetite, bruising, immune suppression, and more.* So the risks are high. What are the benefits? There have been many studies showing the relative ineffectiveness of chemo in treating cancer. One of the more respected published articles showed that <u>chemo works in about 2% of all cancer patients</u>.[4] Yet chemo is given to nearly 2/3 of cancer patients. And <u>chemo may even cause the cancer to spread or metastasize.</u>[5]

As a percentage of total annual deaths in America, cancer has escalated from 1% in 1900 to 24% of today's deaths. Many experts have been quick to explain away this frightening trend by claiming that our aging population is responsible for the increase in cancer incidence--older people are more likely to get cancer. But aging does not entirely explain our epidemic proportions of cancer in America.

TIME FOR EXAMINING OPTIONS

The purpose of this section is not to blast the National Cancer Institute, but rather to make it blatantly obvious that our current cancer treatment methods are inadequate and incomplete and that we need to examine some options--like nutrition. Also, we need to address the urgent question: "Does nutrition reduce the effectiveness of chemotherapy?" There are two parts to this debate.

1) Does nutrition interfere with chemotherapy? "No."
2) Is chemotherapy effective? The answer is "sometimes."

A growing body of dissidents cite data to refute the NCI's confident numbers. Among the skeptics is John Bailar, MD, PhD, of Harvard University, whose outspoken article in the prestigious *New England Journal of Medicine* ushered in a champion for the many strident critics of the National Cancer Institute[6].

> *"We are losing the war against cancer".*
> *John Bailar, MD, PhD, Harvard University, former editor Journal of the National Cancer Institute, member National Academy of Sciences*

The death rate, age-adjusted death rate, and both crude and age-adjusted incidence rate of cancer continue to climb in spite of efforts by the NCI. Non-whites are excluded from the NCI statistics for vague reasons. Blacks, urban poor, and the 11 million workers exposed to toxic substances have all experienced a dramatic increase in cancer incidence and mortality.

Less than 10% of patients with cancer of the pancreas, liver, stomach, and esophagus will be alive in five years. Bailar wrote a follow up article "Cancer Undefeated" published in the May 1997 edition of the New England Journal of Medicine with similar news. The exception and thin shaft of sunlight in this article indicated a 1% decline in age-adjusted mortality from all cancers from 1991 to 1994. Bailar felt that this almost insignificant improvement may have been due to earlier detection of cancer, not better treatment techniques.

INCREASING INCIDENCE OF CANCER IN AMERICA
not totally due to our aging population

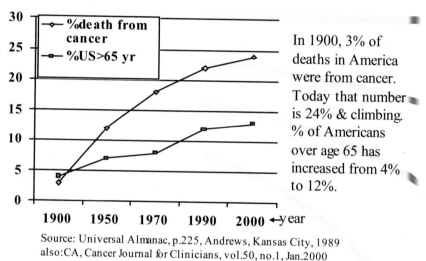

In 1900, 3% of deaths in America were from cancer. Today that number is 24% & climbing. % of Americans over age 65 has increased from 4% to 12%.

Source: Universal Almanac, p.225, Andrews, Kansas City, 1989
also: CA, Cancer Journal for Clinicians, vol.50, no.1, Jan.2000

Perhaps the most tragic "pawns" in this game are the children. The NCI admits to a 28% rise in the incidence of childhood cancers from 1950 through 2005, much of which is due to the ubiquitous presence of environmental pollutants.[7] On the other side of the coin, progress in the 11,000 cases of pediatric oncology has produced cure rates in some forms of childhood cancer of up to 90%, which makes chemotherapy for childhood cancers an NCI victory, of sorts. However, while these patients do survive longer, they have a much higher risk for developing bone cancer later in life as a result of the chemo and/or radiation therapy.[8]

Ulrich Abel, PhD, of the Heidelberg Tumor Center in Germany, has brought the issue to a fever pitch. Abel, a well-respected biostatistics expert, published a controversial 92-page review of the world's literature on survival of chemotherapy-treated cancer patients, showing that chemotherapy alone can help only about 3% of the patients with epithelial cancer (such as breast, lung, colon, and prostate), which kills 80% of total cancer patients.

> *"...a sober and unprejudiced analysis of the literature has rarely revealed any therapeutic success by the [chemotherapy] regimens in question."*[9]

A prominent scientist from the University of Wisconsin, Johan Bjorksten, PhD, has shown that chemotherapy alone destroys the immune system beyond a point of return, which increases the risk for early death from infections and other cancers in these immunologically-naked people.[10] Ralph Moss, PhD, former assistant director of public affairs at Sloan Kettering cancer hospital in New York, has written a thoroughly documented analysis of the history of chemotherapy, showing its troublesome beginning as mustard gas for warfare and its current questionable status as the prevailing treatment for the majority of cancer patients.[11]

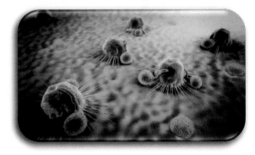

Critics of American cancer treatment point out that the therapy may sometimes be worse than the condition. Researchers reported in the *New England Journal of Medicine* that the risk of developing leukemia from chemotherapy treatment of ovarian cancer outweighs the benefits of the therapy.[12]

Though interest is growing to find patented prescription drugs to bolster the body's immune system, there is an abundance of evidence showing that nutrition enhances the body's immune ability to find and destroy cancer cells, as shown in this medical animation of lymphocytes engulfing cancer cells.

Breast and prostate cancers have recently surfaced in the press as "forgotten cancers", due to their intimate nature. While one out of 20 women in 1950 were hit with breast cancer, today that number is one in eight. Even with early detection and proper treatment, a "cured" breast cancer patient will lose an average of 19 years of lifespan. Breast cancer kills about 42,000 women each year.[13] Lack of faith in cancer treatment has led a few physicians to recommend that some women with a high incidence of breast or ovarian cancer in their family undergo "preventive surgery" to remove these high-risk body parts.[14] Life and health insurance companies now refer to healthy intact women as "with organs" and at high risk, therefore forced to pay higher health insurance premiums.

While Tamoxifen is an estrogen binder that can be of benefit in short-term use for breast cancer patients and it has been touted as a chemo-preventive agent for millions of high-risk breast cancer patients, other data show that long-term tamoxifen use elevates the risk for heart attack,[15] eye,[16] and liver damage[17] and INCREASES the risk of endometrial cancer.[18]

And while breast cancer is tragic, prostate cancer is equally prevalent in men and even more lethal. The NCI spends one fourth the amount on prostate cancer research as on breast cancer research. The prostate specific antigen (PSA) and digital rectal exam are the early screening procedures for prostate cancer. In the majority of the prostate cancers found, the cancer has spread beyond the prostate gland and is difficult to treat. Comparing the outcome of 223 patients with untreated prostate cancer to 58 patients who underwent radical prostatectomy, the 10-year disease-specific survival was 86.8% and 87.9%, respectively. There was essentially no difference in survival between the treated and untreated groups.[19]

According to an extensive review of the literature, there has been no improvement in cancer mortality from 1952 through 1985.[20] These authors state: "Evidence has steadily accrued that [cancer therapy] is essentially a failure." Meanwhile, we spend millions researching molecular biology in a futile quest for a "magic bullet" against cancer.[21] A London physician and researcher has provided statistical backing for his contention that breast cancer screenings in women under age 50 provide no benefit in 99.85% of the premenopausal women tested.[22] A gathering chorus of scientists and clinicians proclaim that success from chemo and radiation therapy has plateaued, and that we need to examine alternative therapies.[23]

A 1971 textbook jointly published by the American Cancer Society and the University of Rochester stated that biopsy of cancer tissue may lead to the spread of cancer.[24] Although encapsulated cancer can be effectively treated with surgery, and 22% of all cancer can be "cured" through surgery[25], 30% or more of surgery patients with favorable prognosis still have cancer recurrences.[26]   A study of 440,000 cancer patients who received chemotherapy or radiation showed that those treated with radiation had a significantly increased risk for a type of leukemia involving cells other than the lymphocytes.[27]   Long-term effects of radiation include birth defects and infertility. Short-term effects include mouth sores and ulcers, which can interfere with the ability to eat, rectal ulcers, fistulas, bladder ulcers, diarrhea, and colitis.

        In a survey of 79 Canadian oncologists, all of them would encourage patients with non-small cell lung cancer to participate in a chemotherapy protocol, yet 58% said that they themselves would not participate in such a therapy and 81% said they would not take cisplatin (a chemo drug) under any circumstances.[28]

        Analysis of over 100 clinical trials using chemotherapy as sole treatment in breast cancer patients found no benefits and significant damage from the chemotherapy in post-menopausal patients.[29] Dr. Rose Kushner pointed out that toxic drugs are "literally making healthy people sick" and are "only of marginal benefit to the vast majority of women who develop breast cancer."[30] Some evidence indicates that chemotherapy actually shortens the life of breast cancer patients.[31]

        According to a psychologist writing in the American Cancer Society Journal, "the side effects of cancer chemotherapy can cause more anxiety and distress than the disease itself."[32]   A well-recognized side effect of chemotherapy is suppression of bone marrow, which produces the white blood cells that fight infection. This common immune suppression leads to the all-too-common death from infection.[33]

        According to the literature that comes with each chemotherapeutic agent, methotrexate may be "hepatotoxic" (damaging to the liver) and suppresses immune function. Adriamycin can cause "serious irreversible myocardial toxicity (damage to heart) with delayed congestive heart failure often unresponsive to any cardiac supportive therapy." Cytoxan can cause "secondary malignancies" (cancer from its use). It is widely known among health care professionals that just working around chemotherapy agents can cause birth defects.[34]

In spite of $200 billion in research at the NCI and billions more spent in private industry, there have been few new chemotherapy drugs discovered in the past 20 years.[35] Not even NCI official Dr. Daniel Ihde can conjure up any enthusiasm for the failure of chemotherapy drugs against lung cancer.[36] Given the limited successes in traditional cancer treatment, it is not surprising that over 60% of all American cancer patients seek "alternative therapies".

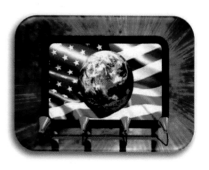

Biological therapies, such as interferon and interleukin, are extremely toxic, with treatment requiring weeks of hospitalization, usually in intensive therapy, with multiple transfusions, severe bleeding, shock, and confusion as common side effects.[37] Interferon causes rapid onset of fever, chills, and severe muscle contractions that may require morphine.[38]

WHERE DID WE GO WRONG?

There is a lot of finger-pointing since the war on cancer has been so heavily criticized. For starters, it would be easy to blame bread mold, from which springs penicillin, which was discovered by Alexander Fleming in 1928 and gave us hope that there was a "magic bullet" against every disease. We now see the hazards in the excessive use of antibiotics to disrupt the microbiome in the human gut, laying the stage for many diseases, including cancer and autoimmune diseases.

Another scapegoat is good old patriotic pride. After all, it was the Americans who rode in to World Wars I and II to rescue the world. Americans stepped in to finish the Panama Canal after the French had failed. Americans threw enough money at the Manhattan Project to develop a war-ending nuclear bomb and again bought our way to the moon in a massive and expensive effort from NASA scientists. Americans have more patents and Nobel laureates than any other nation on earth. We had good reasons to be confident of buying a cure for cancer.

Some of our problems lie in scientific research models. Using animals with induced leukemia, a non-localized disease of the blood-forming organs, is not a realistic representation of how well a cancer drug will work against a solid human tumor. We have also made the erroneous assumption that "no detectable cancer" means no cancer. A million cancer cells are undetectable by even the most sensitive medical equipment. A billion cancer cells become a tiny and nearly undetectable "lump".[39] When the surgeon says: "We think we got it all."--that is when the war on cancer must become an invisible battle involving the patient's well-nourished immune system.

We also have wrongly guessed that "response rate", or shrinkage of the tumor, is synonymous with cure. As mentioned, chemotherapy works on cancer cells like pesticides work on insects. Spraying pesticides on a field of plants may kill 99% of the bugs in the field, but the few insects that survive this baptism of poison have a unique genetic advantage to resist the toxicity of the pesticide. These "super bugs" then reproduce even more rapidly without competition, since the pesticides killed off biological predators in the field and reduced the fertility of the soil for an overall drop in plant health. Similarly, blasting a typically malnourished cancer patient with bolus (high dose once per week) injections of chemotherapy alone may elicit an initial shrinkage of the tumor, but the few tumor cells that survive this poison become resistant to therapy and may even accelerate the course of the disease in the now immune-suppressed patient. Meanwhile, the once marginally malnourished patient becomes clinically malnourished, since nausea becomes a prominent symptom in bolus chemo usage. An expert in cancer at Duke University, Dr. John Grant, has estimated that 40% or more of cancer patients actually die from malnutrition.[40]

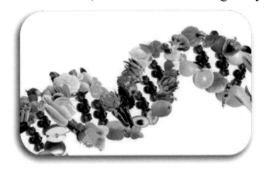

We also made the mistake of becoming enamored with a few tools that we thought could eradicate cancer. We focused all of our energies in these three areas and ridiculed or even outlawed any new ideas. The real reason for our failure lies in our error in thinking. The wellness and illness of our bodies are almost entirely dependent on what we eat, think, drink, breathe, and how we move. These forces shape our general metabolism, which is the sum total of bodily processes. Our metabolism then either favors or discourages the growth of both infectious and degenerative diseases. Cancer is a degenerative disease of abnormal metabolism throughout the body--not just a regionalized lump or bump.

Our health is composed of a delicate interplay of nutrients consumed and toxins expelled, coupled with mental and spiritual forces that influence metabolism. We are a product of our genes, lifestyle, and environment. Mounting evidence shows us that lifestyle and nutrition can turn on and off oncogenes. We are not dumb automobiles to be taken to the mechanic and fixed. We are physical and metaphysical beings who must become part of the cure, just as surely as we are a part of the disease process. Healing is a joint effort between patient, clinician, and that mysterious and wonderful force which most of us take for granted. The days of "magic bullet" cures are over. The days of cooperative efforts between patient and clinician are here to stay.

SHIFTING THE CANCER PARADIGM
MUST WE KILL TO CURE?

Journal of Clinical Oncology (ASCO), vol.13, no.4, p.801, Apr.1995
H. Schipper, CR Goh, TL Wang

"the limits of the [cancer killing] model seem to have been reached"

"consider cancer as potentially reversible"

"killing strategies may be counterproductive because they impair host response and drive the already defective regulatory process [of the cancer cell] toward further aberrancy."

"[chemotherapy] treatment strategies have been based on the log-cell kill hypothesis, derived from leukemia cells in culture...but is rarely seen in nature and only sustained under stringent conditions"

"remission does not predict cure...the failure of adjuvant therapies to flatten disease-free survival curves"

"conventional antineoplastic approaches will play a role as debulkers, ...the strategy will change to one of reregulation."

MUST WE KILL TO CURE?

In the official journal of the American Society of Clinical Oncologists, researchers showed the limitations of the cancer killing model of chemo. These authors suggested that cancer treatment will shift to one of "re-regulation", change the way the body works and revert the cancer back to healthy tissue. That is exactly what optimal nutrition can do.

ONLY TEAMWORK WILL BEAT CANCER

Cancer is the number one or two cause of death in America, depending on how you crunch numbers. We need teamwork in cancer treatment because of the formidable "Predator" that we face. We cannot discard any cancer therapy, no matter how strange or perpendicular to medical theories, unless that therapy does not work.

There are no "magic bullets" against cancer, nor can we anticipate such a development within our lifetime. We need to use restrained chemo, radiation, hyperthermia, and surgery to debulk the tumors, which can remove 10 or 20 trillion cancer cells and give the cancer patient's system a fighting chance. At the same time, we need to re-regulate the cancer back toward healthy cooperation in the body with agents like intravenous vitamin C and protease enzymes.[41] Then we need to apply nutrition and other naturopathic fields to bolster "non-specific host defense mechanisms" in the cancer patient to reverse the underlying cause of the disease. 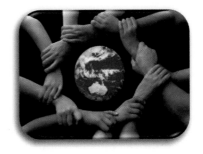 This threefold approach, reduction of tumor burden without harming the patient, re-regulating the cancer to convert to normal healthy tissue, and nourishing the patient's recuperative powers, will be the humane and clinically effective cancer treatment of the new millennium.

Chemotherapy can be useful, especially for certain types of cancer and when administered in fractionated dose or via intra-arterial infusion to a therapeutically-nourished patient. Radiation therapy has its place, especially as the highly-targeted brachytherapy or intensity modulated radiation therapy (IMRT). Surgery has its place, especially when the tumor has been encapsulated and can be removed without bursting the collagen envelope. Hyperthermia can be extremely valuable. Combinations of these traditional therapies are becoming better accepted in medical circles. Later in this book, you will see the synergism in creative combinations of conventional and unconventional cancer therapies, such as quercetin (a bioflavonoid) with heat therapy, or niacin with radiation therapy. The take-home lesson here is: "Just because traditional medicine has failed to develop an unconditional cure for cancer doesn't mean that we should categorically reject all traditional approaches."

Comprehensive cancer treatment uses traditional cancer therapies to reduce the tumor burden, while concurrently building up the "terrain" of the cancer patient to fight the cancer on a microscopic level. That is the "one-two punch" that will eventually bring the predator of cancer to its knees.

For more information on how your body can fight cancer go to GettingHealthier.com.

PATIENT PROFILE:

Ann E. Fonfa, annieappleseedpr@aol.com

I was diagnosed with breast cancer in January 1993. Because of extreme Multiple Chemical Sensitivity, I ended up refusing chemotherapy, had no radiation and no hormonal therapy. The main things I changed, was what I ate, becoming a 100% organic vegan, exercising daily for an hour, and starting on dietary supplements.

I found Dr. Quillin's book very early on thankfully. There was no Internet but a book with the exciting and satisfying title of Beating Cancer With Nutrition, meant so much to me. I even shared the information with other women in my support group who were going through conventional treatments. Some of them were brave enough to add these ideas to their own protocols and received benefits. I have always been grateful for the wisdom Dr. Quillin imparted which made me feel confident in the path I chose.

My own outcome was completely different than everyone else as I continued to have small tumors (largest was 1.5 cm). Amazingly all but the first were growing slower than normal cells and from the first recurrence onward I was told not to take chemotherapy. Eventually I met a Chinese Herbalist who prescribed an herbal protocol for me, which despite his initial request to only do his herbs, I added to my existing program. MRI-proven free of cancer in September 2001. I share all information about my protocols and evidence-based ideas on getting and staying well during treatment and after via **Annie Appleseed Project**, the all-volunteer nonprofit I founded. We also host annual conferences. 26 years after my diagnosis, I am still in remission.

ENDNOTES

[1] https://www.amazon.com/War-Cancer-Anatomy-Failure-Blueprint/dp/1402036183

[2]. Ingram, B., Medical Tribune, vol.33, no.4, p.1, Feb.1992

[3] https://academic.oup.com/jnci/article/97/5/330/2544115

[4] https://www.ncbi.nlm.nih.gov/pubmed/15630849

[5] https://stm.sciencemag.org/content/9/397/eaan0026

[6]. Bailar, JC, New England Journal of Medicine, vol.314, p.1226, May 1986

[7]. Epstein, SS, and Moss, RW, The Cancer Chronicles, p.5, Autumn 1991

[8]. Weiss, R., Science News, p.165, Sept.12, 1987

[9]. Abel, U., CHEMOTHERAPY OF ADVANCED EPITHELIAL CANCER: A Critical Survey, Hippokrates Verlag Stuttgart, 1990

[10]. Bjorksten, J, LONGEVITY, p.22, JAB Publ., Charleston, SC, 1987

[11]. Moss, RW, QUESTIONING CHEMOTHERAPY, Equinox Press, NYC, 1995

[12]. Kaldor, JM, et al., New England Journal of Medicine, vol.322, no.1, p.1, Jan.1990

[13]. Neuman, E, New York Times, Insight, p.7, Feb.9, 1992

[14]. Bartimus, T., Tulsa World, p.B3, Dec.22, 1991

[15]. Nakagawa, T., et al., Angiology, vol.45, p.333, May 1994

[16]. Pavlidis, NA, et al., Cancer, vol.69, p.2961, 1992

[17]. Catherino, WH, et al., Drug Safety, vol.8, p.381, 1993

[18]. Seoud, MAF, et al., Obstetrics & Gynecology, vol.82, p.165, Aug.1993

[19]. Johansson, JE, et al., Journal American Medical Association, vol.267, p.2191, Apr.22, 1992

[20]. Temple, NJ, et al., Journal Royal Society Medicine, vol.84, p.95, 1991

[21]. Temple, NJ, et al., Journal Royal Society of Medicine, vol.84, p.95, Feb.1991

[22]. Shaffer, M., Medical Tribune, p.4, Mar.26, 1992

[23]. Hollander, S., et al., Journal of Medicine, vol.21, p.143, 1990

[24]. Rubin, P., (ed), CLINICAL ONCOLOGY FOR MEDICAL STUDENTS AND PHYSICIANS: A MULTI-DISCIPLINARY APPROACH, 3rd edition, Univ. Rochester, 1971

[25]. American Cancer Society, "Modern cancer treatment" in CANCER BOOK, Doubleday, NY, 1986

[26]. National Cancer Institute, Update: Primary treatment is not enough for early stage breast cancer, Office of Cancer Communications, May 18, 1988

[27]. Curtis, RE, et al., Journal National Cancer Institute, p.72, Mar.1984

[28]. Ginsberg, RJ, et al., Cancer of the lung, in: DeVita, CANCER PRINCIPLES AND PRACTICES OF ONCOLOGY, Lippincott, Philadelphia, p.673, 1993

[29]. New England Journal Medicine, Feb.18, 1988; see also Boffey, PM, New York Times, Sept.13, 1985

[30]. Kushner, R., CA-Cancer Journal for Clinicians, p.34, Nov.1984

[31]. Powles, TJ, et al., Lancet, p.580, Mar.15, 1980

[32]. Redd, WH, CA-Cancer Journal for Clinicians, p.138, May1988

[33]. Whitley, RJ, et al., Pediatric Annals, vol.12, p.6, June 1983; see also Cancer Book, ibid.

[34]. Jones, RB, et al., California Journal of American Cancer Society, vol.33, no.5, p.262, 1983

[35]. Hollander, S., and Gordon, M., Journal of Medicine, vol.21, no.3, p.143, 1990

[36]. Ihde, DC, Annals of Internal Medicine, vol.115, no.9, p.737, Nov.1991

[37]. Moertel, CG, Journal American Medical Association, vol.256, p.3141, Dec.12, 1986

[38]. Hood, LE, American Journal Nursing, p.459, Apr.1987

[39]. Dollinger, M., EVERYONE'S GUIDE TO CANCER THERAPY, p.2, Somerville, Kansas City, 1990

[40]. Grant, JP, Nutrition, vol.6, no.4, p.6S, July 1990 supl

[41]. Hoffman, EJ, CANCER AND THE SEARCH FOR SELECTIVE BIOCHEMICAL INHIBITORS, CRC Press, Boca Raton, FL, 1999

Chapter 5

UNDERSTANDING
YOUR CANCER

Knowing What Questions to Ask Your Doctor

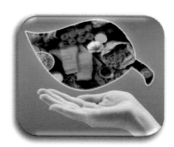

Each patient carries his own doctor inside him.
Albert Schweitzer, MD, Nobel laureate 1940

WHAT'S AHEAD?
Cancer is a collection of abnormal cells. This chapter will help you to understand:
✓ how cancer is diagnosed and classified
✓ how to ask your doctor the right questions
✓ how to make sure that you have the right doctor for your cancer
✓ how to understand your doctor's discussions with you.

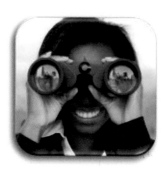

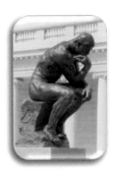

The diagnosis of cancer can be a scary thing. To maintain some sense of control in your treatment process, it helps to understand how doctors diagnose, classify, and treat cancers. This chapter is a very basic, but extremely valuable, guide to putting you in charge of your cancer treatment team. Think. Know. Ask the right questions. Find the right doctor. Choose the right therapies. And you stand a much better chance of a favorable outcome from your cancer.

HOW DOES CANCER START IN YOUR BODY?

Your body contains about 37 trillion cells working in harmony to keep you well. These amazing "non-specific host defense mechanisms" function smoothly in most of us for most of our lives. Part of this process of living involves cell replication, or the "copying" of a cell to make two new cells. The cell tears its DNA in half, copies the DNA for both sides of the torn halves, then creates new cells that can continue the work of life. This cell replication process can create defective new cells, which can eventually become cancer, or tumor.

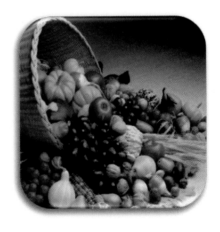

Researchers find that each of us carries the seeds of our own destruction in our DNA, called oncogenes, or genetic messages that can turn on and trigger a cancer. Think of genes as "loading the gun" and lifestyle, such as nutrition, "pulling the trigger" on this gun. Meaning, just because your family has a tendency toward cancer, does not mean that you are doomed to get cancer. Lifestyle is at least 90% responsible for cancer, while genes play a 5-10% role. This is good news, because it means that you can do something about "silencing" these oncogenes through lifestyle. Most of this book is dedicated to "re-regulating" your body out of cancer mode and into healthy mode. Nutrients can affect the DNA in elegant and helpful ways for the cancer patient.

BENIGN VS MALIGNANT TUMORS

Tumors do not always threaten our lives. Some tumors, such as freckles, moles, and fatty lumps in the skin, do not invade the rest of the body, and hence do not cause death.

Malignant tumors differ in at least two respects:

1) they put down roots and begin to burrow into the tissue of your body

2) they spread through the body by generating enzymes that break down your tissue and also send out "seed" cells to start a new colony somewhere else in your body.

Rarely does anyone die from a lump or a bump tumor. It is the spreading, or metastasizing, that does the damage. While different cancers in different parts of the body behave somewhat differently, almost all cancers share the common features of being abnormal cells that spread throughout the body and lay down roots to penetrate healthy tissue. These common features allow your body to fight cancer with common mechanisms, regardless of where the cancer started in your body.

HOW CANCER SPREADS

Usually, the cancer begins in one spot in the body and spreads via various means. Rarely, several cancers begin in different parts of the body and spread.

Direct extension. Tumors can lay down roots and burrow into the tissue nearby, like carrots growing into the earth.

Travelling through the blood (hematogenous spreading). As a tumor grows beyond 1/4 inch in diameter (about 7 millimeters), it needs a blood supply to bring nutrients and carry away waste products. This form of metastasis involves the tumor sending out "seed" cells into the bloodstream to attach somewhere in the body and begin a new tumor.

Through the lymphatic system. Your body has two separate blood vessel systems. One is the pumping of red blood cells by the heart through 60,000 miles of arteries and

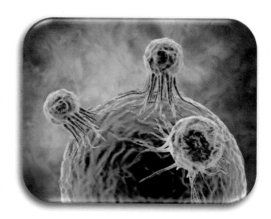

veins. The other network involves the much smaller lymphatic vessels, which carry lymph, a milky liquid that is full of immune cells for battle against invaders, as well as toxins and waste products for elimination. The lymphatic system joins the blood circulation of veins at the thoracic duct, in the left side of the neck. Some cancers spread through the lymphatic system, which is why your doctor may choose to remove a lymph node near the cancer to see if it contains malignant tissue.

This score card gives your doctor an idea of how far advanced the cancer has spread. Some doctors inject a blue dye into the tumor, then remove the lymph node nearest the tumor, called sentinel node, for the pathologist to look at under the microscope.

DIFFERENT KINDS OF TUMORS

Based on three broad categories (Where is the tumor growing? How fast is it growing? How big has it already grown?), doctors assign a category to the cancer.

Carcinomas. These tumors grow in the tissues that line internal organs (epithelium). Most carcinomas grow in an organ that secretes something. Lung tissue secretes mucus, breast tissue secretes milk, prostate tissue secretes a milky fluid that contributes to sperm semen, and pancreas tissue secretes digestive juices.

Sarcomas. These cancers develop in supporting or connective tissue, such as muscles, tendons, bones, nerves, or blood vessels. A carcinoma may eventually develop a sarcoma, depending on the site of metastasis.

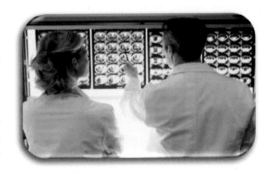

Lymphomas and leukemias. These tumors develop in the lymph glands or bone marrow. Lymphomas (aka lymphosarcomas) develop in the lymph glands, which are small bean-shaped "bus depots" that are spaced regularly throughout the lymphatic vessels. Lymphomas are generally divided into Hodgkin's or non-Hodgkin's lymphomas.

Add the organ name. Body parts are named in Latin and Greek root names. Hence, bone cancer might be osteo (bone) sarcoma. Stomach cancer might be called gastric carcinoma, etc.

MEASURING THE RATE OF GROWTH

Whenever possible, the surgeon removes a section of the tumor and sends it to a doctor who specializes in tissue examinations (pathologist) for assessment on "how fast is this cancer growing?"

Well-differentiated tumors. If the tumor tissue looks similar to the surrounding tissue of healthy cells, then it is called well-differentiated.

Undifferentiated tumors. Other tumor cells look very different and primitive compared to the surrounding healthy tissue and are called poorly differentiated or undifferentiated. In general, undifferentiated tumors grow faster and have a poorer prognosis than well-differentiated tumors.

High grade. A poorly differentiated, fast growing, aggressive tumor is called high grade, while a well-differentiated, slow growing, and less aggressive tumor is called low grade.

DEFINING THE STAGE OF CANCER

By assessing where the cancer is growing, and how fast, and how fast it is spreading, doctors have developed a system of deciding which protocol (precise plan for therapy) to put you on.

The TNM system of defining stage of cancer has been embraced by many oncologists throughout the world. T stands for Tumor size. N stands for Number of lymph nodes found positive with cancer. And M stands for the presence and degree of Metastasis. T0 means that the entire tumor was removed 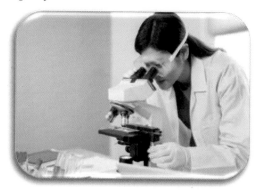 through the biopsy surgical procedure. T1 is a smaller size tumor, with T2, T3, and T4 being larger tumors. N0 means that there were no lymph nodes found with cancer. N1, N2, and N3 indicate increasing involvement of regional lymph nodes with the cancer. M0 means no metastases found. M1 means that metastases were found. So, for example, a breast cancer diagnosis might come back T2 (tumor is 2.5 centimeters=1 inch in diameter), N1 (one lymph node near breast cancer found with malignant cells), and M0 (no evidence of metastasis).

Other oncologists speak of Stage 1 (no metastasis) through stage 2A then B, through stage 3A then B, and culminating in stage 4 (considerable metastasis) cancers.

HOW CANCER IS DIAGNOSED

While early diagnosis of cancer is crucial for improved outcome, most people still do not involve themselves in routine cancer screening techniques. Hence, most cancer patients come to their doctor with a lump, or bump, or soreness, or blood in the stools or urine as the first sign of a health problem.

Physical exam is the starting point for many cancer patients, examining lymph nodes for signs of swelling, Pap smear for cervical cancer, digital rectal exam for prostate cancer, and so on.

Blood tests. There are markers in the blood that can be non-specific indicators of cancer somewhere in the body: alkaline phosphatase (elevated in bone and liver disease), SGOT and SGPT (elevated in liver damage), bilirubin (elevated in liver disease), and LDH (lactate dehydrogenase) elevated in many cancers and indicating how much anaerobic (lacking oxygen) metabolism is going on in the body. Uric acid is elevated in gout and cancers of the blood and lymph nodes. Creatinine and BUN (blood urea nitrogen) are elevated in kidney disease. Calcium is elevated in cancers that have spread to the bone.

Tumor markers. It is useful for the doctor to track substances in the blood that relate to the cancer getting better or worse. None of these tumor markers are perfect. All include a certain percentage of false positive (the test came back positive, but you don't have that cancer) and false negative (the test came back negative, but you do have cancer).

- CEA, or carcinoembryonic antigen, may be elevated in cancers of the colon, breast, lung, and pancreas.
- CA-125 elevated in cancers of the ovary and uterus.
- CA 19-9 elevated in gastrointestinal tract cancers, such as colon, pancreas, stomach, and liver.
- CA 15-3 elevated in breast cancer.
- AFP, or alpha fetal protein, elevated in liver and testis cancer.
- HCG, or human chorionic gonadotropin, elevated in pregnancy and cancers of the testis, ovary, and lung.
- PAP, or prostatic acid phosphatase, elevated in prostate cancer.
- PSA, or prostate specific antigen, elevated in prostate cancer.
- Serum protein electrophoresis, elevated in multiple myeloma.

Testing blood, urine, feces, and spinal fluid may be part of your doctor's exam.

Imaging techniques. Modern medicine has developed some fabulous devices for finding the cancer. What used to require an autopsy can now be done with reasonable accuracy on healthy or sick patients.

X-ray (radiography) can see through tissue and identify differences in the density of tissue, such as a tumor versus healthy tissue. Depending on where your radiologist is examining, the patient may have to consume lightly radioactive material (barium) to add contrast to the diagnosis. X-ray can easily tell the difference between bone and soft flesh. However, in order to determine soft tissue cancers, new techniques, such as nuclear scans, CT (computerized tomography), MRI (magnetic resonance imaging), and ultra sound may be

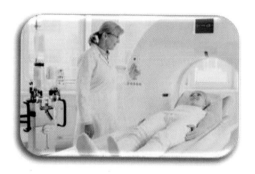

used. PET (positron emission tomography) scans require the doctor to inject radioactively-labeled glucose into the blood stream, then use a "geiger counter"-like device to locate the glucose, because cancer is a sugar feeder, taking up more than its share of sugar in the bloodstream.

The best technique, if possible, is to see the cancer, using a scope. Rigid, thin telescopes can be inserted in various regions of the body to find cancers. A bronchoscope would help examine the lungs. A cytoscope would examine the urethra and bladder. Flexible fiber optic telescopes can not only look inside the body's cavities, but also take out tissue samples for later examination. An endoscope can look into the stomach or colon for signs of cancer.

Biopsy. By taking a sample of the suspect tissue, the doctor can have a pathologist examine the tumor for staging and deciding what protocol to offer the patient. Incisional biopsy involves cutting into the tumor, removing part of it, then stitching the area closed. Excisional biopsy involves removing the entire tumor. It is during the biopsy process that some doctors send the tissue to a lab for determining what forms of chemo might kill this cancer. This process is called "in vitro chemo sensitivity testing" or "ex vivo apoptosis". See RationalTherapeutics.com for more information on this valuable technique for eliminating useless chemo agents and focusing on potentially valuable chemo agents.

YOUR CANCER DOCTOR TEAM

ONCOLOGIST: A Medical Doctor (MD) or Doctor of Osteopathy (DO) who has specialized training in cancer and its treatments with chemotherapy.

RADIOLOGIST: An MD or DO with specialized training in diagnostic use of X-rays and other assessment tools, such as MRI and CT scans.

RADIATION ONCOLOGIST, or radiotherapist: An MD or DO with specialized training in the therapeutic use of radiation to treat cancer or palliate cancer symptoms.

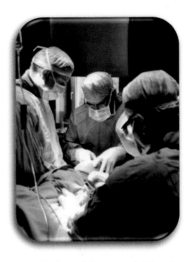

SURGICAL ONCOLOGIST: An MD or DO with specialized training in the surgical removal of cancer masses.

PAIN MANAGEMENT SPECIALIST: An MD or DO with specialized training in dealing with the pain that can accompany cancer. It is imperative that patients get adequate pain management. Whether Tylenol or codeine or morphine, whatever it takes to provide reasonable comfort, is crucial for the recovery of the cancer patient.

INTERNIST: An MD or DO trained in internal medicine or the biochemistry of the body and how to adjust problems that arise.

WHAT ABOUT YOUR CANCER?

While there are nearly 200 different cancers, there are only three main categories:

- ◆ carcinoma, such as breast, lung, colon, and prostate
- ◆ sarcomas, which are found in the connective tissue
- ◆ leukemias and lymphomas, which originate in the blood, bone marrow, and lymph nodes

Of the 1.7 million Americans who will be newly diagnosed with cancer this year, and of the 46 main cancers that are tracked, over 50% of these cancer patients will have one of the more common cancers:

- ◆ Colon/rectum 144,000 per year
- ◆ Lung 228,000
- ◆ Breast 240,000
- ◆ Prostate 240,000

Yet, each of these cancer diagnoses have something in common: the cancer is an abnormal growth that could consume the patient through malnutrition, organ failure, or infection. Nutrition can improve outcome in nearly all cancer patients who are undergoing medical therapies.

PATIENT PROFILE: SURVIVING KIDNEY CANCER
M.M. was diagnosed with renal cell carcinoma stage 4. She took thalidomide and interferon for nearly 2 years, then stopped these medications due to side effects, which included vomiting, headaches, and neuropathy (numb and painful hands and feet). M.M. used the nutrition guidelines in this book along with mistletoe and dendritic cell therapy to shrink her tumor by 30%. She was given 6 months to live, yet has survived 3 years, although she still has tumor burden. Her quality of life is good. M.M. says that "we are all terminal. Just try to make a difference in someone else's life."

For more information on how your body can fight cancer go to GettingHealthier.com.

Chapter 6

CONVENTIONAL CANCER TREATMENTS

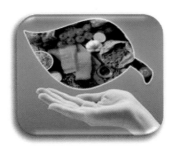

"Nature to be commanded must be obeyed.
Francis Bacon, founder of modern science, circa 1600

WHAT'S AHEAD?
- ✓ Conventional treatments for cancer include chemo, radiation, and surgery.
- ✓ None of these therapies are a universal fix for all cancer patients.
- ✓ See the chapter on Rational Cancer Treatments for more therapies to consider.

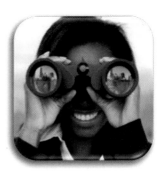

CONVENTIONAL THERAPIES

Chemotherapy is a spin-off product from the chemical warfare of World Wars I and II and is now given to 75% of all American cancer patients. Yale University pharmacologists who were working on a government project during World War II to develop an antidote for mustard gas noted that bone marrow and lymphoid tissue were heavily damaged by these poisons. That observation led to experiments in which mustard gas was injected into mice with lymphomas (cancer of the lymph glands) and produced remission. In 1943, researchers found that mustard gas had a similar effect on human Hodgkin's disease.[1] Chemo has also become a useful agent against testicular cancer, which is now 92% curable. Most proponents of chemo now recognize the limitations of using chemo as the sole therapy against many types of cancer.

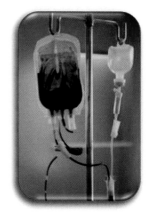

Shortly after these initial exciting discoveries, progress on chemo cures quickly plateaued and forced the innovative thinkers into creative combinations of various chemo drugs, which is now the accepted practice. In the 1980s, oncologists began using chemo by "fractionated drip infusion" in the hospital rather than one large (bolus) injection in the doctor's office. The fractionated method was not only more effective against the cancer, but also less toxic for the patient. Think of the difference in toxicity between taking two glasses of wine with dinner each night, or guzzling all 14 glasses at one time at the end of the week. Also, fractionated drip infusion is more likely to catch the cancer cells in their growth phase, while bolus injections are a random guess to coincide with the growth phase of cancer.

In the next evolutionary step, borrowing from technology developed for heart disease, oncologists began using catheters (thin tubes) that could be inserted into an artery (called intra-arterial infusion) to deliver chemo at the site of the tumor, once again improving response and reducing overall toxicity.

Radiation therapy is given to about 60% of all cancer patients. In 1896, a French physicist, Marie Curie discovered radium, a radioactive metal. For her brilliance, Madam Curie was eventually awarded two Nobel prizes and was considered one of the founders of radiation therapy and the nuclear age. For her unprotected use of radioactive materials, she eventually died while still young of leukemia.

Cancer patients were soon being treated with a new technique developed by the German physicist, Wilhelm Roentgen, called radiation therapy. This technique relies on regional destruction of unwanted tissue through ionizing radiation that disrupts the DNA of all bombarded cells. Radiation therapy can be externally or internally originated, high or low dose, and delivered with uncanny computer-assisted precision to the site of the tumor.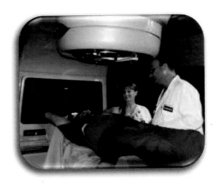

Brachytherapy, or interstitial radiation therapy, places the source of radiation directly into the tumor, as an implanted seed. New techniques use radiation in combination with heat therapy (hyperthermia). Intensity modulated radiation therapy (IMRT) has the potential of being more destructive on the tumor and less harmful to the patient.

Surgery is the first treatment of choice for about 67% of cancer patients. By 1600 B.C., Egyptian physicians were excising tumors using knives or red-hot irons.[2] By physically removing the obvious tumor, physicians feel that they have the best chance for overall success. Unfortunately, many tumors are so entwined with delicate body organs, such as brain and liver, that the tumor cannot be resected (cut out). Another concern is that partial removal of a cancer mass may open the once-encapsulated tumor to spread, like opening a sack of dandelion seeds on your lawn.

Biological therapies, as with most other discoveries, were the product of accidents being observed by a bright mind. William B. Coley, MD, a New York cancer surgeon, scoured the hospital records around 1880 looking for some clue as to why only a minority of patients survived cancer surgery. He found that a high percentage of survivors had developed an infection shortly after the surgery to remove the cancer. This observation led Dr. Coley to inject a wide variety of bacteria, known as Coley's cocktail, into his cancer patients, who then underwent the feverish recovery phase, with noteworthy cancer cures produced. Infections were found to induce the immune system into a higher state of activity, which then helped to destroy tumors. From this crude beginning, molecular biologists have found brilliant ways of producing injectable amounts of the immune factors that can fight cancer.

Biological therapies attempt to fine-tune and focus the immune system into a more vigorous attack on the cancer. Lymphokines are basically "bullets" produced by the immune system to kill invading cells, such as cancer. Lymphokine-activated killer (LAK) cells are incubated in the laboratory in the presence of a stimulator (interleukin-2) and then injected back into the cancer patient's body for an improved immune response.[3]

Interferon, interleukin, monoclonal antibodies, and tumor necrosis factor are among the leading contenders as biological therapies against cancer. The downside of biological therapies is that most forms have extremely toxic side effects.

Heat Therapy (hyperthermia). Cancer cells seem to be more vulnerable to heat than normal healthy cells. Since the time of Hippocrates and the Egyptian Pharaohs, heat therapy has been valued. Experts have shown that applying heat to the patient elevates immune responses. Temperatures of 42 degrees Celsius or 107 degrees Fahrenheit will kill most cancer cells, but can be quite stressful on the patient also. Could it be that exercise induces regular "hyperthermia" to kill off cancer cells before they can become a problem?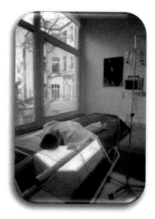

Whole body hyperthermia involves a very sophisticated hot tub device, general anesthesia, and medical supervision. Regional hyperthermia can involve either a miniature waterbed-like device applied to the tumor or focused microwaves. Hyperthermia can be useful by itself, or used synergistically to improve the response to chemo and radiation therapy. German oncologist, Friedrich Douwes, MD, has reported superb results using hyperthermia (website: klinik-st-georg.de). American hyperthermia units are found throughout the country.

PATIENT PROFILE

J.B. was diagnosed with stage 4 prostate cancer in 2010. He underwent surgery, radiation and other treatments recommended by his Oncologist, but none of it worked. He says, "My doctors were killing me. My Oncologist and Urologist kept giving me more drugs, I was feeling bad, and there was pain. I did not want to live like a human skeleton living in a wheelchair." He heard Dr. Quillin at The Truth About Cancer and read Beating Cancer with Nutrition. J.B. resonated with what PQ had to say. He had an initial phone consultation with PQ late 2015. J.B. keeps Beating Cancer with Nutrition handy and refers to it often. "Beating Cancer with Nutrition is doable," he said. He has changed his diet, eats more natural foods, and drinks organic juices. J.B. has turned to Mind Body Medicine and believes he can heal himself. While his PSA is often a little high, he is still here, feels good and energetic. He goes to the gym 3x week, swims and walks regularly. J.B. is now 9 years beyond his diagnosis of a very poor prognostic cancer.

For more information on how your body can fight cancer go to GettingHealthier.com.

ENDNOTES

[1]. Romm, S, Washington Post, p.Z14, Jan.9, 1990

[2]. Herman, R., Washington Post, p.Z14, Dec.3, 1991

[3]. Boly, W, Hippocrates, p.38, Jan.1989

Chapter 7

MALNUTRITION AMONG CANCER PATIENTS

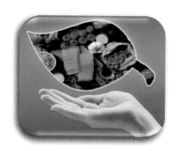

"The western diet is fertilizer for cancer."
David Servan-Schreiber, MD, PhD
author ANTI-CANCER: A NEW WAY OF LIFE

WHAT'S AHEAD?

✓ At least 20% of Americans are clinically malnourished, with 70% being sub-clinically malnourished (less obvious), and the remaining "chosen few" 10% in good to optimal health.

✓ Once these malnourished people get sick, the malnutrition oftentimes gets worse through higher nutrient needs and lower intake

✓ Once at the hospital, malnutrition escalates another notch

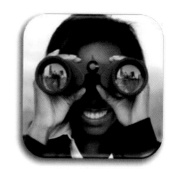

> ✓ Cancer is one of the more serious wasting diseases known
> ✓ A malnourished cancer patient suffers a reduction in quality and quantity of life, with higher incidences of complications and death
> ✓ The only solution for malnutrition is optimal nutrition

Howard Hughes, the multi-billionaire, died of malnutrition. In his later years, Hughes became paranoid of germs and would not eat. When Hughes died at age 70, he was only recognizable through his fingerprints. While over 1 billion people in the world are obese, 800 million are in the death grips of starvation.

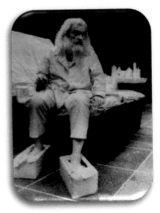

92% of Americans do not get the RDA for the established essential nutrients. All of this is malnutrition. And once a person gets diagnosed with cancer, malnutrition becomes much more common and lethal. This chapter is dedicated to preventing and reversing the malnutrition that kills at least 40% of cancer patients.

MALNUTRITION IN THE LAND OF PLENTY?

It is hard to believe that there can be malnutrition in this agriculturally abundant nation of ours--but there is. At the time of the Revolutionary War, 96% of Americans farmed while only 4% worked at other trades. Tractors and harvesting-combines became part of an agricultural revolution that allowed the 2% of Americans who now farm to feed the rest of us. We grow enough food in this country to feed ourselves, to make half of us overweight, to throw away enough food to feed 50 million people daily, to ship food overseas as a major export, and to store enough food in government surplus bins to feed Americans for a year if all farmers quit today. With so much food available, how can Americans be malnourished?

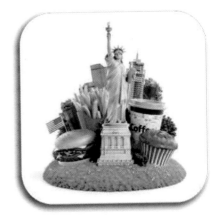

The answer is: poor food choices. Americans choose their food based upon taste, cost, convenience, and psychological gratification--thus ignoring the main reason that we eat, which is to provide our body cells with the raw materials to grow, repair, and fuel our bodies. The most commonly eaten foods in America are white bread, coffee, and hot dogs. Based upon our food abundance, Americans could be the best nourished nation on record. But we are far from it.

CAUSES OF NUTRIENT DEFICIENCIES:

There are many reasons for developing malnutrition:

♦ We don't eat well due to poor food choices, loss of appetite, discomfort in the gastrointestinal region, or consuming nutritionally bankrupt "junk food"; many people just don't get enough nutrients into their stomachs.

♦ We don't absorb nutrients due to loss of digestive functions (including low hydrochloric acid or enzyme output), allergy, "leaky gut", or intestinal infections, like yeast overgrowth.

♦ We don't keep enough nutrients due to increased excretion or loss of nutrients because of diarrhea, vomiting, or drug interactions.

♦ We don't get enough nutrients due to increased requirements caused by fever, disease, alcohol, or drug interactions.

♦ Anyone who is confused about why we spend so much on medical care with such poor results in cancer treatment might glean some wisdom by reading what sells best in American grocery stores.

♦ Overwhelming evidence from both government and independent scientific surveys shows that many Americans are low in their intake of:[1]

VITAMINS: A, D, E, C, B-6, riboflavin, folacin, pantothenic acid

MINERALS: calcium, potassium, magnesium, zinc, iron, chromium, selenium; and possibly molybdenum and vanadium. With many common micronutrient deficiencies in the Western diet, it makes sense that a major study in Australia found that regular use of vitamin supplements was a protective factor against colon cancer.[2]

MACRONUTRIENTS: fiber, complex carbohydrates, plant protein, special fatty acids (EPA, GLA, ALA), clean water.

Meanwhile, we also eat alarmingly high amounts of: fat, salt, sugar, cholesterol, alcohol, caffeine, food additives, and toxins.

This combination of too much of the wrong things along with not enough of the right things has created epidemic proportions of degenerative diseases in this country. The Surgeon General, Department of Health and Human Services, Center for Disease Control, National Academy of Sciences, American Medical Association, Academy of Nutrition and Dietetics, and most other major public health agencies agree that diet is a major contributor to our most common health problems, including cancer.

Americans have deviated so far from our ancestral diet as to be laughable. Drs. Shostak, Eaton, and Connor studied the diets of indigenous people around the world, those not influenced by processed foods. They published their findings as the "paleolithic diet" in an article in the New England Journal of Medicine and a book. Our hunter-gatherer ancestors ate less sodium (salt), more potassium (from plant food), more calcium (from bones), much more fiber (from plant foods), much more vitamin C (from plant foods), no refined carbohydrates (from white flour and sugar), and more protein (from free range animals, high in essential fats).

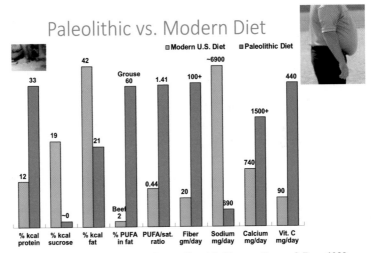

Source: Paleolithic Prescription by Eaton, Shostak, Konner, Harper & Row, 1988

The typical diet of the cancer patient is high in fat, while being low in fiber and vegetables--"meat, potatoes, and gravy" is what many of my patients lived on. Data collected by the United States Department of Agriculture from over 11,000 Americans showed that on any given day:

- ◆ 41% did not eat any fruit
- ◆ 82% did not eat cruciferous vegetables
- ◆ 72% did not eat vitamin C-rich fruits or vegetables
- ◆ 80% did not eat vitamin A-rich fruits or vegetables
- ◆ 84% did not eat high fiber grain food, like bread or cereal[3]

At the world-famous San Diego Safari Park, experts spend an incredible amount of time and money replicating the diet of that animal in its native environment, because that's how you keep the animals healthy. Humans ignore this obvious link to our ancestral past. Not surprisingly, 88% of Americans suffer from some metabolic disease, often due to malnutrition.

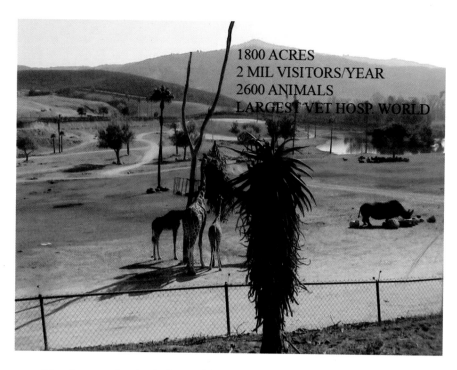

1800 ACRES
2 MIL VISITORS/YEAR
2600 ANIMALS
LARGEST VET HOSP. WORLD

The human body is incredibly resilient, which sometimes works to our disadvantage. No one dies on the first cigarette inhaled, or the first drunken evening, or the first decade of unhealthy eating. We misconstrue the fact that we survived this ordeal to mean we can do it forever. Not so. Malnutrition can be as blatant as the starving babies in third world countries, but malnutrition can also be much more subtle.

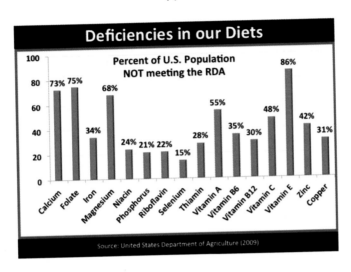

Deficiencies in our Diets

Percent of U.S. Population NOT meeting the RDA

Source: United States Department of Agriculture (2009)

SEQUENCE IN DEVELOPING NUTRIENT DEFICIENCY

- ◆ 1) *Preliminary.* Reduction of tissue stores and depression of urinary excretion.
- ◆ 2) *Biochemical.* Reduction of enzyme activity due to insufficient coenzymes (vitamins). Urinary excretion at minimum levels.
- ◆ 3) *Physiological.* Behavioral effects, such as insomnia or somnolence. Irritability accompanied by loss of appetite and reduced body weight. Modified drug metabolism and reduced immune capabilities.
- ◆ 4) *Clinical.* Classical deficiency syndromes as recognized by the scientific pioneers in the developmental phases of nutrition science.
- ◆ 5) *Terminal.* Severe tissue pathology resulting in imminent death.

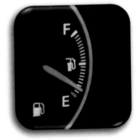

BAD MATH. While there are 118 elements in the periodic table, or the building blocks of the planet earth and you, about 83 of these are considered essential/useful for human or plant health. Yet only 3 of these elements (Nitrogen, Potassium K, Phosphorus) are added to the soil in agribusiness. There has been a dramatic decline in the mineral content of food grown on American soil due to this bad math. Americans are deficient in magnesium, selenium, chromium, vanadium, lithium, strontium, and more. Malnutrition at macro and micro levels can lead to cancer. Restoring human health requires attention to the missing nutrients in the American diet.

ELEMENTS REQUIRED FOR HUMAN HEALTH

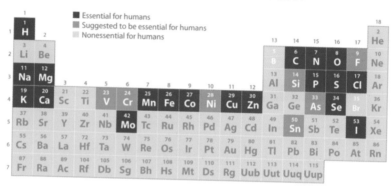

83 elements possibly involved in human and plant health
MAJOR ELEMENTS: H, C, O
major elements in agriculture: N, P, K
minor elements in agriculture: Mg, Ca, S, Na, Cl
trace elements in agriculture: B, Cu, Mn, Mb, Zn, I, Co, Se
64 elements remaining unimportant?

It was the Framingham study done by Harvard University that proclaimed: "Our way of life is related to our way of death." Typical hospital food continues or even worsens malnutrition. While many Americans are overfed, the majority are also poorly nourished. If proper nutrition could prevent from 30% to 90% of all cancer, then doesn't it seem foolish to continue feeding the cancer patient the same diet that helped to induce cancer in the first place?

MALNUTRITION AMONG CANCER PATIENTS

From 25%-50% of hospital patients suffer from protein calorie malnutrition. Protein calorie malnutrition leads to increases in mortality and surgical failure, with a reduction in immunity, wound healing, cardiac output, response to chemo and radiation therapy, and plasma protein synthesis, and generally induces weakness and apathy. Many patients are malnourished before entering the hospital, and another 10% become malnourished once in the hospital. Nutrition support, as peripheral parenteral nutrition, has been shown to reduce the length of hospital stay by 30%. Weight loss leads to a decrease in patient survival. Common nutrient deficiencies, as determined by experts at M.D. Anderson Hospital in Houston, include protein calorie, thiamin, riboflavin, niacin, folate, and K.

Nutrition therapy has two distinct phases:

1) Take the clinically malnourished patient and bring him/her up to "normal" status.

2) Take the "normal" sub-clinically malnourished person and bring him/her up to "optimal" functioning. For at least the few nutrients tested thus far, there appears to be a "dose-dependent" response--more than RDA levels of intake provide for more than "normal" immune functions.

Not only is malnutrition common in the "normal" American, but malnutrition is extremely common in the cancer patient. A theory has persisted for decades that one could starve the tumor out of the host. That just ain't so. The tumor is quite resistant to starvation, and most studies find more harm to the host than to the tumor in either selective or blanket nutrient 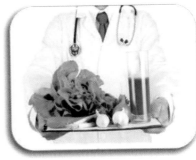 deficiencies.[4] Pure malnutrition (cachexia) is responsible for at least 22% and up to 67% of all cancer deaths. Up to 80% of all cancer patients have reduced levels of serum albumin, which is a leading indicator of protein and calorie malnutrition.[5] Dietary protein restriction in the cancer patient does not affect the composition or growth rate of the tumor, but does restrict the patient's well-being.[6]

A commonly used anti-cancer drug is methotrexate, which interferes with folate (a B vitamin) metabolism. Many scientists guessed that folate in the diet might accelerate cancer growth. Not so. Depriving animals of folate in the diet allowed their tumors to grow anyway.[7] Actually, in starved animals, the tumors grew more rapidly than in fed animals, indicating the parasitic tenacity of cancer in the host.[8] Other studies have found that a low folate environment can trigger "brittle" DNA to fuel cancer metastasis.

There is some evidence that tumors are not as flexible as healthy host tissue in using fuel. A low carbohydrate parenteral formula may have the ability to slow down tumor growth by selectively starving the cancer cells.[9] Overall, the research shows that starvation provokes host wasting while tumor growth continues unabated.[10] Weight loss drastically increases the mortality rate for most types of cancer, while also lowering the response to chemotherapy.[11]

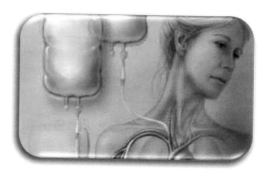

Parenteral feeding improves tolerance to chemotherapeutic agents and immune responses.[12] Of 28 children with advanced malignant disease, 18 received parenteral feeding for 28 days with resultant improvements in weight gain, increased serum albumin and transferrin, and major benefits in immune functions. In comparing cancer patients on TPN versus those trying to nourish themselves by oral intake of food, TPN provided major improvements in calorie, protein, and nutrient intake, but did not encourage tumor growth. Malnourished cancer patients who were provided TPN had a mortality rate of 11%, while the group without TPN feeding had a 100% mortality rate.[13] Pre-operative TPN in patients undergoing surgery for GI cancer provided general reduction in the incidence of wound infection, pneumonia, major complications, and mortality.[14] Patients who were the most malnourished experienced a 33% mortality and 46% morbidity (problems and illness) rate, while those patients who were properly nourished had a 3% mortality rate with an 8% morbidity rate. In 49 patients with lung cancer receiving chemotherapy with or without TPN, complete remission was achieved in 85% of the TPN group versus 59% of the non-TPN group.[15] A TPN formula that was higher in protein, especially branched chain amino acids, was able to provide better nitrogen balance in the 21 adults tested than the conventional 8.5% amino acid TPN formula.[16]

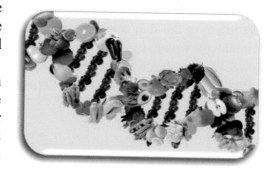

A finely-tuned nutrition formula can also nourish the patient while starving tumor cells. Enteral (oral) formulas fortified with arginine, fish oil, and RNA have been shown to stimulate the immune system, accelerate wound repair, and reduce tumor burden in both animals and humans.

In 20 adult hospitalized patients on TPN, the mean daily vitamin C needs were 975 mg, which is over 16 times the RDA, with the range being 350-2250 mg.[17] Of the 139 lung cancer patients studied, most tested deficient or scorbutic (clinical vitamin C deficiency).[18] Another study of cancer patients found that 46% tested scorbutic, while 76% were below acceptable levels for serum ascorbate.[19] Experts now recommend the value of nutritional supplements, especially in patients who require prolonged TPN support.[20] The Recommended Dietary Allowance (RDA) is inadequate for many healthy people and nearly all sick people.

DRAGON-SLAYER SHAKE

Many people with chemo nausea can drink this shake when nothing else sounds appetizing. Shakes can be a quick and easy breakfast or meal substitute. Depending on your calorie requirements, use this shake in addition to or instead of a meal. See the chapter on anti-cancer foods for details and ingredients for this invaluable food supplement.

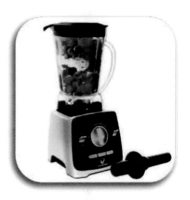

PATIENT PROFILE

J.H. was a wasting 38 year old male with advanced lymphoma when he was admitted to our hospital as a medical emergency, having failed prior therapies. He was dying more from malnutrition than the cancer. We put him on total parenteral nutrition, with a disease-specific formula that is higher in protein and fats and lower in glucose than standard TPN formulas. Within a month, he was able to eat solid foods. He rebounded from his malnutrition so that he could resume chemo. Within 6 months he was disease-free. Eight years later, still in remission

For more information on how your body can fight cancer go to GettingHealthier.com.

ENDNOTES

[1]. Quillin, P., HEALING NUTRIENTS, p.43, Vintage Books, NY, 1989

[2]. Kune, GA, and Kune, S., Nutrition and Cancer, vol.9, p.1, 1987

[3]. Patterson, BH, and Block, G., American Journal of Public Health, vol.78, p.282, Mar.1988

[4]. Axelrod, AE, and Traketelis, AC, Vitamins and Hormones, vol.22, p.591, 1964

[5]. Dreizen, S., et al., Postgraduate Medicine, vol.87, no.1, p.163, Jan.1990

[6]. Lowry, SF, et al., Surgical Forum, vol.28, p.143, 1977

[7]. Nichol, CA, Cancer Research, vol.29, p.2422, 1969

[8]. Norton, JA, et al., Cancer, vol.45, p.2934, 1980

[9]. Dematrakopoulos, GE, and Brennan, MF, Cancer Research, (sup.),vol.42, p.756, Feb.1982

[10]. Goodgame, JT, et al., American Journal of Clinical Nutrition, vol.32, p.2277, 1979

[11]. Dewys, WD, et al., American Journal of Medicine, vol.69, p.491, Oct.1980

[12]. Eys, JV, Cancer, vol.43, p.2030, 1979

[13]. Harvey, KB, et al., Cancer, vol.43, p.2065, 1979

[14]. Muller, JM, et al., Lancet, p.68, Jan.9, 1982

[15]. Valdivieso, M., et al., Cancer Treatment Reports, vol.65, sup.5, p.145, 1981

[16]. Gazzaniga, AB, et al., Archives of Surgery, vol. 123, p.1275, 1988

[17]. Abrahamian, V., et al., Journal of Parenteral and Enteral Nutrition, vol.7, no.5, p.465, 1983

[18]. Anthony, HM, et al., British Journal of Cancer, vol.46, p.354, 1982

[19]. Cheraskin, E., Journal of Alternative Medicine, p.18, Feb.1986

[20]. Hoffman, FA, Cancer, vol.55, 1 sup.1, p.295, Jan.1, 1985

Chapter 8

MAKING CHEMO AND RADIATION MORE EFFECTIVE

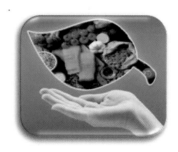

Modern medicine is based on a lie.
Dale Bredesen, MD,
author of bestselling book THE END OF ALZHEIMER'S

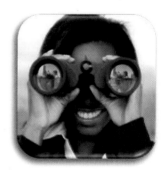

WHAT'S AHEAD?

Nutrients can improve cancer treatment by:
- ✓ protecting the patient from the damaging effects of chemotherapy and radiation while allowing these therapies to kill the tumor
- ✓ bolstering host defense mechanisms, like the immune system

Cancer patients often feel like a child in a wicked divorce custody battle. The oncologist tells the patient "Don't take that nutrition therapy. It is nothing more than expensive urine. And it will reduce the effectiveness of my chemo and radiation therapies." The nutritionist tells the same patient "Don't take that poisonous chemo or radiation therapy. It will do you no good." In fact, when the oncologist and nutritionist work together, both are more successful at helping the cancer patient. Nutrients make medical therapy more toxic to the tumor and less toxic to the patient.

Properly nourished patients experience less nausea, malaise, immune suppression, hair loss, and organ toxicity than patients on routine oncology programs. Antioxidants like beta carotene, vitamin C, vitamin E, glutathione, and selenium appear to enhance the effectiveness of chemo, radiation, and hyperthermia, while minimizing damage to the patient's normal cells; thus making therapy more of a "selective toxin." An optimally-nourished cancer patient can better tolerate the rigors of cytotoxic therapy.

Charles Simone, MD has published a peer reviewed meta-analysis of the world's literature on supplement use during chemo and radiation.[1] Analyzing 50 clinical trials involving 8,500 cancer patients, nutrients were found to enhance outcome in cancer patients treated with chemo and radiation.

In a separate review of the world's peer reviewed scientific literature, Keith Block, MD examined 33 studies involving 2,400 cancer patients and found that antioxidant supplements reduced the toxicity of the chemo allowing patients to complete their treatment cycles; and there was no reduction in tumor kill from the chemo.[2]

Roots of Chemo

"All is fair in love and war." Mustard gas (aka nerve gas) was used as a weapon in World War I. For even the horrors of war, mustard gas was deemed unethical. Mustard gas had profound effects on reducing bone marrow cells that develop into blood cells in soldiers exposed.[3] Yet, from that basis, the field of chemotherapy developed.

It is puzzling why oncologists will readily prescribe a drug antioxidant (like Mesna) to reduce the toxicity of chemo and enhance outcome, yet balk at giving an even more safe and inexpensive nutrient antioxidant.[4]

In many of my patients, using nutrition supplements while undergoing chemo and radiation has had a profound effect on improving patient quality of life and minimizing "collateral damage" to the patient's body. Oncologists often prescribe chemo to the "therapeutic brink of death", meaning the patient's immune system is so compromised that death by infection is very possible. By using nutrition supplements in conjunction with chemo and radiation, tumor kill is unaffected while the patient's immune system remains intact.

Free Radicals Vs. Antioxidants

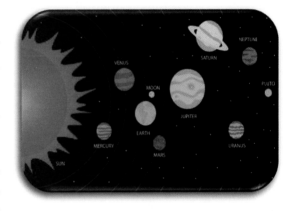

Linus Pauling, PhD, earned one of his Nobel prizes in chemistry in the 1950s by discovering how atoms bond together to become molecules. Picture the sun with Earth, Saturn, and Mars among other planets orbiting around the sun. Atoms and molecules are a tiny rendition of our solar system. Electrons orbit the nucleus of an atom just like planets orbit around the sun in our solar system. Atoms bond together, such as hydrogen with oxygen to yield water, by sharing electrons, as if two suns came close together and shared planets or moons to keep in balance and to be complete.

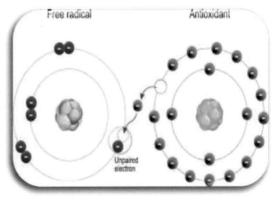

Now imagine if a planet was missing from a solar system. There is an imbalance in forces that makes this solar system unstable. Free radicals, or pro-oxidants, are like unstable solar systems, because they lack a planet in their outer orbit. Free radicals will grab a planet from a nearby solar system to make that solar system now unstable. And on it goes in domino fashion, disrupting solar systems (or atoms and molecules) until tissue damage occurs and cancer or premature aging sets in. Though there are many variations of pro-oxidants and antioxidants, the theme is always the same: pro-oxidants can destroy tissue, while antioxidants can protect tissue. Humans generate pro-oxidants in our immune system to kill invaders, like cancer. We also generate pro-oxidants in the process of metabolizing our food...not only unavoidable, but essential functions. So free radicals are only bad if they are destroying tissue that needs to be spared.

Oxygen, hydrogen peroxide (which we constantly create inside of our bodies as part of living), air pollution (ozone), tobacco smoke, most chemotherapy drugs, radiation therapy, and alcohol are among the more common and noteworthy free radicals in life. Chemo and radiation are free radicals that work by, hopefully, killing more cancer cells than healthy cells. We are constantly "rusting" from within, just like a nail rusts outside. We can slow down this rusting with antioxidants, such as vitamin C and lipoic acid, but we cannot stop it.

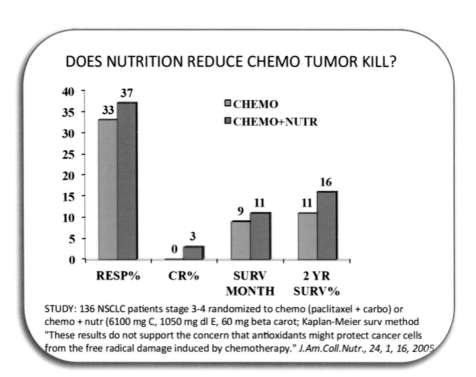

DOES NUTRITION REDUCE CHEMO TUMOR KILL?

STUDY: 136 NSCLC patients stage 3-4 randomized to chemo (paclitaxel + carbo) or chemo + nutr (6100 mg C, 1050 mg dl E, 60 mg beta carot; Kaplan-Meier surv method "These results do not support the concern that antioxidants might protect cancer cells from the free radical damage induced by chemotherapy." *J.Am.Coll.Nutr., 24, 1, 16, 2005*

Basically, free radicals are electron (planet) thieves, and antioxidants, such as vitamin C, are electron donors. Antioxidants perform like a sacrificial warrior, giving up their life so that your tissue is not harmed. However, in an anaerobic environment, such as cancer, antioxidants can become pro-oxidants.

Researchers "assume" that antioxidant nutrients (such as coenzyme Q, glutathione, and vitamin E) will reduce the tumor kill rate from chemo and radiation. In simplistic chemistry, one might think this to be true. However, in test tubes (in vitro), in animals, and in human cancer patients, such is not the case. Since cancer is usually an oxygen-deprived tissue, or anaerobic cell, the cancer cell has very poor mechanisms for absorbing proper amounts of antioxidants. A cancer cell has no more use for antioxidants than a gopher needs sunglasses. The exception is vitamin C, which becomes a selective toxin against cancer without harming the patient.

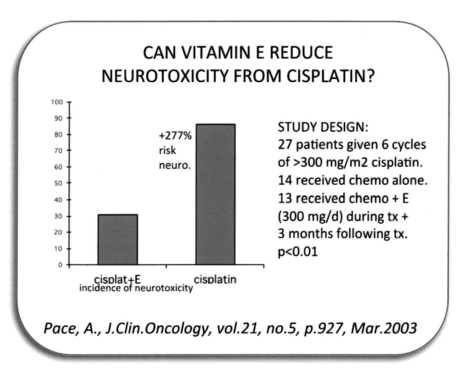

CAN VITAMIN E REDUCE NEUROTOXICITY FROM CISPLATIN?

+277% risk neuro.

STUDY DESIGN:
27 patients given 6 cycles of >300 mg/m2 cisplatin.
14 received chemo alone.
13 received chemo + E (300 mg/d) during tx + 3 months following tx.
p<0.01

cisplat+E   cisplatin
incidence of neurotoxicity

Pace, A., J.Clin.Oncology, vol.21, no.5, p.927, Mar.2003

Cancer cells are primarily anaerobic (meaning "without oxygen") cells. With the exception of vitamin C, cancer cells do not absorb nor use antioxidants the same way that healthy aerobic cells do. Vitamin C (ascorbic acid) is nearly identical in chemical structure to glucose, which is the favored fuel for cancer cells. When researchers found that radioactively labeled ascorbic acid was preferentially absorbed by implanted tumors in animals, they admitted that this effect takes place because cancer has many more glucose receptors on the cell surface than healthy normal cells. The vitamin C is gulped by the cancer cells, then becomes toxic because <u>cancer cells cannot generate catalase</u> to protect themselves against the hydrogen peroxide generated by vitamin C.[5]

VITAMIN K. While in simplistic theory, vitamin K might inhibit the effectiveness of anticoagulant therapy (coumadin), actually vitamin K seems to augment the anti-neoplastic activity of coumadin. In a study with human rheumatoid arthritis patients being given methotrexate, folic acid supplements did not reduce the antiproliferative therapeutic value of methotrexate.[6] In one study, patients with mouth cancer who were pre-treated with injections of K-3 prior to radiation therapy doubled their odds (20% vs. 39%) for 5-year survival and disease-free status.[7] Animals with implanted tumors had greatly improved anti-cancer effects from all chemotherapy drugs tested when vitamins K and C were given in combination.[8] In cultured leukemia cells, vitamins K and E added to the chemotherapy drugs of 5FU (fluorouracil) and leucovorin provided a 300% improvement in growth inhibition when compared to 5FU by itself.[9] Animals given methotrexate and K-3 had improvements in cancer reversal, with no increase in toxicity to the host tissue.[10]

VITAMIN C. There is compelling evidence that <u>high dose intravenous vitamin C</u> has a central role in cancer treatment.[11] High dose IVC as sole therapy has often been shown to be <u>effective in advanced cancer patients</u>.[12] Researchers from the NCI and other institutions have reported that in 2008 there were 172 doctors who <u>administered IVC to over 12,000</u> patients with remarkably few side effects and good clinical outcomes.[13] Tumor-bearing mice fed high doses of vitamin C (antioxidant) along with adriamycin (pro-oxidant) had a prolonged life and no reduction in the tumor-killing capacity of adriamycin.[14] Lung cancer patients who were provided antioxidant nutrients prior to, during, and after radiation and chemotherapy had enhanced tumor destruction and significantly longer life span.[15] Tumor-bearing mice fed high doses of vitamin C experienced an increased tolerance to radiation therapy without reduction in the tumor-killing capacity of the radiation.[16]

FISH OIL. A special fat in fish (eicosapentaenoic acid, EPA) improves tumor kill in hyperthermia and chemotherapy by altering cancer cell membranes for increased vulnerability.[17] EPA increases the ability of adriamycin to kill cultured leukemia cells.[18] Tumors in EPA-fed animals are more responsive to Mitomycin C and doxorubicin (chemo drugs).[19]

EPA and another special fat from plants (gamma linolenic acid, GLA) were selectively toxic to human tumor cell lines while also enhancing the cytotoxic effects of chemotherapy.[20] When <u>fish oil was given along with chemo</u> in patients with non-small cell lung cancer, the one year survival rate was nearly double (60% vs. 38%) in the fish oil group.[21]

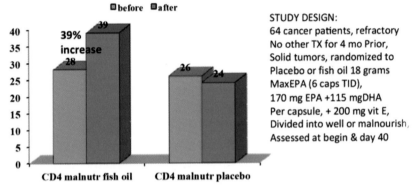

DOES FISH OIL SUPPLEMENTATION AS SOLE THERAPY IMPROVE OUTCOME IN REFRACTORY PATIENTS WITH SOLID TUMORS

"...consider alternative, less toxic treatment approaches..."

STUDY DESIGN:
64 cancer patients, refractory
No other TX for 4 mo Prior,
Solid tumors, randomized to
Placebo or fish oil 18 grams
MaxEPA (6 caps TID),
170 mg EPA +115 mgDHA
Per capsule, + 200 mg vit E,
Divided into well or malnourish,
Assessed at begin & day 40

"Omega 3 prolonged survival of all patients...resulted in significant (p<0.025) increase in survival for all patients compared with placebo"
Gogos, et al., Cancer, vol.82, p.395, 1998

VITAMIN A & BETA-CAROTENE. There is a synergistic benefit of using vitamin A with carotenoids in patients who are being treated with chemo, radiation, and surgery for common malignancies.[22] Beta-carotene and vitamin A together provided a significant improvement in outcome in animals treated with radiation for induced cancers.[23]

VITAMIN E. Vitamin E protects the body against the potentially damaging effects of iron (pro-oxidant) and fish oil. Vitamin E deficiency, which is common in cancer patients, will accentuate the cardiotoxic effects of adriamycin.[24] The worse the vitamin E deficiency in animals, the greater the heart damage from adriamycin.[25] Patients undergoing chemo, radiation, and bone marrow transplant for cancer treatment had markedly depressed levels of serum antioxidants, including vitamin E.[26] Vitamin E protects animals against a potent carcinogen, DMBA.[27]

Vitamin E supplements prevented the glucose-raising effects of a chemo drug, doxorubicin,[28] while improving the tumor-kill rate of doxorubicin.[29] Vitamin E modifies the carcinogenic effect of daunomycin (chemo drug) in animals.[30] One study found that vitamin E supplements (300 mg/day) could reduce the neurotoxicity commonly caused by cisplatin (a chemo drug) from 86% of patients getting the placebo and cisplatin down to 31% of the patients getting vitamin E and cisplatin, which is a 55% reduction in tingling and painful nerves. There was no loss in tumor kill rate from the cisplatin.

NIACIN. Niacin supplements in animals were able to reduce the cardiotoxicity of adriamycin while not interfering with its tumor-killing capacity.[31] Niacin combined with aspirin in 106 bladder cancer patients receiving surgery and radiation therapy provided for a substantial improvement in 5-year survival (72% vs. 27%) over the control group.[32] Niacin seems to make radiation therapy more effective at killing hypoxic cancer cells.[33] Loading radiation patients with 500 mg to 6,000 mg of niacin has been shown to be safe and is one of the most effective agents known to eliminate acute hypoxia in solid malignancies.[34]

SELENIUM. Selenium-deficient animals have more heart damage from the chemo drug, adriamycin.[35] Supplements of selenium and vitamin E in humans did not reduce the efficacy of the chemo drugs against ovarian and cervical cancer.[36] Animals with implanted tumors who were then treated with selenium and cisplatin (chemo drug) had reduced toxicity to the drug with no change in anti-cancer activity.[37] Selenium supplements helped repair DNA damage from a carcinogen in animals.[38] Selenium was selectively toxic to human leukemia cells in culture.[39]

CARNITINE. Carnitine may help the cancer patient by protecting the heart against the damaging effects of adriamycin.[40]

QUERCETIN. Quercetin reduces the toxicity and carcinogenic capacity of substances in the body[41], yet at the same time may enhance the tumor-killing capacity of cisplatin.[42] Quercetin significantly increased the tumor-kill rate of hyperthermia (heat therapy) in cultured cancer cells.[43] See the chapter on minor dietary constituents for more info on quercetin.

GINSENG. Panax ginseng was able to enhance the uptake of mitomycin (an antibiotic and anti-cancer drug) into the cancer cells for increased tumor kill.[44]

PUTTING IT ALL TOGETHER

Finnish oncologists used high doses of nutrients along with chemo and radiation for lung cancer patients. Normally, lung cancer is a "poor prognostic" malignancy, with a 1% expected survival at 30 months under normal treatment. In this study, however, 8 of the 18 patients (44%) that were given nutrition supplements were still alive 6 years after therapy.[45]

NUTRITION IMPROVES OUTCOME IN MEDICALLY TREATED LUNG CANCER PATIENTS

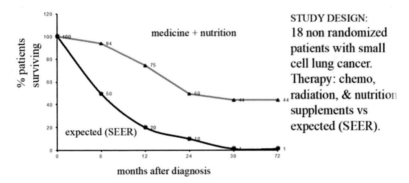

STUDY DESIGN: 18 non randomized patients with small cell lung cancer. Therapy: chemo, radiation, & nutrition supplements vs expected (SEER).

"No side effects observed (from nutrients)." "Surviving patients started AOX treatment earlier than those who succumbed." "AOX treatment should start as early as possible in combination with chemotherapy and/or radiation." Jaakkola, K., et al., Anticancer Research, vol.12, p.599, 1992

In a non-randomized clinical trial, Drs. Hoffer and Pauling instructed patients to follow a reasonable cancer diet (unprocessed foods low in fat, dairy, and sugar), coupled with therapeutic doses of vitamins and minerals.[46] All 129 patients in this study received concomitant oncology care. The control group of 31 patients who did not receive nutrition support lived an average of less than 6 months. The group of 98 cancer patients who did receive the diet and supplement program were categorized into 3 groups:

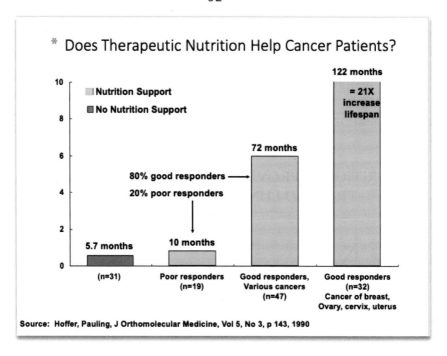

Source: Hoffer, Pauling, J Orthomolecular Medicine, Vol 5, No 3, p 143, 1990

- ◆ Poor responders (n=19) or 20% of treated group. Average lifespan of 10 months, or a 75% improvement over the control group.
- ◆ Good responders (n=47), who had various cancers, including leukemia, lung, liver, and pancreas; had an average lifespan of 72 months (6 years) or a 1,200% improvement in lifespan.
- ◆ Good female responders (n=32), with involvement of reproductive areas (breast, cervix, ovary, uterus); had an average lifespan of over 10 years, or a 2,100% improvement in lifespan. Many were still alive at the end of the study.

Oncologists at West Virginia Medical School randomized 65 patients with transitional cell carcinoma of the bladder into either the "one-per-day" vitamin supplement providing the RDA, or into a group which received the RDA supplement plus 40,000 iu of vitamin A, 100 mg of B-6, 2,000 mg of vitamin C, 400 iu of vitamin E, and 90 mg of zinc. At 10 months, tumor recurrence was 80% in the control group (RDA supplement) and 40% in the experimental "megavitamin" group. Five year projected tumor recurrence was 91% for controls and 41% for "megavitamin" patients. Essentially, high dose nutrients cut tumor recurrence in half.[47]

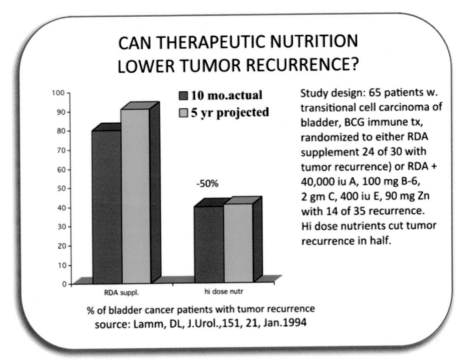

CAN THERAPEUTIC NUTRITION LOWER TUMOR RECURRENCE?

■ 10 mo.actual
□ 5 yr projected

-50%

Study design: 65 patients w. transitional cell carcinoma of bladder, BCG immune tx, randomized to either RDA supplement 24 of 30 with tumor recurrence) or RDA + 40,000 iu A, 100 mg B-6, 2 gm C, 400 iu E, 90 mg Zn with 14 of 35 recurrence. Hi dose nutrients cut tumor recurrence in half.

% of bladder cancer patients with tumor recurrence
source: Lamm, DL, J.Urol.,151, 21, Jan.1994

Lung cancer patients given a basic multi vitamin supplement after surgery for their lung cancer had a nearly 400% longer lifespan than those not given the vitamins.

Chemo and radiation can damage the heart of the patient leading to complications after cancer treatment. Multiple antioxidants (vitamins E, C and N-acetyl cysteine) were able to dramatically reduce the damage to the heart during chemo and radiation.

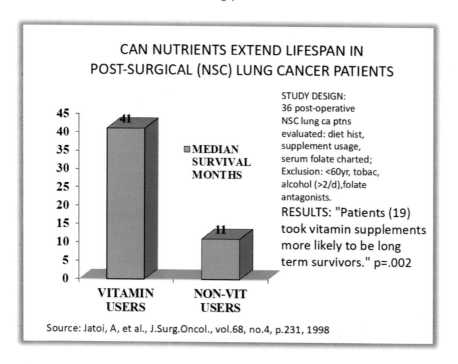

CAN NUTRIENTS EXTEND LIFESPAN IN
POST-SURGICAL (NSC) LUNG CANCER PATIENTS

STUDY DESIGN:
36 post-operative
NSC lung ca ptns
evaluated: diet hist,
supplement usage,
serum folate charted;
Exclusion: <60yr, tobac,
alcohol (>2/d),folate
antagonists.

RESULTS: "Patients (19)
took vitamin supplements
more likely to be long
term survivors." p=.002

Source: Jatoi, A, et al., J.Surg.Oncol., vol.68, no.4, p.231, 1998

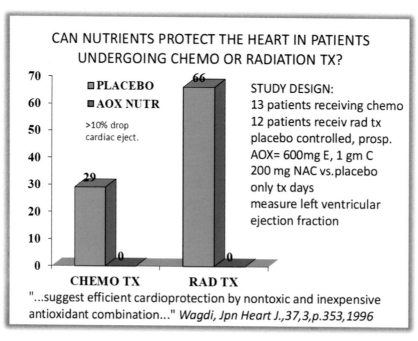

CAN NUTRIENTS PROTECT THE HEART IN PATIENTS
UNDERGOING CHEMO OR RADIATION TX?

STUDY DESIGN:
13 patients receiving chemo
12 patients receiv rad tx
placebo controlled, prosp.
AOX= 600mg E, 1 gm C
200 mg NAC vs.placebo
only tx days
measure left ventricular
ejection fraction

"...suggest efficient cardioprotection by nontoxic and inexpensive
antioxidant combination..." Wagdi, Jpn Heart J.,37,3,p.353,1996

IN SUMMARY: Given the abundance of information supporting the aggressive use of nutrients throughout chemo and radiation, it appears to be illogical and inhumane to ignore or even ban nutrients from the comprehensive cancer treatment regimen.

PATIENT PROFILE: BEAT PANCREATIC CANCER

RM was diagnosed with advanced adenocarcinoma of the pancreas in August 1996 at the age of 53. His lifestyle was unhealthy. He was obese and on cholesterol lowering drugs. His doctors admitted that this cancer was a "poor prognostic" cancer, meaning very few people beat the condition. RM underwent surgery (Whipple), chemo, and radiation. He felt sorry for himself briefly, then realized that he was going to do everything in his power to beat this cancer, including a fighting spirit. RM followed the advice in BEATING CANCER WITH NUTRITION, including food, supplements, and eating your way through the nausea of intra-arterial infusion chemo. He kept the subclavian port (medical device that allows doctors to inject chemo into the vein near the neck) in place for another 7 years to remind himself of his newfound healthier lifestyle. As of February 2010, and at 66 years of age, RM was in complete remission, travels the world, feels great, and doesn't worry anymore. Cancer has brought RM a newfound sense of "life is short and precious, savor it, and do not worry your way through it." His doctors were very pleased and surprised at RM's admirable outcome.

For more information on how your body can fight cancer go to GettingHealthier.com

ENDNOTES

1. https://www.ncbi.nlm.nih.gov/pubmed/17405678
2. https://www.ncbi.nlm.nih.gov/pubmed/18623084
3. https://www.cancer.org/cancer/cancer-basics/history-of-cancer/cancer-treatment-chemo.html#:~:text=Evolution%20of%20Cancer%20Treatments%3A%20Chemotherapy,that%20develop%20into%20blood%20cells.
4. https://europepmc.org/article/med/1899489
5. https://www.ncbi.nlm.nih.gov/pmc/articles/PMC5106370/
6. Leeb, BF, Clin.Exper.Rheum, 13,459,1995
7. Krishanamurthi, S., et al., Radiology, vol.99, p.409, 1971
8. Taper, HS, et al., Int.J.Cancer, vol.40, p.575, 1987
9. Waxman, S., et al., Eur.J.Cancer Clin.Oncol., vol.18, p.685, 1982
10. Gold, J., Cancer Treatment Reports, vol.70, p.1433, Dec.1986
11. http://ar.iiarjournals.org/content/29/3/809.short
12. https://www.cmaj.ca/content/174/7/937?sid=c4b05
13. https://journals.plos.org/plosone/article/file?type=printable&id=10.1371/journal.pone.0011414
14. Shimpo,K, Am.J.Clin.Nutr.54,1298S,1991
15. Jaakkola, K. Anticancer Res., 12, 599, 1992
16. Okunieff, P, Am.J.Clin.Nutr.54, 1281S, 1991
17. Burns, CP, et al., Nutrition Reviews, vol.48, p.233, June 1990
18. Guffy, MM, et al., Cancer Research, vol.44, p.1863, 1984
19. Cannizzo, F., et al., Cancer Research, vol.49, p.3961, 1981
20. Begin, ME, et al., J.Nat.Cancer Inst., vol.77, p.1053, 1986
21. https://acsjournals.onlinelibrary.wiley.com/doi/full/10.1002/cncr.25933
22. Santamaria, L., et al., Nutrients and Cancer Prevention, p.299, Prasad, Humana Press, 1990
23. Seifter, E., et al., J.Nat.Cancer Inst., vol.71, p.409, 1983
24. Singal, PK, et al., Mol.Cell.Biochem., vol.84, p.163, 1988
25. Singal, PK, et al., Molecular Cellular Biochem., vol.84, p.163, 1988
26. Clemens, MR, et al., Am.J.Clin.Nutr., vol.51, p.216, 1990
27. Shklar, G., et al., J.Oral Pathol.Med., vol.19, p.60, 1990
28. Geetha, A., et al., J.Biosci., vol.14, p.243, 1989
29. Geetha, A., et al., Current Science, vol.64, p.318, Mar.1993
30. Wang, YM, Molecular Inter Nutr.Cancer, p.369, , Arnott, MS, (eds), Raven Press, NY, 1982
31. Schmitt-Graff, A., et al, Pathol.Res.Pract., vol.181, p.168, 1986
32. Popov, AI, Med.Radiol. Mosk., vol.32, p.42, 1987
33. Kjellen, E., et al., Radiother.Oncol., vol.22, p.81, 1991
34. Horsman, MR, Radiotherapy Oncology, vol.22, p.79, 1991
35. Coudray, C., et al., Basic Res.Cardiol., vol.87, p.173, 1992
36. Sundstrom, H., et al., Carcinogenesis, vol.10, p.273, 1989
37. Ohkawa, K., et al., Br.J.Cancer, vol.58, p.38, 1988
38. Lawson, T., et al.,Chem.Biol.Interactions, vol.45, p.95, 1983
39. Milner, JA, et al., Cancer Research, vol.41, p.1652, 1981
40. Furitano, G, et al., Drugs Exp.Clin.Res., vol.10, p.107, 1984
41. Wood, AW, et al., in PLANT FLAVONOIDS IN BIOLOGY, p.197, Cody, V. (eds), Liss, NY, 1986
42. Scambia, G., et al., Anticancer Drugs, vol.1, p.45, 1990
43. Kim, JH, et al., Cancer Research, vol.44, p.102, Jan.1984
44. Kubo, M., et al., Planta Med, vol.58, p.424, 1992
45. Jaakkola, K., et al., Treatment with antioxidant and other nutrients in combination with chemotherapy and irradiation in patients with lung cancer, Anticancer Res 12,599-606, 1992
46. Hoffer, A, Pauling, L, J Orthomolecular Med, 5:3:143-154, 1990
47. Lamm, DL, et al., Megadose vitamin in bladder cancer, J Urol, 151:21-26, 1994

Chapter 9

NUTRITION THERAPY IMPROVES IMMUNE FUNCTIONS

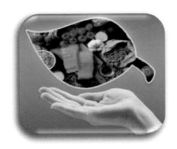

"Nature alone cures."
Florence Nightingale, founder of modern nursing, circa 1900

WHAT'S AHEAD?

Your immune system consists of 20 trillion specialized "warrior" cells in your body that are responsible for killing lethal invaders, such as cancer, yeast, bacteria, and virus. The immune system is heavily dependent on your nutritional status to be able to detect and destroy cancer cells.

✓ sugar slows the immune system to a crawl
✓ protein, calories, vitamins, minerals, amino acids, food extracts, fatty acids, and other nutrition components feed the immune system

When your oncologist says "We think we got it all," what he or she is really saying is "We have destroyed all DETECTABLE cancer cells, and now it is up to your immune system to find and destroy the cancer cells that are inevitably remaining in your body." A billion cancer cells are about the size of the page number at the top of this page. We must rely on the capabilities of the 20 trillion cells that compose an intact immune system to destroy the undetectable cancer cells that remain after medical therapy. There is an abundance of data linking nutrient intake to the quality and quantity of immune factors that fight cancer.[1]

YOUR IMMUNE SYSTEM: THE FIREWALL BETWEEN YOU AND DEATH

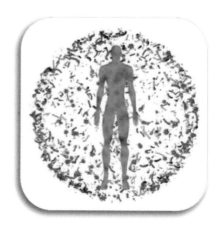

In the classic science fiction story, WAR OF THE WORLDS, author H.G. Wells spins a yarn of a very advanced Martian civilization with unstoppable war weapons to take over the earth. Spoiler alert: in the end, the Martians die from the microbes that are found in our routine air supply, because the Martians had refined their own climate on Mars to be free of germs, hence their immune systems atrophied, and they could not tolerate our routine pathogens in the air.

By one estimate, there are about 100,000 virus and bacteria pathogens per cubic meter of air that we breath.[2] Swimming in this sea of pathogens as we do, it should not be surprising that pneumonia (lung infection) kills about 50,000 Americans annually, most of them older and immune compromised.[3] The Center for Disease Control estimates that 56,000 Americans die annually from the flu, another viral upper respiratory disease.[4]

And that's just the job of the immune system for outside invaders. Inside invaders (cancer, infections) are another battle altogether. Bruce Ames, PhD from UC Berkeley estimated that each cell in your body endures 5,000-10,000 DNA hits, or potentially cancer causing reactions per day.[5] The immune system is partially responsible for correcting these cancer causing hits.

The link between the vitality of your immune system and <u>nutrient intake</u> has long been established.[6] We could overwhelm our reader with the abundance of data linking a <u>healthy diet to a healthy immune system</u>.[7] But we will summarize thousands of pages of concrete scientific information and hundreds of peer reviewed articles into this short and simple chapter. Here is the soundbite: "optimal nutrition delivers an optimal immune system."

The greatest catastrophe to strike the planet earth was the Black Plague, often depicted as death riding on a pale stallion. Sweeping over Europe, Asia, and North Africa, before the plague was done in 1351 somewhere between 75 and 200 million people were killed, by some estimates 60% of Europe. More than 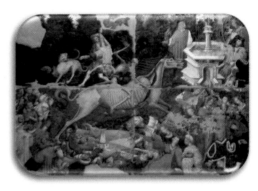 coincidentally, the Plague rode in on the coattails of the Crusades, wars fought when Christians from Europe sought to take Jerusalem from Muslims. Mix many people from many lands, add in the stress of war, and the common malnutrition that occurs when the farmers go to war and you have the makings of the Plague. In 1918 the Spanish Flu killed about 50 million people worldwide on the coattails of World War I.

As of this writing, the Covid plague of 2020 has infected 18 million people worldwide with 695,000 deaths, or 0.009% of global population. As we age the immune system weakens in many people (aka immune senescence), which is why the vast majority of cancer patients and COVID victims are older. The state of Pennsylvania found the average age of COVID victims to be 80, with 2/3 occurring in nursing homes. Underlying conditions of obesity, diabetes, heart disease, medications all increase risk factors for COVID mortality. Both COVID and cancer strike the weakened immune systems. In a surprise to the aggressive vaccination community, the <u>flu vaccine increased the risk for COVID infection by 36%</u>.[8] The purpose of this chapter is to get your immune system up to the challenge of reversing your cancer.

RECOGNIZE SELF FROM NON-SELF

Imagine being a special-forces cop in downtown New York City. There are millions of people of all different sizes, shapes, colors, languages, manner of dress, and movement. Most are good people. Some are bad people. Some are terrorists with very evil intentions. Your job is to find the bad guys and get rid of them. No easy chore. That is what your immune system is trying to do in your body: recognize self from non-self. Good guys from bad guys. Patriots from traitors. Your immune system's job is to eliminate cancer.

The immune system of the average American is "running on empty". Causes for this problem include toxic burden, sleep deprivation, stress, no exercise, poor diet, multiple nutrient deficiencies, unbridled use of antibiotics and vaccinations, and less breast feeding.

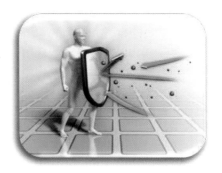

Most experts now agree to the "surveillance" theory of cancer. Cells in your body are duplicating all day every day at a blinding pace. This process of growth is fraught with peril. When cells are not copied exactly as they should be, then an emergency call goes out to the immune system to find and destroy this abnormal saboteur cell. This process occurs frequently in most people throughout their lives. Fortunately, only 42% of Americans will actually develop detectable cancer, yet most experts agree that everyone gets cancer about six times per lifetime with one cancer cell sprouting up in everyone each day. It is the surveillance of an alert and capable immune system that defends most of us from cancer.

A healthy adult body includes around 37 trillion cells of which 20 trillion cells are immune factors. Among the primary aspects of the immune system are:

- ◆ **Birth place.** The bone marrow generates most immune cells, primarily in the long bones, especially the ribs.
- ◆ **Maturation.** Bone immune cells (B-cells) move into the thymus gland for maturation and activation, and are then called "T" cells.
- ◆ **Gastrointestinal (GI) tract.** 70% or more of the immune system surrounds the GI tract as lymph nodes, not only to absorb fat soluble nutrients (like essential fatty acids) and to protect against bacterial

translocation (crossing of the intestinal barrier into the bloodstream by disease-causing bacteria), but also to stimulate the production of various immunoglobulins (IgA etc.) A healthy gut is a critical aspect of a healthy immune system.

◆ **Filtering.** The immune cells move through the lymphatic ducts, not unlike the blood moving through the arteries and veins. Dead immune cells and invaders are filtered out of this "freeway" system in the spleen and lymph nodes.

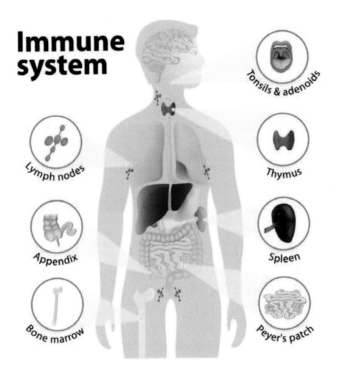

✓ **Quantity.** There are many factors that can influence the sheer numbers of immune warriors.

✓ **Quality.** Not all immune cells have the same level of ferocity against an invading tumor cell. Some immune cells become confused about "who to shoot at" and end up creating an autoimmune response (often called an allergic response), which imbalances the immune system and detracts from the critical task of killing cancer cells. Some nutrients provide the immune warriors with a protective coating, like an asbestos suit, so that the immune cell is not destroyed in the process of killing a cancer cell with some "napalm". Some nutrients provide the immune cells with more "napalm" or "bullets" in the form of granulocytes and nitric oxide.

Many nutrition factors affect the ability of the immune system to recognize and destroy cancer cells and invading bacteria. In the cancer patient, for a variety of reasons, the immune system has not done its work.

IMMUNE SYSTEM: internal warriors

- Enhanced by:
- Vitamins: A, C, E, B-6
- Minerals: Zn, Cr, Se
- Quasi-vit: CoQ, EPA, GLA
- Amino acids: arg, gluta
- Herbals: astragalus, Cat's claw, Pau D'arco
- Foods: yogurt, cartilage, garlic, enzymes, green leafy, shark oil,colostrum
- Positive emotions: love

- Reduced by:
- Toxic metals: Cd, Pb, Hg
- VOC: PCB, benzene
- Sugar: glycemic index
- Omega 3:6 ratio, 1:1; 1:16
- Stress: depression

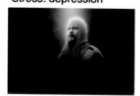

WE ARE GOING TO BOLSTER YOUR IMMUNE ARMY WITH IMPROVED:

♦ **quantity** by producing more natural killer cells, tumor necrosis factor, lymphocytes, interleukin, and interferon.

♦ **quality** by:

1) reducing the ability of cancer cells to hide from the immune system. A healthy immune system will attack and destroy any cells that do not have the "secret pass code" of host DNA. Both the fetus and cancer are able to survive by creating a hormone, HCG, which allows the fetus to hide from the immune system. Tumor necrosis factor (TNF), which is specifically made by the immune system to kill cancer cells, is like a sword. TNF-inhibitor is produced in the presence of HCG and is like putting a sheath on the sword. Digestive enzymes and vitamins E and A help to clear away the "stealth" coating on the tumor and improve tumor recognition by the immune system.

2) Providing antioxidants. We can put special shielding on the immune soldiers so that when they douse a cancer cell with deadly chemicals, the immune soldier is protected and can go on to kill other cancer cells. Otherwise, you seriously restrict the "bag limit" of any given immune soldier.

DEAL WITH YOUR ALLERGIES

Depending on whose projections you believe, somewhere between 4% and 10% of Americans have food allergies. Your immune system cannot fully direct its energies toward destroying cancer cells if it spends too much time erroneously destroying your dinner. Food allergies are caused by food proteins being absorbed into the bloodstream, then your immune system attacking the food as if it were an invading bacteria. Many food allergies can be caused by a leaky gut, which may be caused by yeast overgrowth.

From 25% to 50% of the population suffer from allergies, which can come from foods that we eat (ingestant), air particles that we breath (inhalant), or substances on our skin (contact). Allergies can cause an amazing array of diseases, including immune problems, arthritis, diabetes, heart disease, mental illness, and more.

Some people have transient food allergies, that come and go along with the pollen seasons. Because of this trend, some allergists subscribe to the "rain barrel" theory, in which you only have allergic reactions when the rain barrel is overflowing, such as combining allergies with stress.

Allergies are common, complex to diagnose, difficult to treat, and closely related to a variety of diseases, including cancer. A primitive and not terribly accurate way to find allergies involves the hypoallergenic diet. For 4 days, eat nothing but a hypoallergenic diet of rice, apples, carrots, pears, lamb, turkey, olive, and black tea. If you find relief from any particular symptoms, then add back a new food every four days and record the results. The most common allergenic foods are milk, wheat, beef, eggs, corn, peanut, soybeans, chicken, fish, nuts, mollusks, and shellfish. To resolve food allergies, work with your nutritionally oriented doctor.

NUTRIENTS AFFECT THE IMMUNE SYSTEM

There is an abundance of scientific documentation linking nutrient intake with immune quality and quantity. This is a very crucial issue for the cancer patient.

Many nutrients taken orally can provide pharmacological changes in immune function in humans. Protein, arginine, glutamine, omega-6 and omega-3 fats, iron, zinc, vitamins E, C, and A have all been proven to modulate immune functions.[9]

Vitamin A deficiency causes reduced immune response while beta-carotene supplements stimulate immune responses.[10] Vitamin A (retinol) improves immune response to fungal infections.[11] In developing countries, vitamin A deficiency causes the blindness of 250,000 to 500,000 children annually.[12] Oral doses of vitamin A at 200,000 iu (40 times the Recommended Daily Allowance) lowered measles mortality by 80% in children in developing countries with no side effects.[13] Vitamin A and synthetic derivatives have been used worldwide to treat and prevent various cancers.[14]

Vitamin B-6 has been used to prevent and treat cancer and as a blood marker that determines outcome in cancer treatment.[15] B-6 supplements (50 mg/day) provided a measurable improvement in immune functions (T3 and T4 lymphocytes) for 11 healthy, well-fed older adults.[16]

Various B vitamins have been linked to the proper functioning of antibody response and cellular immunity.

Folate deficiency decreases mitogenesis, or the normal division of cells. Folate deficiency increases the risk for various cancers.[17]

Deficiency of vitamin C impairs phagocyte functions (immune cells that gobble invaders) and cellular immunity. Intravenous vitamin C is a viable cancer treatment option.[18]

Vitamin E deficiency decreases antibody response to T-dependent antigens, all of which gets worse with the addition of a selenium deficiency. Vitamin E succinate is a viable cancer treatment agent[19].[20]

While iron deficiency can blunt immune functions, iron excess can increase the risk for cancer.[21] Iron presents an interesting case: 1) because it is one of the most common nutritional deficiency problem worldwide, 2) because low levels of iron will depress the immune system, and 3) because high levels of iron will stimulate both bacterial and tumor growth. Iron intake needs to be well regulated...not too much, and not too little.

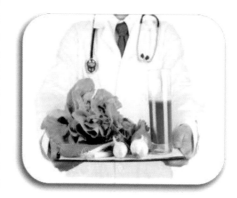

Zinc exerts a major influence on the immune system. Lymphocyte function is seriously depressed, and lymphoid tissues undergo general atrophy in zinc-deficient individuals. The lymphocytes in zinc-deficient animals quickly lose their killing abilities (cytotoxicity) and engulfing talents (phagocytosis) for tumor cells and bacteria. Natural killer cell and neutrophil activity is also reduced. Zinc has become a proven therapeutic agent in treating advanced COVID[22] patients.[23]

Copper plays a key role in the production of superoxide dismutase and cytochrome systems in the mitochondria. Hence, a deficiency of copper is manifested in a depressed immune system, specifically reduced microbicidal activity of granulocytes.

Selenium works in conjunction with vitamin E to shield host cells from lipid peroxidation. Humoral immune response is depressed in selenium deficient animals. Selenium and vitamin E deficiencies lead to increased incidence of enteric (intestinal) lesions. Lymphocyte proliferation (making more warriors) is reduced in selenium deficiency. The theory is that selenium and vitamin E help to provide the host immune cells with some type of "bullet-proof plating" against the toxins used on foreign cells. Hence, one immune body can live on to destroy many invaders if enough vitamin E and selenium allow for these critical chemical shields.

In magnesium deficiency, all immunoglobulins (except IgE) are reduced, along with the number of antibody forming cells. Magnesium is crucial for lymphocyte growth (involvement in protein metabolism) and transformation in response to mitogens. Prolonged magnesium deficiency in animals leads to the development of lymphomas and leukemia.

Iodine plays an important role in the microbicidal activity of polymorphonuclear leukocytes. Activated neutrophils may use the conversion of iodide to iodine to generate free radicals for killing foreign invaders. Iodine is one of the more common deficiencies worldwide. Iodine has the unusual role in nature of being essential to humans and lethal to most microbes, but not your friendly gut microbes.

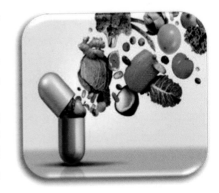

Boron prevents osteoporosis, yet is still not considered an essential mineral in human nutrition. <u>Boron deficiency in soil is a worldwide</u> problem with boron soil amendments dramatically enhancing plant growth.[24] Boron has shown activity in <u>preventing and reversing cancer</u>.[25] In a human study, the more boron in the diet, the lower the <u>risk for prostate cancer</u>.[26]

Toxic trace minerals, like mercury, cadmium, arsenic, and lead all blunt the immune system.

The quality and quantity of fat in the diet play a major role in dictating the health of the immune system. Since fat directly affects prostaglandin pathways, and prostaglandins (depending on the pathway) can either depress or enhance immune function, fat intake is crucial in encouraging a healthy immune system.

There are many foods and supplements that can have a favorable impact on the immune system. Much of this book is dedicated to reinforcing your immune system to recognize and destroy your cancer using nutrition as a key modality.

BOTTOM LINE

Your health, vitality, longevity, and ability to prevent and reverse cancer or infections is directly tied to the ability of your immune system to recognize "self" from "non-self", which is heavily dependent on your nutritional status.

PATIENT PROFILE: REVERSING KIDNEY CANCER:

C.H. was diagnosed with renal cell carcinoma stage 4 that had spread to his liver and spleen. All 3 oncologists said that C.H. had less than 6 months to live with no chance of recovery. C.H.'s daughters gathered the information in this book to create a diet, supplement, and detoxification program. Within a few weeks, his pain was significantly less and his pain medications could be reduced. "The doctor was amazed and said the patient's tumors are shrinking and there has been no new tumor growth in 2 months." Six months after his initial diagnosis C.H. is in good spirits, out of pain, and has much less tumor burden than the beginning. "Thank you for writing your wonderful book," states the daughters who provided their father with his nutrition program.

For more information on how your body can fight cancer go to GettingHealthier.com.

ENDNOTES

[1]. Bendich, A, Chandra, RK (eds), Micronutrients and Immune Function, New York Academy of Sciences, 1990, p.587

[2] https://www.ncbi.nlm.nih.gov/pmc/articles/PMC4515362/

[3] https://www.cdc.gov/dotw/pneumonia/index.html

[4] https://www.webmd.com/cold-and-flu/qa/how-many-people-die-from-the-flu-each-year-and-how-is-it-prevented

[5] http://toxicology.usu.edu/endnote/Endogenous_DNA_damage.pdf

[6] https://www.ncbi.nlm.nih.gov/pmc/articles/PMC6212925/

[7] https://www.ncbi.nlm.nih.gov/pmc/articles/PMC6723551/

[8] https://pubmed.ncbi.nlm.nih.gov/31607599/

[9]. Alexander, JW, et al., Critical Care Medicine, vol.18, p.S159, 1990

[10]. Rhodes, J., and Oliver, S., Immunology, vol.40, p.467, 1980

[11] https://link.springer.com/article/10.1007/s00430-014-0351-4

[12] https://www.who.int/nutrition/topics/vad/en/

[13] https://www.cochranelibrary.com/cdsr/doi/10.1002/14651858.CD001479.pub3/abstract

[14] https://www.sciencedirect.com/science/article/abs/pii/S0899900700004366

[15] https://www.nature.com/articles/onc2012623/

[16]. Talbott, MC, et al., American Journal of Clinical Nutrition, vol.46, p.659, 1987

[17] https://cebp.aacrjournals.org/content/13/4/511.short

[18] http://ar.iiarjournals.org/content/29/3/809.short

[19] https://www.nature.com/articles/6601360

[20] https://www.tandfonline.com/doi/abs/10.1080/07315724.2003.10719283

[21]. Cerutti, PA, Science, vol.227, p.375, 1985

[22] https://www.sciencedirect.com/science/article/pii/S0306987720306435

[23] https://www.spandidos-publications.com/10.3892/ijmm.2020.4575

[24] https://www.sciencedirect.com/science/article/pii/S006521130860142X

[25] https://www.ingentaconnect.com/content/ben/acamc/2010/00000010/00000004/art00009

[26] https://www.spandidos-publications.com/or/11/4/887#

Chapter 10

SUGAR FEEDS CANCER

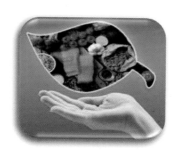

"Our way of life is related to our way of death."
Framingham Study, Harvard University

WHAT'S AHEAD?
Cancer cells feed almost exclusively on sugar.
You can slow tumor growth by:
- ✓ eating a diet that lowers blood and gut sugar, including intermittent fasting
- ✓ exercise to burn up any extra glucose in the blood
- ✓ taking supplements such as chromium, CLA, cinnamon, and gymnema
- ✓ using medications, if necessary, for better control of diabetes

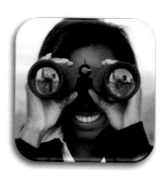

A moth is attracted to bright light, which can be its own demise if the bright light is a flame. Two hundred years ago Americans consumed about 2 pounds/year of sugar. Today that <u>number is 150 pounds of refined sugar</u> per year, mostly in the form of sucrose (white sugar) and corn syrup. [1] Our incidence of obesity, diabetes, and many cancers has escalated parallel to our rise in sugar intake. We consume 15 billion gallons of soft drinks, 2.7 billion Krispy Cremes, and 500 million Twinkies per year. IHOP alone serves more than 700 million pancakes per year. Our appetite for sugar is like a hummingbird sucking on sweet food all day long. Problem is, we are not exercising like a hummingbird.

A special region of our tongue is exclusively reserved for finding and appreciating sweet foods. This makes good sense. Sweet foods are more likely to have carbohydrates for nourishment and less likely to be poisonous, such as some bitter plants. Our hunter-gatherer ancestors were hard pressed to find sweet foods, and thus their bodies were forced to make glucose out of proteins

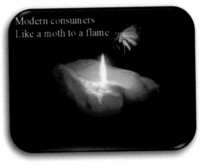

Modern consumers
Like a moth to a flame

in the body. However, once mankind developed the technology for growing and concentrating refined sugars in unimaginable levels, that sweet tooth of ours has become our enemy within. That sweet tooth leads us on to greater and greater heights of sugar intake like a moth drawn to a flame.

Cut back dramatically on total sweetener intake: either caloric or non-caloric. By doing so, you will begin to taste the flavors of the food and begin to lose that sweetness craving. Once you have cut back your intake of caloric sugars from the current average of 150 pounds per year per person to a more reasonable 20 pounds per year and have removed all aspartame (NutraSweet) from your diet, then choose from the preferred sweeteners listed below.

The alphabet of sugars:
Disaccharide means 2 sugar molecules together, like table sugar, or sucrose.
Monosaccharide means 1 sugar molecule, like fructose in honey or fruits.
glucose + fructose=sucrose (table sugar)
glucose + glucose=maltose
glucose + galactose=lactose (milk sugar)

SUGAR & CANCER
PET scan maps tumors via rad.label GLUCOSE
FDG (fluorodeoxy-glucose)

Cancer cells demonstrate a 3-5 fold increase in glucose uptake compared to healthy cells. *Cancer Research, vol.42, p.7565, Feb.1982* Malignant cells produce up to 30 times more lactic acid than normal counterparts. *Med.Hypotheses, vol.40, p.235, 1993*

1. Control blood glucose through diet, intermittent fasting, supplements, exercise, stress reduction, medication.
2. ?Use of insulin? to lower blood glucose or increase cancer cell permeability to chemotherapy. Insulin Poten.Therapy
3. Elevate blood glucose (IV dextrose) to 400 mg%, then use hyperthermia, chemo, rad tx: Systemic Ca Multi-Step Tx
4. High dose glucose IV potentiates anti-neoplastic tx.
5. Hydrazine sulfate inhibits PEP-CK

CALORIC SWEETENERS
contain 4 kcal per gram & can cause cavities

SUGAR: Based upon federal laws passed after World War II to protect the California and Hawaii sugar industry, a "sugar" must have at least 96% of all other plant matter stripped from it in order to be called sugar. 90% of the bulk of cane sugar is fiber, protein, and other matter. All of this is lost in the sugar refining process. Therefore, turbinado sugar, brown sugar, and other health food store sugars are virtually identical to white sugar in nutrient density and glycemic index.

Barley malt is a mild natural sweetener made from barley sprouts that is less sweet and less hazardous on blood glucose levels than other sweeteners listed here, yet very expensive.

Blackstrap molasses: what's left over at the bottom of the barrel from the sugar refining industry. Molasses contains the concentrated vitamins and minerals that were once in the cane sugar, though it still can create havoc with blood glucose levels and has an unusual wild taste. It has more calcium than milk, more iron than eggs, and is a rich source of potassium.

Brown sugar can be made by blending white sugar with molasses. Little advantage over white sugar.

Corn syrup is commercial glucose from cornstarch with some sucrose syrup added. Very refined food, with a very high glycemic index.

Date sugar is ground and dried dates from desert climates. Tasty whole food, but high glycemic index.

Fructose is found in many fruits, honey, and as pure crystalline fructose. It is slowly absorbed in the intestinal tract, and requires the liver to convert fructose to glucose for body use. Glycemic index of 20. Very useful for diabetics. While a roomful of PhDs from agribusiness have tried to convince the consumer that fructose from high fructose corn syrup (added to most processed foods) is the same as the fructose found in fruit, the scientific evidence says otherwise. More on the health merits of fruit later in this chapter.

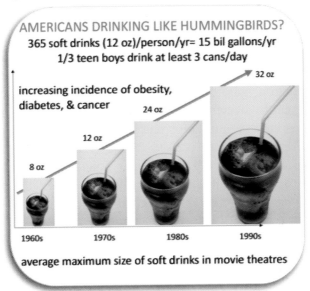

GLUCOSE/dextrose: Here is the gold currency of sugar in the blood. Glucose is usually extracted from corn syrup and is rapidly absorbed from the intestines into the bloodstream. Foods high in glucose (watermelon, parsnips) or starches easily digested into glucose (like rice cakes or white bread) can create rapid and dangerous rises in blood glucose.

Gymnema sylvestre is a valuable herb that can block the taste of sugar in the mouth. Using gymnema tea with those occasional sweet snacks can help to reduce the amount of sugar that you crave.

Honey is formed when bees partially digest nectar from flowers. Honey has well documented value as an antiseptic, antibiotic, and stomach calming food. Honey from your nearby vicinity can help with allergies and is a real food vs. the "cadaver" state of most other highly refined caloric sweeteners. Honey varies in taste and content based on the hives and flowers in your region. Honey is usually about 31% glucose, 38% fructose, 18% water, 9% other sugars, and 2% sucrose. Yet, honey, in excess, can create problems with glycemic index and weight. Once honey has been heated, which neutralizes many of its benefits, the honey will become more water-like. Rich honey is thick and organically-raised.

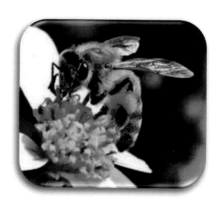

Lactose (milk sugar). About <u>65% of adults are lactose intolerant</u> and therefore do not digest this sugar well, which then generates intestinal cramps, constipation, gas, or diarrhea.[2] In yogurt, the lactose has been fermented by healthy bacteria into lactic acid, hence the slightly tart taste. People who are lactose intolerant can usually consume yogurt with no problem.

Maltitol is a relatively new sugar found in health food stores. Made from corn, maltitol has a better glycemic index than sucrose and 25% fewer calories per gram. However, it is expensive and not as sweet as table sugar.

Maple syrup is concentrated sweetener from the sap of sugar maple trees. It requires 30-40 gallons of sap to make 1 gallon of maple syrup. Unless the product is labelled "pure" maple syrup, then it is probably diluted with corn syrup to cut the cost. Though the flavor is unique, the glycemic index is little better than white sugar.

Rice syrup is made by culturing rice with digestive enzymes to break down the starch into glucose. Tasty whole food, but high glycemic index.

Sorghum molasses is the concentrated juice from the sorghum plant, a cereal grain. Has a lighter flavor than blackstrap molasses.

Sucanat: trade name that means "SUgar CAne NATural" and comes from ground up organically grown sugar cane. 85% is sugar, with the balance of 15% being fiber, vitamins, minerals, amino acids, and molasses. Though Sucanat is a whole food, it is more expensive and provides a minor advantage in nutrient density and glycemic index vs white table sugar.

Sucrose is basic table sugar and merits a special discussion here. It was around 600 AD that Persians began growing and refining sugar cane into something similar to our white table sugar. Since then, sugar has been a pivotal point in history, wars, taxes, and even the Declaration of Independence of the United States of America. The immoral trade route that connected the continents of Europe, Africa, and North America for centuries involved slaves from Africa to work the sugar cane plantations in the Caribbean, then bring the sugar, molasses, and rum to Europe and back to Africa for more trade.

Long before the Boston Tea Party, the Molasses Act of 1733 put British rulers in the crosshairs of American colonists. At the time of the Revolutionary War, the average annual consumption of molasses rum was 4 gallons per man, woman, and child. One could argue that the

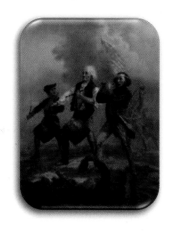

enthusiastic consumption of sugar and its by-products have been instrumental in bringing us the "diseases of civilization", including tuberculosis, diabetes, heart disease, many forms of cancer (which is a sugar-feeder), various mental disorders (including hyperactivity), and more. Suffice it to say that sucrose is more of a drug than a food. Consume it with caution.

Turbinado sugar is raw sugar that has been washed of its molasses content in a centrifuge. Basically, it is over-priced white sugar.

CALORIC BUT NON-CARIOGENIC
contain 4 kcal per gram and cannot cause cavities

Sorbitol is derived from corn, absorbed slowly, requires little insulin, and is used in many foods for diabetics. Probably safe, but may cause diarrhea in some sensitive individuals. Use in moderation.

Xylitol (Xylitol.com) is extracted from birchwood chips and used in chewing gum. May reduce cavities by neutralizing the acids in the mouth. Use in moderation.

Tagatose (Naturlose.com) is the new kid on the block among sugar substitutes. Tagatose is nearly identical (C-4 epimer) to D-fructose, the common simple sugar found in many fruits. Tagatose has full GRAS (generally regarded as safe) approval from the FDA. Tagatose provides only 37% of the calories found in an equal amount of sucrose, has a mild laxative effect and seems to have no toxicity. Currently, tagatose can only be found in mixed products, but may soon be available by itself as a sugar substitute.

NON-CALORIC SWEETENERS
no calories & no cavities

Stevia, or stevioside, is extracted from a sweetening herb, stevia rebaudiana, and does not have either calories or a long and checkered past like many of the other artificial sweeteners listed here. Stevia was commercialized in the 1970s by a Japanese firm and still enjoys over 40% of the food sweetener market in both South America and Asia. Stevia has been used as a natural sweetener for over 1,500 years in South America. The herb is actually beneficial for people with poorly regulated blood glucose, though the concentrated extract, stevioside, sold in health food stores, does not retain these healing properties. Stevioside and stevia are the safest and most recommended of the artificial sweeteners available today.

Splenda, or sucralose, is a relatively new artificial sweetener invented in 1976, patented by a subsidiary of Johnson & Johnson, and approved by the Food and Drug Administration in 1998. Splenda is made from sugar, is stable in cooking, tastes like sugar, but cannot cause dental caries and does not raise blood sugar. Splenda has a molecule that is slightly different in shape from normal table sugar and has a chlorine atom added. __Splenda has been implicated__ in causing migraines, negatively affecting the gut microflora, and possibly increasing the risk for some cancers.[3] Avoid it.

Aspartame provides us with a classical example of how the FDA is not protecting the American consumer, but rather creating extremely profitable monopolies for those who can afford the $150-800 million investment required to pass the "safety tests". Aspartame, Equal, or NutraSweet (trademark of the NutraSweet Company) is consumed by over 100 million people in the US alone. It is 180 times sweeter than table sugar, is included in over 1,200 products in America, and was approved by the FDA in 1981. Over a billion pounds of aspartame are used annually in the US.

I will spare you the detailed accounts of how aspartame has been linked to our 250% rise in brain cancer since its approval[4], or the double blind study by psychiatrists that was halted because aspartame created such blatant depression in the test subjects[5], or the study showing that aspartame caused headaches in a double blind trial[6], or the fact that of the 2800 FDA approved food additives, 80% of all complaints are regarding aspartame.[7] Aspartame breaks down after long term storage, heating, and in the body into wood alcohol (methyl alcohol) and dangerous isomers of the amino acid phenylalanine.

Researcher Richard Wurtman, MD of MIT cautioned the FDA on the approval of aspartame, noting the rise in brain tumors among animals fed aspartame. Along with the meteoric rise in the consumption of aspartame has come a parallel rise in the incidence of both obesity and morbid obesity (people who are dangerously overweight). Avoid it.

Saccharin is a chemical derivative of petroleum and toluene, a solvent used to reduce the knocking in automobile engines.[8] Saccharin was found to increase the incidence of bladder cancer in animals, but under pressure from lobbyists, the FDA allowed saccharin to remain on the market with a warning label. Avoid it.

Acesulfame K, sold as Sunette or Sweet One, was approved by the FDA in 1988 as a sugar substitute. Early studies show that Acesulfame may cause cancer: "Acesulfame K...might be carcinogenic." David Rall, MD, PhD, Assistant Surgeon General of America. Avoid it.

DOES SUGAR (GLUCOSE) FEED CANCER CELLS?

Nobel laureate (1931 Medicine) Otto Warburg, MD, PhD, first discovered that <u>cancer cells have a fundamental difference in energy metabolism</u> [9] <u>compared to healthy undifferentiated cells</u>.[10] Cancer cells ferment glucose anaerobically. [11] Since Warburg's pivotal study published in *Science* in 1956, many other researchers have corroborated his conclusions.

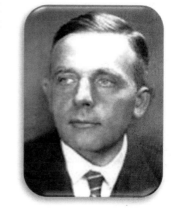

"A frequent characteristic of many malignant tumors is an increase in anaerobic glycolysis, that is the conversion of glucose to lactate, when compared to normal tissues."

"The high rate of glucose consumption by malignant cells, their heavy dependence on the inefficient glycolytic mode for energy production, their increased energy expenditures, and the susceptibility to carbohydrate deprivation prompted several attempts to exploit the tumoricidal potential of manipulations interfering with carbohydrate and/or energy metabolism, hoping that such interventions could preferentially impair the malignant cells."[12]

"**In normoglycemic hosts the in vivo consumption of glucose by neoplastic tissues was found to be very high**. Cerebral tissue is reported to use from 0.23 to 0.57 gm of glucose per hour per 100 gm wet brain and rates as one of the highest consumers among the normal tissues. However, hepatomas and fibrosarcomas consumed roughly as much glucose as the brain does and carcinomas about twice as much."[13]

"**The glucose utilization rate in neoplastic tissues, unlike in host tissues, is high**. Glucose, in fact, is the preferred energy substrate, utilized mainly via the anaerobic glycolytic pathway. The large amount of lactate produced by this process is then transported to the liver where it is converted to glucose, thus contributing to further increase host's energy wasting."[14]

Elevated Lactate Levels. "Our laboratory has been interested in the metabolic derangements of cancer, particularly lactate overproduction, in view of our work linking lactate overproduction in obesity to insulin resistance…Thus, in all four studies listed above, lactate levels were 27-83% higher in cancer patients than in related controls."[15]

Lower Ph Through Lactic Acid Accumulation. Since cancer cells use glucose through anaerobic fermentation, then lactic acid must accumulate as the inefficient by-product of energy metabolism. Human tumors were implanted in rats, which were then given IV solutions of glucose. pH in the tumor tissue was reduced to an average of 6.43, given the logarithmic scale of hydrogen ions in pH measurement, "This pH value corresponds to a ten-fold increase in H^+ ion activity in tumor tissue as compared to arterial blood."[16] By lowering pH in tumor cells, we can effectively create a selective systemic therapy which will kill cancer cells and not healthy tissue.

"After IV glucose, tumor acidification occurred in 9 out of 10 patients…Larger tumors tended to exhibit a greater decrease in pH…We conclude that IV and IV + oral glucose administration are equally effective at inducing tumor acute acidification."[17]

Elevated Blood Glucose May Suppress Immune Functions. Ten healthy human volunteers were assessed for fasting blood glucose levels and tumor engulfing ability of neutrophils. "Oral 100 gm portions of carbohydrates from glucose, fructose, sucrose, honey, or orange juice all significantly decreased the capacity of neutrophils to engulf bacteria as measured by the slide technique. Starch ingestion did not have this effect."[18]

Insulin-Cancer Relationship. "Insulin is a major anabolic hormone in mammals and its involvement in malignancies is well documented."[19] Diabetics have a <u>much higher risk for cancer</u>.[20]

Epidemiological Evidence. "Risk associated with the intake of sugars, independent of other energy sources, is more than doubled [for biliary tract cancer]".[21] "In older women, a strong correlation was found between breast cancer mortality and sugar consumption…"[22]

THE SUGAR-CANCER LINK

At the world-famous Sloan-Kettering Cancer hospital in New York City, researchers found that tumors sucked up radioactively-labeled vitamin C like thirsty sponges because cancer cells thought they were getting their favorite fuel, glucose, which is nearly identical in chemical structure to vitamin C. Meanwhile, across the globe in a modern clinic in Germany, oncologists were injecting glucose into cancer patients to activate the cancer growth, then whack the cancer with intensive chemo, radiation, or hyperthermia. Their results have doubled 5-year survival for these patients undergoing Systemic Cancer Multistep Therapy.

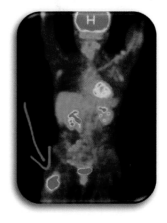

In most major cancer hospitals around the world, oncologists use a $2 million device, called a PET scan (positron emission tomography), which detects cancer by finding hot spots of sugar feeding cells in the body. All of these world-class scientists are using the same principle: sugar feeds cancer. When we can lower blood glucose, we can slow cancer growth.

Professor Seyfried of Boston College and Yale University has written a medical textbook showing the strong link between cancer and glucose: CANCER AS A METABOLIC DISEASE. Researchers at

Harvard University have developed a special Total Parenteral Nutrition formula for cancer patients that uses much less sugar (glucose) and more protein and fats. The net result of this "disease-specific" formula for starving cancer patients is to feed the immune system and not the cancer.

CONTROL BLOOD AND GUT GLUCOSE TO CONTROL CANCER

>Simple sugars,not starches,impaired neutrophil phagocytosis.
Sanchez, A., et al., American Journal Clinical Nutrition, vol.26, p.180, 1973
>Comparing 50 colorectal cancer patients to healthy controls, cancer patients ate more sugar and fat than the healthy people.
Bristol, JB, et al., Proceedings American Association of Cancer Research, vol.26, p.206, Mar.1985
>In a 40 country epidemiological study, sugar consumption predicts
(0.73 correl) breast cancer. *Hems, G., Br.J.Cancer, vol.37, p.974, 1978*
>Animals were fed isocaloric diets of sugar or starch carbohydrates. The group eating more sugar developed significantly more mammary tumors than the starch-fed group. *Hoehn, SK, et al., Nutrition & Cancer, vol.1, no.3, p.27, Spring 1979*
>Animals w.implanted breast cancer survived longest with diet that lowered blood glucose. *Santisteban, Biochem.& Biophys Res. Comm., vol.132, no.3, p.1174, 1985*
>Insulin is a major anabolic hormone in mammals and its involvement in malignancies is well documented. *Yam, D., Med.Hypotheses, vol.38, p.111, 1992*

Tumors are primarily obligate glucose metabolizers, meaning "sugar feeders".[23] The average American consumes 20% of calories from refined white sugar, which is more of a drug than a food. We also manifest poor glucose tolerance due to stress, obesity, low chromium and fiber intake, and sedentary lifestyles. Blood glucose is basically there to feed the brain and other glucose-dependent organs, while also supplying fuel for muscle movement.

When we sit all day, the sugar in our blood is like a teenager with nothing to do--trouble is bound to happen. Elevated sugar levels in the blood will "tan" proteins (glycosylation), which makes immune cells and red blood cells less capable of doing their jobs. Elevated sugar in the blood has a number of ways in which it promotes cancer:

- ♦ While fish oil (EPA) and borage oil (GLA) have a favorable impact on cancer, these potent fatty acids are neutralized when the blood glucose levels are kept high.
- ♦ Cancer cells feed directly on blood glucose, like a fermenting yeast organism. Elevating blood glucose in a cancer patient is like throwing gasoline on a smoldering fire.
- ♦ Elevating blood glucose levels suppresses the immune system

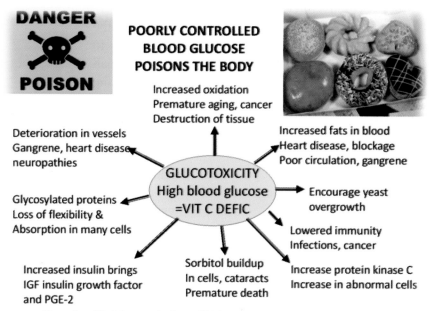

DANGER POISON

POORLY CONTROLLED BLOOD GLUCOSE POISONS THE BODY

Increased oxidation
Premature aging, cancer
Destruction of tissue

Deterioration in vessels
Gangrene, heart disease,
neuropathies

Increased fats in blood
Heart disease, blockage
Poor circulation, gangrene

GLUCOTOXICITY
High blood glucose
=VIT C DEFIC

Glycosylated proteins
Loss of flexibility &
Absorption in many cells

Encourage yeast
overgrowth

Lowered immunity
Infections, cancer

Increased insulin brings
IGF insulin growth factor
and PGE-2

Sorbitol buildup
In cells, cataracts
Premature death

Increase protein kinase C
Increase in abnormal cells

Mooradian, AD, Advances in Care of Diabetes, vol.15, no.2, p.255, May 1999

Cancer cells primarily use glucose for fuel. This inefficient pathway for energy metabolism yields only 5% of the ATP energy available in food, which is one of the reasons why 40% of cancer patients die from malnutrition or cachexia. Cancer therapies need to regulate blood glucose levels via diet, intermittent fasting, supplements, enteral and parenteral solutions for cachectic patients, medication, exercise, gradual weight loss, stress reduction, etc. The role of glucose in the growth and metastasis of cancer cells can be utilized to help the cancer patient with such therapies as:

- diets designed with glycemic index in mind to regulate rises in blood glucose, hence selectively starving the cancer cells
- low glucose total parenteral nutrition (TPN) solution
- positron emission tomography (PET) assays of tumor progress
- hydrazine sulfate to inhibit gluconeogenesis in cancer cells
- avocado extract (mannoheptulose), which inhibits glucose uptake in cancer cells
- Systemic Cancer Multistep Therapy, which injects glucose into the cancer patient to initiate malignancy growth, then uses hyperthermia to selectively destroy tumor tissue.

DOES FRUIT FEED CANCER CELLS?

Given the abundant scientific data supporting the sugar-cancer link, many people have been quick to discourage the consumption of fruit. Throughout human history, fruit has been the ultimate health food, until the paleo and keto diet trends set in. There is abundant misinformation that fruits are harmful since fruits contain natural sugars. While the Paleolithic and ketogenic diets have their place, they have eliminated or seriously reduced the most powerful anticancer food groups: fruit, whole grains, legumes.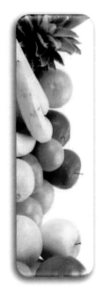

In fact, ALL scientific evidence shows that whole fruits are an important part of anyone's diet, especially the cancer patient. Whole fruits are a rich mixture of vitamins, minerals, bioflavonoids, carotenoids, pectin, fiber, potassium, and promising anti-cancer agents, such as ficin in figs and phytoalexins in red fruits. The antioxidant capacity (ORAC) and laxative effect of most fruits is therapeutic for the body.

In one study, Harvard researchers followed 75,000 women for 24 years and found that 2 servings of peaches per week lowered the risk for breast cancer by 40%.[24] In another study, Harvard researchers studied 44,000 men in Hawaii. The more fruit they ate, the lower the risk for cancer; in a dose dependent fashion.[25] For more information on the health merits of whole fruit see the chapter on foods with anti-cancer activity.

Fruit: Primal Human Food

Fact is, fruit, eggs, and insects were the original caveman food, when intelligence and tools limited what was available to eat. Red and green fruits and vegetables, garlic and cabbage family contain phytoalexins, which have powerful anti-cancer and anti-fungal activity. Here is where you begin to appreciate the brilliant design of nature. Fruit contains sugar, which fungus and insects would love to eat. Hence, fruits could only survive by producing substances that inhibit fungal growth, insects, etc. Is cancer a fungal infection? More on that later.

BOTTOM LINE Eat more fruit, especially organic, biodynamic, whole colorful fruit.

INTERMITTENT FASTING

This therapy may be one of the more crucial ways of beating cancer. Inadvertent fasting has been with the human race since the dawn of time. We are built to fast. Our ancestors suffered through endless periods of fasting, famine, and other issues with their food supply. Humans have adapted to require frequent times of no food intake. Most religions include fasting as part of the annual rituals because it became obvious that fasting improves health. Then, along came the modern food supply with dehydration, freezing, refrigeration, and canning. Slice, dice, chop, and blend until the food has a shelf life of forever and is no longer recognizable as a real food. Fast no more. The feast is here. And so are the epidemic levels of disease, including obesity, heart disease, cancer, diabetes, kidney disease, etc..

The domino of poor health starts like this. We eat. The body needs to digest that food and prepare for processing, receiving, and metabolizing the food. Insulin is secreted by the pancreas to allow glucose into the cells for the 100,000 chemical reactions that take place per second per cell. But the food intake is constant, just like the flow of insulin is constant, which creates insulin resistance on the cell membranes. The "noise" of constant eating, glucose, and insulin creates "deafness" or insulin resistance. So the body makes more insulin, which is an essential yet perilous hormone in the body. Excess insulin, such as is found in all type 2 diabetics and most Americans, causes weight gain, fat storage, inflammation, and a higher risk for cancer.

The benefits of fasting are extraordinary. Your humble author found out the easy way. I practice what I preach. I live a healthy lifestyle. Am fit, trim, active. Yet for years my fasting blood glucose was in the 90-105 mg% range, which is pre-diabetic. HbA1C (glycosylated hemoglobin, a more accurate measure of chronic blood glucose) was 5.9, which is okay, but not 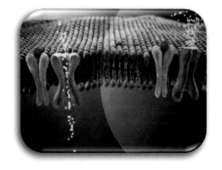 great. Tried everything. Every diet, including Paleolithic and ketogenic, many different supplements. Nothing worked. Then I tried intermittent fasting (IF), by limiting my feeding "window" to 8 hours per day (e.g. eating from 10 am to 6 pm) and water fasting one day a week. Within 3 weeks on this program my fasting blood glucose dropped to 67 mg% and I felt great.

There is abundant data showing the <u>mental and physical benefits of IF</u>. For 2 million years of adaptation, humans faced chronic food scarcity. These cave dwellers were physically fit enough to catch and kill an animal or the human died. They consumed abundant plant food with naturally occurring pesticides that eventually became protective against aging and cancer. We now eat too much and too often and the wrong foods. We are obese and unfit, and avoid any food that does not taste like ice cream or soda. And that lifestyle is killing advanced civilizations by the millions.

IF is being used by the best and brightest business people and athletes to <u>sharpen mental clarity</u> with "bio-hacking". IF has been shown to <u>lower the risk for</u> Alzheimer's disease, cognitive decline, and increase lifespan. IF gives the digestive tract a break, allowing for regeneration of cells. IF offers a <u>wealth of benefits</u> with zero cost. What does it cost to skip eating for 24 hours? Nothing. But since the biggest advertisers on TV are food and drugs companies who would all suffer revenue loss if broad portions of the population embraced IF, then you are not going to see articles on TV about this extremely important topic.

HOW DOES IT WORK?

Think of your ancestors 20,000 years ago. Life was tough. Food supply was undependable. Predators were everywhere. If caveman and cavewoman went a week without food, then the adaptive forces of nature kicked in to generate a process of autophagy (auto=self, phagy=to eat). Your body begins this critical process of scavenging marginal cells to create newer, younger, faster, smarter cells. Nature is telling caveman, "you better get smart and fast enough to find food, or you are going to die." That is what IF does for us.

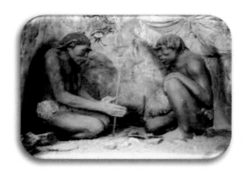

HOW DOES IT HELP CANCER PATIENTS?

Dietary restriction (DR) is the strategy of eating less calories, say dropping your intake from the necessary 2000 kcal/d to 1200 kcal/d, which eventually leads to some weight loss. But the long term benefits of DR have been mixed. There are a dozen good books for the public on the benefits of IF, starting with Jason Fung, MD THE OBESITY CODE. Dr. Fung is a diabetologist who found the treadmill of treating diabetics with renal failure discouraging. Upon research, Dr. Fung found that he could reverse/cure most type 2 diabetes with simple fasting. Now Dr. Fung is using IF to help prevent and reverse cancer.[26]

Meanwhile, IF has been shown to be a quick therapy to lower insulin like growth factor (IGF-1) which is a major accelerator of cancer growth. IF enhances success rates with chemo and radiation. Ketogenic and Paleolithic diets have their merits, but the inconvenient truth is that your body can generate glucose from protein, fat, or stored glycogen. By improving insulin sensitivity, you lower blood glucose and IGF...which is a major victory in your pursuit of healing.

On the other hand, you cannot starve a parasite out of a host. You cannot starve a cancer out of the cancer patient. But you can make the cellular environment inhospitable for the cancer. Do not undertake excessive fasting without medical advice. Up to 40% of cancer patients actually die from malnutrition, which is due to the effects of cancer, many chemicals created by cancer cells, chemo and radiation, depression, and loss of appetite. Hence, the goal is to use strategic IF to make the body hostile toward cancer cells, while feeding the cancer patient adequate calories and protein to be able to maintain strength and host defense mechanisms.

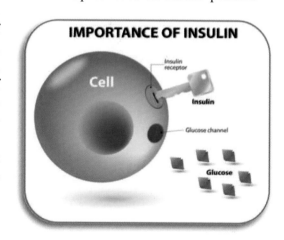

WHAT TO DO?

Take one day a week and eat no food, no calories, just water and tea. On the six days per week that you do eat, narrow your feeding "window" to 8 hours daily, such as from 10 am to 6 pm and eat enough to maintain optimal weight and strength. You not only are making it very uncomfortable for your cancer cells, but also rejuvenating your body and mind for the longer and smarter life that you will enjoy. On a risk to benefit to cost ratio, it doesn't get any better than IF.

ACTION PLAN: STARVE CANCER CELLS

DIET AND EXERCISE TO LOWER BLOOD AND GUT GLUCOSE. Eat foods low in glycemic index. Avoid the whites: sugar, flour, rice, potatoes. Make sure that you get the nutrients which help us to metabolize glucose, including B vitamins, magnesium, chromium, vanadium. Exercise daily to keep muscle tone, which becomes a great way of lowering blood glucose through muscle mass.

HYDRAZINE SULFATE. Since cancer cells derive most of their energy from anaerobic glycolysis, Joseph Gold, MD, developed hydrazine sulfate to inhibit the excessive gluconeogenesis that occurs in cancer patients. Hydrazine inhibits the enzyme phosphoenol pyruvate carboxykinase (PEP-CK), and in placebo-controlled clinical trials at UCLA, hydrazine was proven to slow and reverse cachexia in advanced cancer patients.[27] Studies with hydrazine sulfate as a therapy for cancer have been disappointing. Hydrazine is available online.

IV GLUCOSE WITH HYPERTHERMIA. Since cancer growth can be accelerated with intravenous glucose solutions, researchers in Germany have developed a technique, Systemic Cancer Multistep Therapy (SCMT), in which the cancer patient is given injections of glucose to elevate blood glucose to around 400 mg%, which generates a substantial reduction in pH in all malignant tissues due to lactic acid formation, then the patient is given whole body hyperthermia (42°C core temp.). Patients may then be treated with chemotherapy and radiation, which are optional. Five year survival in these SCMT treated patients increased by 25-50%, and complete regression of tumor increased by 30-50%.[28]

LOW GLUCOSE TOTAL PARENTERAL NUTRITION (TPN) SOLUTION. When a cancer patient cannot eat enough food to prevent lean tissue wasting, nutrients may be injected into a port implanted in the sub-clavian artery. Since "tumors appear to be obligate glucose utilizers..."[29], we can capitalize on the differences in energy metabolism between healthy and differentiated malignant cells by providing starving cancer patients with TPN solutions that are relatively low in glucose and higher in amino acids and lipids.[30] Many starving cancer patients are offered either no nutrition support or the standard TPN solution developed for intensive care units with 70% of kcal from glucose (dextrose). Disappointing results have been found when using standard high glucose TPN solutions for cachectic cancer patients.[31]

TUMOR HYPOXIA AND TREATMENT RESISTANCE. "...tumor hypoxia is present in at least one third of cancers in the clinical setting."[32] "Tumors differ from normal tissues because there is not enough oxygen to meet demand, even under baseline conditions."[33] Since solid tumors can develop pockets of hypoxic tissue that are particularly resistant to radiotherapy, a unique protocol using vitamin B-1 niacin (to improve aerobic energy metabolism) has been used by Jae Ho Kim, MD, PhD, at Ford Hospital in Detroit with noteworthy successes.

DOES BLOOD SUGAR IMPACT BREAST CA SURVIVAL?

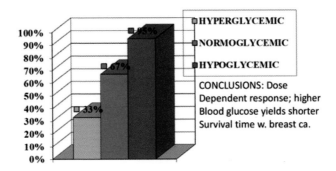

STUDY DESIGN: Mice (BALB/C) placed on 3 different diets
to alter blood glucose then injected with aggressive mammary tumor
(expect 50% survival at 60 days). Sucrose used to raise blood glucose.
Survival after 70 days was 8 of 24 (hyper), 16 of 24 (normo) & 19 of 20 (hypo).
Santisteban, GA, Biochem.& Biophys Res. Comm., vol.132, no.3, p.1174, Nov.198

Animals were injected with an aggressive strain of breast cancer, then fed diets that would provide either 1) hypoglycemia, 2) normoglycemia, or 3) hyperglycemia. There was a dose-dependent response in which the lower the blood glucose, the greater the survival percentage at 70 days.[34]

Glycemic index is a scientific approach to measuring the role of dietary carbohydrates in blood glucose levels and was developed in 1981 by Dr. David Jenkins. Though glycemic index does not take into consideration "nutrient density", it is a useful means of helping people to select foods that will create a more favorable blood glucose level. Given a choice, eat the food with a lower glycemic index.

ORAL GLUCOSE TOLERANCE CURVES

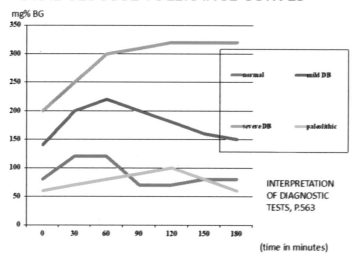

INTERPRETATION
OF DIAGNOSTIC
TESTS, P.563

PATIENT PROFILE:

A.J. was diagnosed in 2014 with mesothelioma, aka asbestiosis. A.J. had been given a very poor prognosis by his doctors. A.J. had a consultation with PQ in 2016. A.J. consulted an oncologist and family doctor specializing in functional and integrative medicine. Since his consultation with PQ, he now eats a clean diet, mostly plant-based with bone broth and occasional high-quality meats. Initially he juiced, for about 1 year, then switched to smoothies and included the whole plant, not just the juice. He has added several supplements to his diet.

A.J. believes his inquisitive mind has helped him on his road to recovery. Initially it was all doom and gloom, and depressing, but PQ was uplifting and explained how nutrition is powerful in healing the body. A.J. continues to monitor his blood work, and continues to dig to find the underlying cause when blood work is a little off. Today he is in remission.

ENDNOTES

[1] https://www.dhhs.nh.gov/dphs/nhp/documents/sugar.pdf

[2] https://ghr.nlm.nih.gov/condition/lactose-intolerance#statistics

[3] https://www.womenshealthnetwork.com/nutrition/the-dangers-of-splenda-and-other-artificial-sweeteners.aspx

[4] . Olney, JW, et al., J.Neuropathol.Exp.Neurol., vol.55, p.1115, 1996

[5] . Walton, RG, et al., Biol.Psychiatry, vol.34, p.13, 1993

[6] . VanDen Eeden, SK, et al., Neurology, vol.44, p.1787, Oct.1994

[7] . Roberts, HJ, ASPARTAME: IS IT SAFE?, p.12, Charles Press, Philadelphia, 1990

[8] . Page, LR, HEALTHY HEALING, p.199, Healthy Healing Publ, 1996

[9] https://link.springer.com/article/10.1007/s10863-007-9086-x

[10] https://www.ingentaconnect.com/content/ben/acamc/2008/00000008/00000003/art00006

[11] . Warburg, O., Science, vol.123, no.3191, p.309, Feb.1956

[12] . Demetrakopoulos, GE, Cancer Research, vol.42, p.756S, Feb.1982

[13] . Gullino, PM, Cancer Research, vol.27, p.1031, June 1967

[14] . Rossi-Fanelli, F., J.Parenteral Enteral Nutr., vol.15, p.680, 1991

[15] .Digirolamo, M., in DIET AND CANCER: MARKERS, PREVENTION, AND TREATMENT, p.203, Plenum Press, NY, 1994

[16] Volk, T., Br.J.Cancer, vol.68, p.492, 1993

[17] . Leeper, DB, Int.J.Hyperthermia, vol.14, no.3, p.257, 1998

[18] . Sanchez, A., Amer.J.Clin.Nutr., vol.26, p.1180, Nov.1973

[19] . Yam, D., Medical Hypotheses, vol.38, p.111, 1992

[20] https://www.nature.com/articles/6605240

[21] . Moerman, CJ, Int.J.Epidemiology, vol.22, no.2, p.207, 1993

[22] . Seeley,S.,, Med.Hypotheses, vol.11, p.319, 1983

[23] . Rothkopf, M, Fuel utilization in neoplastic disease: implications for the use of nutritional support in cancer patients, Nutrition, supp, 6:4:14-16S, 1990

[24] https://link.springer.com/article/10.1007/s10549-013-2484-3

[25] http://cancerres.aacrjournals.org/content/58/3/442

[26] https://www.amazon.com/Cancer-Code-Wellness-Book-ebook/dp/B084VRNSCN/ref=sr_1_15?crid=1DHOKUI0PSJK3&dchild=1&keywords=jason+fung&qid=1589839520&sprefix=jason+fung%2Caps%2C236&sr=8-15

[27] https://acsjournals.onlinelibrary.wiley.com/doi/abs/10.1002/1097-0142(19870201)59:3%3C406::AID-CNCR2820590309%3E3.0.CO;2-W

[28] . von Ardenne, M., Strahlentherapie und Onkologie, vol.170, p.581, 1994

[29] . Rothkopf, M, Nutrition, vol.6, no.4, p.14S, July 1990 supp

[30] . Tuttle-Newhall, JE, Cancer & Nutrition, in ADJUVANT NUTRITION IN CANCER TREATMENT, Quillin, P (ed), p.145, Cancer Treatment Research Foundation, Arlington Heights, IL 1994

[31] . Sakurai, Y, Japanese J. Surgery, vol.28, p.247, 1998

[32] . Vaupel, P., Int.J.Rad.OncologyBiol.Phys., vol.42, no.4, p.843, 1998

[33] . Gulledge, CJ, Anticancer Research, vol.16, p.741, 1996

[34] . Santisteban, GA, Biochem. & Biophys.Res.Comm., vol.132, no.3, p.1174, Nov.1985

GLYCEMIC INDEX (Brand-Miller, J. et al., Glucose Revolution, Marlow, NY 1999:
how fast does the carbohydrate food get into the blood compared to glucose (=100)

	Bread/Grain	Vegetables	Fruit	Legumes	Dairy	Beverages	Snack Food
90-100		parsnip, baked white potato	dried dates (103)				glucose, maltose (105)
80-89	corn flakes, crispbread	red skinned potato					
70-79	raisin bran, vanilla wafers, graham crackers, waffles, white & wheat bread, bagel, cocoa krispies	french fries, pumpkin	watermelon	broad beans		Gatorade	corn chips, Life Savers, Skittles Fruit Chews
60-69	taco shells, shredded wheat, arrowroot cookies, shortbread	beets, new potatoes	cantaloupe, pineapple, raisins		ice cream	soft drink syrup, Fanta	sucrose (white sugar), Mars almond bar
50-59	all bran, whole wheat, buckwheat, brown & white rice, blueberry muffin, pita & sourdough bread	sweet corn, sweet potato, yam	banana, kiwi, mango, papaya				Power bar, potato chips, honey, popcorn
40-49	noodles, sponge cake, spaghetti, oatmeal, banana bread	carrots, green peas	grapes, orange	baked beans		orange juice, apple juice	chocolate, Twix Cookie, Snickers, lactose
30-39	pasta fettuccine, ravioli		apple, apricot, pear, plum	butter beans, chick peas (garbanzo), lentils, navy beans	low fat yogurt, skim milk, chocolate milk		
20-29			cherries, grapefruit	kidney beans	whole milk		fructose
10-19				soybeans			peanuts

Chapter 11

NUTRIENTS AS BIOLOGICAL RESPONSE MODIFIERS

The Power of Nutritional Synergism

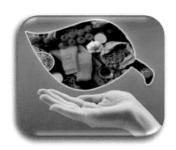

Synergism: the action of two or more substances to achieve an effect of which each is individually incapable

---

WHAT'S AHEAD?

Synergism means that 1 + 1 = 3 or 500, greater than what would be expected. Nutrients work together in an elegant symphony to heal the body from cancer. There is no one "magic bullet" nutrient against cancer, since we need 50 essential nutrients and probably hundreds of other nutrition factors for optimal health.

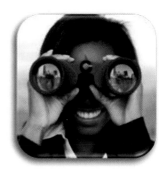

An average of 3 high school football players each year die from heat stroke. Big men exercising hard in the heat of summer without enough water. Water becomes the life-saving biological response modifier for those men. In December of 1971 Richard Nixon launched the "war on cancer" with a promise of a cure for a major cancer by the Bicentennial of 1976. Researchers began an earnest quest for a "magic bullet" or <u>biological response modifier</u> to cure cancer. We still don't have a cure for any major cancer, but we do know a lot more about cancer and how the body can defend itself. Nature provides us with a host of BRMs to prevent and reverse cancer. It is about time that we started harnessing these incredible agents.

HOW CAN NUTRIENTS AFFECT THE CANCER PROCESS?

Shklar, G., Alternative & Complementary Therapies, vol.2, no.3, p.156, May 1996
-inhibit angiogenesis
-dysregulate mutant p53 oncogene
-alter immune cytokines
Schwartz, JL, Cancer Prevention Intl., vol.3, p.37, 1997
-upregulate DNA repair
-augment programmed cell death (apoptosis)
Prasad, KN, et al., Arch.Otolaryngol.Head Neck Surg., vol.119, p.1133, Oct.1993
-regulate gene expression
-induce growth inhibition in cancer
-alter cell differentiation
Lupulescu, A., Intl.J.Vit.Nutr.Res., vol.63, p.3, 1993
-A, C, E regulators of cell differentiation, membrane biogenesis, DNA synthesis
-A, C, E may be cytotoxic and cytostatic in certain cell system
-affect oncogenes
Poppel, GV, et al., Cancer Letters, vol.114, p.195, 1997
-immune stimulation
-enhancement of cell to cell communication, defuse carcinogens, etc.

Certain nutrients, like selenium, vitamin K, vitamin E succinate, and the fatty acid EPA, appear to have the ability to slow down the unregulated growth of cancer. Various nutrition factors, including vitamin A, D, folacin, bioflavonoids, and soybeans, have been shown to alter the genetic expression of tumors. Many of the following chapters in this book address the use of foods and supplements as BRMs against cancer.

There are two primary lessons to be learned in nutritional synergism:

1) Enhanced effects.

✓ **Nutrient & nutrient combinations** augment each other to achieve greater healing capacity. Either vitamin C or essential fatty acids were able to inhibit the growth of melanoma in culture, yet when combined, their anti-cancer activity was much stronger.[1]

✓ **Nutrient & medicine combinations** help to protect the patient while selectively destroying the cancer cells. Maitake D-fraction inhibited tumor growth by 80%, while the drug Mitomycin C inhibited tumor growth by 45%. Yet when both were given together, but at half the dosage for each, tumor inhibition was 98%.

2) Lower doses are required when nutrients are used synergistically. In animals with implanted tumors, vitamin C and B-12 together provided for significant tumor regression and 50% survival of the treated group, while all of the animals not receiving C and B-12 died by the 19th day.[2] C and B-12 seemed to form a cobalt-ascorbate compound that selectively shut down tumor growth. When vitamin C and K were added to cancer cells in culture, the dosage required to kill cancer cells dropped by 98% compared to the dosage required by either of these vitamins alone.[3] Combining vitamins C and K-3 against cultured human breast cancer cells allowed for inhibition of the cancer growth at doses 90-98% less than what was required if only one of these vitamins was used against the cancer.[4]

No one and nothing operates in isolation. Both 20th century research and our multi-billion dollar pharmaceutical-based medical system are rooted in the concept of using a single agent to treat a single symptom. Unfortunately, life is much more complicated than that.

NEGATIVE SYNERGISM OF TOXINS

We know that barbiturates have a certain toxicity on the liver, which is synergistically enhanced when alcohol is consumed at the same time. We know that tobacco brings a major risk for lung cancer, as does asbestos exposure, yet when a person is exposed to both, there is a 500% greater risk for lung cancer than would have been expected by adding the two risks (1+1=2). Scientists recently found that pesticides amplify one another's toxicity by 500-1,000 fold.[5] Thus, 1+1=500. This discovery of synergistic toxicity presents the chilling possibility that the 1.2 billion pounds of pesticides sprayed on our domestic food supply may not be as safe as we once thought. Eat organic or "no spray" whenever possible.

In 1976, a study examined animals that were fed 2% of their diet as either red dye, sodium cyclamate, or an emulsifier--all approved at the time by the Food and Drug Administration. Animals fed one food additive showed no harmful effects. Animals fed two of the food additives exhibited balding scruffy fur, diarrhea, and retarded weight gain. Animals fed all three additives all died within 2 weeks.[6]

The take-home lesson is that poisons probably amplify another's toxicity in logarithmic fashion. The cavalier spirit with which Americans have nonchalantly discarded wastes and intentionally added toxins to our air, food, and water supply makes synergistic toxicity a likely explanation for why 42% of Americans living today will be diagnosed with cancer.

POSITIVE SYNERGISM OF NUTRIENTS

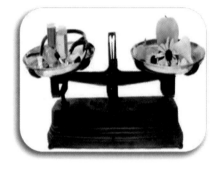

While the prospects of synergistic toxicity are daunting, the prospects of synergistic nutritional healing may be the key to solving many of our health problems. Perusing any biochemistry textbook, we find an abundance of synergistic nutritional relationships: calcium with magnesium with potassium with sodium, vitamin E with selenium, polyunsaturated fats with vitamin E, protein with B-6, and so on.

Antioxidants have surfaced as the "fire extinguishers" that minimize the cellular damage from reactive oxygen species, or free radicals. Yet, these antioxidants work in a hierarchy, not unlike a game of "hot potato", trying to pass along the unpaired electron until the energy dissipates. In this hierarchy, vitamin C recharges vitamin E.

Biologists find this complex hierarchy of antioxidants consists of 8,000 bioflavonoids; 800 carotenoids; known essential vitamins, such as C and E; conditionally essential vitamins, such as lipoic acid and coenzyme Q; and endogenously-synthesized antioxidants like superoxide dismutase (SOD) and glutathione peroxidase (GSH-Px).

The possible combinations and permutations of antioxidants in the human body are like trying to figure out M.C. Escher's artwork. When these antioxidants are all in their proper place in optimal amounts, we have a relatively impenetrable barrier against oxidative damage. Researching any one of these nutrients in isolation is overly simplistic and doomed to misleading results.

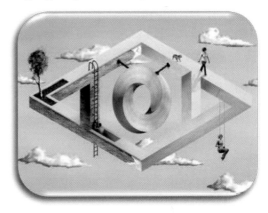

The National Cancer Institute reported in 1994 that beta-carotene supplements provided a slightly elevated risk for lung cancer in heavy smokers. [7] Yet other prominent researchers in nutrition and cancer have published papers showing that antioxidants such as beta-carotene can become pro-oxidants in the wrong biochemical environment, such as the combat zone of free radicals generated by heavy tobacco use.[8] At the International Conference on Nutrition and Cancer, sponsored by the University of California at Irvine, held in July 1997, there were several watershed presentations showing that one nutrient alone may be ineffective or counterproductive, while a host of compatible nutrients in the proper ratio can be extremely effective at slowing or reversing cancer.

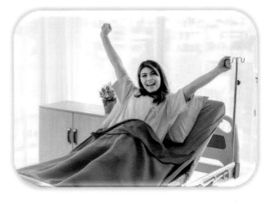

Adjuvant (helpful) nutrition and traditional oncology are synergistic, not antagonistic. While we have detailed the limitations of traditional oncology, there is compelling evidence that nutrition is the missing modality in comprehensive cancer treatment. Restrained tumor killing in combination with changing the cellular environment through nutrition holds promise as 21st century cancer treatment.

NUTRIENTS ALONE CAN REVERSE PRE-CANCEROUS LESIONS

Cancer is not an "on or off" switch. No one goes to bed on Sunday night perfectly healthy and then wakes up Monday morning with stage 4 colon cancer metastasis to the liver. Cancer takes months, and probably years to develop. Research has shown that, in the early stages of cancer cell development, nutrients alone can reverse "pre-malignant" cancers[9], which under the microscope are identical to cancer cells, yet have not invaded beyond their own "turf". As the bowling ball of cancer begins its hazardous deterioration downhill, the body has built-in mechanisms to stop this process, including DNA repair, cell-to-cell communication, macrophage engulfment, tumor necrosis factor, collagen encapsulation, and anti-angiogenesis agents to shut down the making of new blood vessels from the tumor.

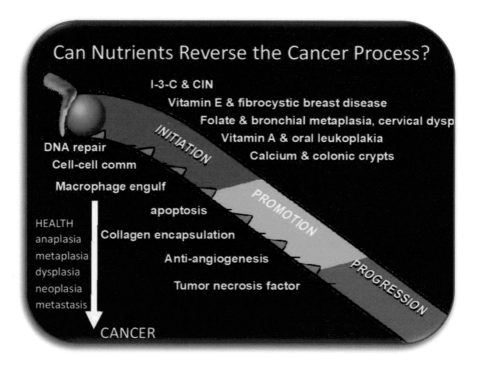

This concept is very pivotal to the notion that nutrition can improve outcome in cancer treatment. For decades, researchers have held the notion that "once the cell turns cancerous, only forceful eradication can help the patient." Maybe not. Pre-cancerous conditions, such as oral leukoplakia, bronchial metaplasia, and colonic crypts, can be reversed by nutrients alone. Once cancer has deteriorated to stage 4 malignancy with extensive metastasis, the patient needs appropriate medical care to selectively reduce tumor burden.

Our 37 trillion cells in the human body are constantly dividing. The DNA, which contains the body's blueprints to make a completely new you, must "unzip" the spiral staircase of chromosomes, then duplicate itself exactly, then "re-zip" the spiral staircase of DNA. This process occurs billions of times daily. The chance for a mistake is quite high, which is why our bodies have many mechanisms in place to correct mistakes in the beginning. Yet, if the mistake cell continues to deteriorate through its many different shades of cancer; including anaplasia, dysplasia, and metaplasia, then the final stage of neoplasia might occur.

As this process is deteriorating, nutrients have been shown to not only arrest the slippery slide toward cancer, but also to reverse the damage and help the body to generate healthy cells from pre-malignant cancers. In high doses:

- folate and B-12 can reverse bronchial metaplasia[10] or cervical dysplasia
- beta-carotene[11] and vitamin A can reverse oral leukoplakia[12]; so can vitamin E[13]
- selenium can reverse pre-cancerous mouth lesions[14]
- vitamin C[15] and calcium can reverse colon polyps[16]
- vitamins A, C, and E reversed colorectal adenomas[17]
- vitamin E can reverse benign breast disease, such as fibrocystic breast disease, which increases the risk for breast cancer by 50-80%[18]
- vitamin E and beta-carotene injected into the tumor reversed mouth cancer in animals.[19]

Pre-malignant and malignant cells look almost identical under the microscope. Since nutrients can reverse pre-malignant cells, it becomes entirely probable that nutrients can help to re-regulate malignant and metastatic cells. Maybe we don't have to kill all the cancer cells in order to cure the cancer patient. The best combination is selective tumor debulking along with re-regulation of the host defense mechanisms through the protocols described throughout this book.

NUTRITIONAL SYNERGISM AGAINST CANCER

Researchers found that all DMBA (tobacco)-exposed animals died. When provided a single chemopreventive nutrient (either selenium, magnesium, vitamin C, or vitamin A), cancer incidence after DMBA exposure was cut in half. When two nutrients were combined, the cancer incidence was cut by 70%; with 3 chemopreventive nutrients the cancer incidence was cut by 80%; and with 4 nutrients the cancer incidence was cut by 88%.[20]

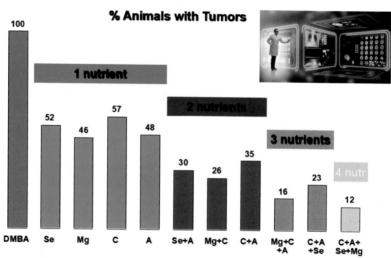

Synergism of Chemopreventive Nutrients

Study design: female rats (15-30/group) exposed to 30 mg total DMBA begin at day 50 after birth, provided nutrient supplements from d 40-240; Rao, AR, et al, Jpn J Ca Res, vol 81, p 1239, Dec 1990

The take home lesson from this chapter is synergism. Do not rely on any one food, nutrition supplement or drug to cure your cancer. The answer to cancer is found in reregulating your body's host defense mechanisms to recognize and destroy the cancer using all of the modalities found throughout this book. Next is to selectively reduce tumor burden through restrained therapies that kill the cancer and not the patient. And finally, provide palliative care for the inevitable symptoms and complications that arise while treating cancer. Together, this synergistic approach will become 21st century cancer treatment with improvements in quality and quantity of life and chances for a complete remission.

PATIENT PROFILE:

K.B. was diagnosed with thyroid cancer in 2014. Her consultation with PQ was August 2015. Prior to diagnosis her diet consisted of low-quality burgers, sodas and sugary foods. K.B. made significant changes to her diet and improved her nutrition and now exercises regularly. K.B has undertaken many natural therapies and believes the immunotherapy (from South America) was very helpful in her recovery. K.B. also takes many supplements daily including fish oil, turmeric, iodine, beta glucan, iv's including with glutathione and vitamin C. K.B. also makes juices, smoothies and plant-based protein drinks almost daily. Today K.B. is in complete remission and feels great.

ENDNOTES

[1] . Gardiner, N, et al., Pros.Leuk., vol.34, p.119, 1988

[2] . Poydock, ME, Am.J.Clin.Nutr., vol.54, p.1261S, 1991

[3] . Noto, V., et al., Cancer, vol.63, p.901, 1989

[4] . Noto, V., et al., Cancer, vol.63, p.901, 1989

[5] . Arnold. SF, et al., Science, vol.272, p.1489, 1996

[6] . Ershoff, BH, Journal of Food Science, vol.41, p.949, 1976

[7] . Alpha tocopherol beta-carotene cancer prevention study group, New England Journal of Medicine, vol.330, p.1029, 1994

[8] . Schwartz, JL, Journal of Nutrition, vol.126, 4 suppl, p.1221S, 1996

[9] Singh, VN, Am.J.Clin.Nutr., vol.53, p.386S, 1991

[10] Heimburger, DC, JAMA, vol.259, no.10, p.1525, Mar.11, 1988

[11] Toma, S., Oncology, vol.49, p.77, 1992

[12] Stich, HF, Am.J.Clin.Nutr., vol.53, p.298S, 1991

[13] Benner, SE, J.National Cancer Institute, vol.85, no.1, p.44, Jan.1993

[14] Toma, S., Cancer Detection & Prevention, vol.15, no.6, p.491, 1991

[15] DeCosse, JJ, Surgery, vol.78, no.5, p.608, Nov.1975

[16] Wargovich, MJ, et al., Gastroenterology, vol.103, p.92, 1992; see also Steinbach, G., Gastroenterology, vol.106, p.1162, 1994

[17] Paganelli, GM, J. National Cancer Institute, vol.84,no.1, p.47, Jan.1992

[18] Krieger, N, American J. Epidemiology, vol.135, no.6, p.619, 1992; see also London, SJ, JAMA, vol.267, no.7, p.941, Feb.1992

[19] Shklar, G., Nutr Cancer, vol.12, p.321, 1989

[20] . Rao, AR, et al., Japanese Journal Cancer Research, vol.81, p.1239, Dec.1990

Chapter 12

FOODS WITH ANTI-CANCER ACTIVITY

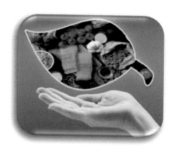

Let food be your medicine and let medicine be your food.
Hippocrates, circa 370 BC

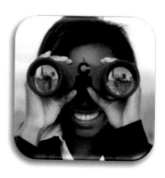

<u>WHAT'S AHEAD?</u>
- ✓ Somewhere between <u>30% to 70% of cancer is driven by poor nutrition.</u>[1]
- ✓ There are foods that can accelerate cancer (high sodium, high sugar, trans fats, too much meat or dairy, excess calories, overcooked meats)
- ✓ And foods that can prevent or even reverse cancer.

Not until the introduction of processed foods did cancer become a common cause of death. Yet even primitive healers noticed the link between diet and cancer. Chinese physicians 2000 years ago wrote: "an immoderate diet will lead to cancer (ye ge)." For most of the 20th century the authorities in government and medicine denied any link between nutrition and cancer. The problem has always been special interest groups. If the FDA,

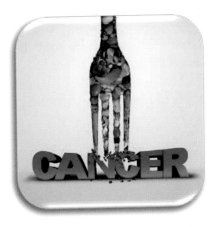

USDA, or AMA discourage the consumption of any food or group, that special interest lobby would assail the report and the people in charge. Which is why it took nearly a hundred years after smoking was known to be harmful before the Surgeon General issued his report in 1964 that smoking was probably not good for you.

In 1982 the National Academy of Sciences issued their report <u>DIET, NUTRITION, AND CANCER</u> [2] with the headlines "spread the good news, cancer may not be as inevitable as death and taxes." By 1991 the Office of Alternative Medicine issued a book NUTRITION IN CANCER TREATMENT which showed that nutrition (food and supplements) "would assume a role as adjuvant therapies in cancer treatment." We are now 30 years beyond that report and most cancer patients are seriously mislead on the subject of nutrition.

Of the <u>$5.8 billion annual budget</u> at the National Cancer Institute, less than 1% is spent on nutrition research. Of the $20 million spent at the NCI to investigate diet and cancer, the following categories were outlined:

1) *Highest* anticancer activity: garlic, soybeans, ginger, licorice, carrots, celery, parsley, parsnips
2) *Moderate* anticancer activity: onion, flaxseed, citrus, turmeric, tomatoes, peppers, brown rice, whole wheat, cruciferous vegetables (broccoli, Brussels sprouts, cabbage, cauliflower)
3) *Modest* anticancer activity: oats, barley, cucumber, medicinal seasonings (mint, rosemary, thyme, oregano, basil)

The <u>American Institute of Cancer Research</u> gathers information to help support cancer patients and cancer prevention.[3] Their website shows foods that have anti-cancer activity:

The following are foods that have demonstrated anti-cancer activity, always to be used in conjunction with your doctor's best care. Recommendations are based on the best studied diet on the planet earth, the Mediterranean diet, which is plant based. See the recipe chapter for practical tips on implementing these foods in the kitchen.

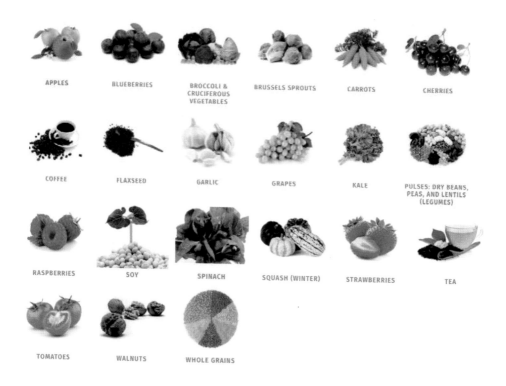

APPLES   BLUEBERRIES   BROCCOLI & CRUCIFEROUS VEGETABLES   BRUSSELS SPROUTS   CARROTS   CHERRIES

COFFEE   FLAXSEED   GARLIC   GRAPES   KALE   PULSES: DRY BEANS, PEAS, AND LENTILS (LEGUMES)

RASPBERRIES   SOY   SPINACH   SQUASH (WINTER)   STRAWBERRIES   TEA

TOMATOES   WALNUTS   WHOLE GRAINS

FOODS AS BIOLOGICAL RESPONSE MODIFIERS

When the National Cancer Institute was given its directives from Richard Nixon in 1971 to "find a cure for a major cancer by 1976", an army of dedicated MDs and PhDs descended on the beltway to find a magic bullet cure, or a "biological response modifier" for cancer…always with the intention of the cure being a patentable and highly profitable drug. Never happened. We are now almost a half century and a trillion dollars spent on research and no major cancer has a cure.

NUTRIENTS AS BIOLOGICAL RESPONSE MODIFIERS
changing the way the body works to reverse cancer

→IMMUNE REGULATORS, ELIMINATE INFECTIONS?
→ALTER GENETIC EXPRESSION OF CANCER
→CELL MEMBRANE DYNAMICS
→DETOXIFICATION
→PH MAINTENANCE, BALANCING PROTONS
→PROOXIDANTS & AOX, BALANCING ELECTRONS
→CELLULAR COMMUNICATIONS (signal cell transduction)
→PROSTAGLANDIN REGULATION
→STEROID HORMONE CONTROL
→ENERGY METABOLISM: AEROBIC VS ANAEROBIC
→PROBIOTICS VS DYSBIOSIS
→ANTI-PROLIFERATIVE AGENTS
→ALTER TUMOR PROTECTIVE MECHANISMS
→APOPTOSIS, PROGRAMMED CELL DEATH

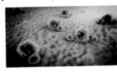
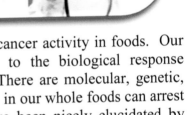

But those bright minds overlooked the anti-cancer activity in foods. Our species survived for 2 million years due to the biological response modifiers in our wholesome food supply. There are molecular, genetic, and biochemical pathways in which nutrients in our whole foods can arrest cancer. These underlying mechanisms have been nicely elucidated by very respected researchers. It's time we started using this miracle formulary of diet as the front-line therapy in the war on cancer.

BIOREGULATORS (examples)

animal	plant	fungal	herbal	mineral	vitamin
BTC	lecithin	PSK	curcumin	Iodine	A
EPA	sesame	Maitake	ginseng	Zinc	D
CLA	GLA	AHCC	kelp	Selenium	folate
whey	kelp	cordycep	ginkgo	Sulfur	niacin
lactoferrin colostrum	bioflav	lentinan	silymarin	Cr/Vd	C

OMNIVORE, VEGAN, CARNIVORE, PALEO, KETO?

While there are compelling reasons to focus on a whole plant food diet, there are also good reasons to include small amounts of free range animal food in the diet.[4] As anthropologists wandered the world in search of answers on humanity's past, there were no vegan groups ever found. Given an option, most people include some animal food in the diet: meat, fish, yogurt, cheese, eggs, etc.

REASONS FOR OMNIVOROUS DIET

CARNIVORE NUTRIENTS	HERBIVORE nutrients
Vitamin A retinol	carotenoids
Vitamin D cholecalciferol	bioflavonoids
Vitamin K2	sterolins (beta sitosterol)
conjugated linoleic acid (CLA)	fiber (butyrate)
eicosapentaenoic acid (EPA)	potassium
cartilage (glycosaminoglycans)	anti-fungals (veg., mushr.,kelp)
carnitine	chlorophyll
glandular extracts	curcumin
CoQ	ellagic acid
B-12	fucoidan (kelp)

minor dietary constituents
conditionally essential nutr.

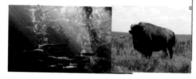

Choose often from the following group of plant foods:

FRUITS: apples, avocado, bananas, cantaloupe, etc.

VEGETABLES: asparagus, broccoli, carrots, cabbage, beets, pigmented potatoes, spinach, etc.

WHOLE GRAINS: amaranth, quinoa, barley, buckwheat, pigmented corn, brown rice, millet, oats, wheat* (unless you have gluten sensitivity)

LEGUMES: peas, beans, chickpeas, lentils, peanuts, etc.

NUTS: walnut, pecan, cashew, pine nut, Brazil nut, coconut

SEEDS: chia, hemp, papaya, poppy, sesame, pumpkin, watermelon, squash

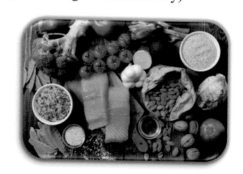

SEAWEED/SEA VEGETABLES: kelp, kombu, wakame, nori, dulse, Irish moss

MUSHROOMS: shiitake, oyster, white button, maitake, Portobello, rei shi

MEDICINAL HERBS/HEALING SPICES: allspice, basil, bay leaf, celery seed, chili, clove, coriander, fennel, mint, mustard, horseradish, turmeric, oregano, sage, thyme, etc.

Choose occasionally from this group of animal foods:

POULTRY: chicken, turkey, eggs

FISH: salmon, sardine, trout, halibut, mahi, halibut, shrimp, lobster, oyster, clam

RED MEAT: grass fed beef, buffalo, goat

DAIRY: yogurt, cheese, cottage cheese, butter

Avoid

Hard liquor, hydrogenated fats, the whites (sugar, flour, potatoes, corn, rice), deep fried anything, overcooked meat (i.e. well done steak on the grill), GMO foods, fake foods

Fruit

Fruit has been the ultimate health food, until the paleo and keto trends set in. For that reason, we are going to spend some time discussing the health merits of fruit. There is abundant misinformation that fruits are harmful since fruits contain natural sugars. While the Paleolithic and ketogenic diets have their place, they have eliminated or seriously reduced the most powerful anticancer food groups: fruit, whole grains, legumes.

Fruits and vegetables were associated with a substantial reduction in risk for heart disease and cancer.[5] In fact, ALL scientific evidence shows that whole fruits are an important part of anyone's diet, especially the cancer patient. Whole fruits are a rich mixture of vitamins, minerals, bioflavonoids, carotenoids, pectin, fiber, potassium, and promising anti-cancer agents, such as ficin in figs and phytoalexins in red fruits. The antioxidant capacity (ORAC) and laxative effect of most fruits is therapeutic for the body.

Since sugar feeds cancer and fruits contain sugars, you might reason that whole fruit is ill advised for many people. Let's look at the evidence.

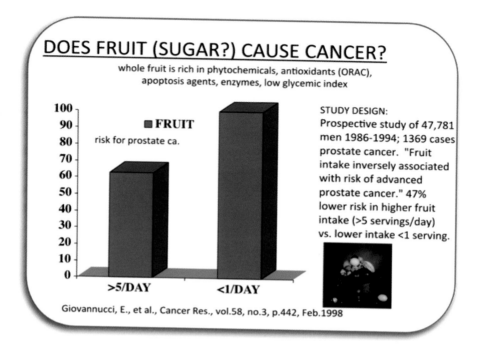

DOES FRUIT (SUGAR?) CAUSE CANCER?

whole fruit is rich in phytochemicals, antioxidants (ORAC), apoptosis agents, enzymes, low glycemic index

■ FRUIT
risk for prostate ca.

>5/DAY   <1/DAY

STUDY DESIGN: Prospective study of 47,781 men 1986-1994; 1369 cases prostate cancer. "Fruit intake inversely associated with risk of advanced prostate cancer." 47% lower risk in higher fruit intake (>5 servings/day) vs. lower intake <1 serving.

Giovannucci, E., et al., Cancer Res., vol.58, no.3, p.442, Feb.1998

Does Fruit Increase Risk for Cancer?

In one study, Harvard researchers followed 75,000 women for 24 years and found that 2 servings of peaches per week lowered the risk for breast cancer by 40%.[6] If that was a drug, it would have been international headlines and peaches would be available only by prescription. In another study, Harvard researchers studied 44,000 men in Hawaii. The more fruit they ate, the lower the risk for prostate cancer; in a dose dependent fashion.[7]

Does Fruit Lower Immune Functions?

In a study of senior citizens in London, researchers found that the more whole fruit these people ate the lower the risk for shingles, a viral infection in the nerves. Those who ate less than one serving of fruit per week had a 300% increase in the risk for shingles compared to those who ate 3 servings of fruit per day.[8]

Does Fruit Promote Diabetes?

In a study examining 3.4 million patient years (patients x years followed) there was a significant decline in type 2 diabetes among those who ate more fruit, particularly grapes, apples, and blueberries. [9] However, fruit juice increased the risk for diabetes. Again, eat whole foods.

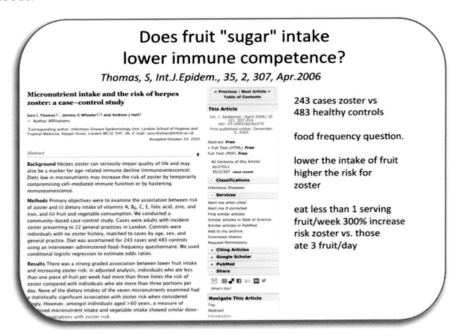

THE ORIGINAL PALEOLITHIC DIET

Fact is, fruit, eggs, and insects were the original caveman food, when intelligence and tools limited what was available to eat. Red and green fruits and vegetables contain phytoalexins, have powerful anti-cancer and anti-fungal activity. Here is where you begin to appreciate the brilliant design of nature. Fruit contains sugar, which fungus and insects would love to eat. Hence, fruits could only survive by producing substances that inhibit fungal growth, and insects, etc. More than coincidentally, fungus and cancer can both be subdued by these anti-fungal compounds. Is cancer a fungal infection? More on that later.

BOTTOM LINE

Eat more fruit, especially organic, biodynamic, whole colorful fruit.

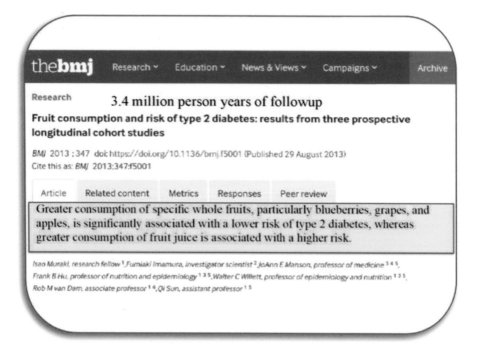

the**bmj**   Research ˅   Education ˅   News & Views ˅   Campaigns ˅   Archive

Research   **3.4 million person years of followup**
Fruit consumption and risk of type 2 diabetes: results from three prospective longitudinal cohort studies

BMJ 2013 ; 347 doi: https://doi.org/10.1136/bmj.f5001 (Published 29 August 2013)
Cite this as: *BMJ* 2013;347:f5001

Article   Related content   Metrics   Responses   Peer review

Greater consumption of specific whole fruits, particularly blueberries, grapes, and apples, is significantly associated with a lower risk of type 2 diabetes, whereas greater consumption of fruit juice is associated with a higher risk.

Isao Muraki, research fellow [1], *Fumiaki Imamura, investigator scientist* [2] *JoAnn E Manson, professor of medicine* [3,4,5],
Frank B Hu, professor of nutrition and epidemiology [1,3,5], *Walter C Willett, professor of epidemiology and nutrition* [1,3,5],
Rob M van Dam, associate professor [1,6], *Qi Sun, assistant professor* [1,5]

Vegetables

This is a food group that receives nearly unanimous approval of nearly any doctor or health group. Asparagus, broccoli, carrots, cabbage, beets, pigmented potatoes, spinach, and more needs to be on your menu often. Try a green smoothie in your blender using spinach, peaches, and coconut milk. Try making roasted vegetables. Recipe is simple. Dice your favorite vegetables into a large blending bowl. Mix 1 cup of olive oil with small amounts of lemon juice, soy sauce, balsamic vinegar, and spices in abundance (see below) in a 2 cup container. Stir the liquid ingredients, then spread over the bowl of mixed vegetables and mix thoroughly. Bake in 400 F oven for 30-40 minutes. Delicious.

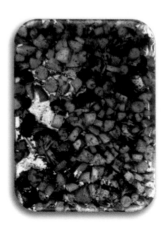

Whole Grains

Whole grains provided the basis for civilization. Our primitive ancestors were hunters and gatherers. They followed the herds. Yet, you cannot have a city until people settle down. It was in the Middle East that wheat was first cultivated, leading to farms, thus leading to cities, and specialization of labor. While the ketogenic and Paleolithic diet advocates have ruled whole grains as "unnecessary", nature and science say otherwise.

The two longest ruling empires on earth, Egyptian and Roman, both made whole wheat their staple in the diet. The wheat we currently eat has been greatly modified in attempts to yield more gluten, which provide texture in making bread. Most modern wheat is genetically modified, then soaked in the herbicide glyphosate, listed as a "probable carcinogen" by the World Health Organization. Their wheat was different than our wheat. When in doubt, avoid wheat/gluten.

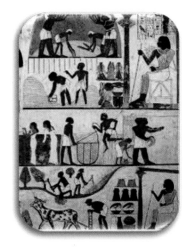

However, it gets complicated. Researchers find that gluten from wheat can interfere with zonulin in the gut that maintains integrity of the intestinal wall. Leaky gut from a "war zone" dysbiosis can lead to various diseases, including auto-immune and cancer.[10] Adding the assaults of the caustic diet of modern society coupled with drugs and stress, our guts are more vulnerable to breakdown.

Yet, whole grains have provided humans with the bulk of calories and protein for centuries. Rice in Asia and South America. Quinoa among the Incas in South America. Corn among the Americas. Whole grains do not provide a complete protein, hence the need to add legumes and vegetables if you are seeking a vegan diet.

Whole grains provide more than just obvious nutrients, but also the prebiotics that your 100 trillion organisms in your gut require. Fiber from whole grains is fermented in the gut by bacteria to form butyrate, which is essential for health of your gut lining. Early nutritionists identified fiber as indigestible, hence useless or counterproductive. Modern science finds that because fiber is indigestible it becomes essential for regularity and health of your gut microbiome.

Research shows that the more whole grains in the diet, the lower the risk for cancer and heart disease. Beta glucans found in oats have shown tremendous health benefits,[11] including stabilizing blood glucose, improving serum lipids, upregulating the immune system through immunoglobulin and NK production. IP6 (inositol hexaphosphate 6) was once considered an anti-nutrient, or harmful, yet now shows promise as a powerful anti-cancer agent[12].

Phytates from grains and legumes should be considered an essential nutrient

International Journal of Food Science and Technology 2002, 37, 769–782

Anti-cancer function of phytic acid

Abulkalam M. Sham...

Department of Pathology,

Summary Inosito...
kingdo...
and its
they a...
experim...
effects

Given the numerous health benefits, its participation in important intracellular biochemical pathways, normal physiological presence in our cells, tissues, plasma, urine, etc., the levels of which fluctuate with intake, epidemiological correlates of deficiency with disease and reversal of those conditions by adequate intake, and safety – all strongly suggest for its inclusion as an essential nutrient

Whole grains are best when steamed or pressure cooked. 3 cups of any whole grain with 6 cups of water in a pressure cooker for 15 minutes will yield a delightful part of your anti-cancer diet. Mix these whole grains with legumes and vegetables, or seafood, poultry and sea vegetables. Then have a party with the healing spices mentioned later.

Lectins merit special note here. There has been considerable interest in the PLANT PARADOX, which states that these commonly present lectins in plant food pose health hazards for humans. Lectins are carbohydrate binding proteins found in most plant food, particularly whole grains and legumes. The proponents of these theories recommend avoiding these foods, and/or selecting white rice over whole grain rice, and/or buying their pills to bind up the lectin in the gut.

Meanwhile, all of the data on lectins shows that they have no adverse effects in humans. In fact, all of the data on the consumption of high lectin foods (whole grains and legumes) actually shows that these foods lower the risk for heart disease, diabetes, cancer, and more.[13] Which is what you would expect with the brilliant designs in Nature. Lectins in plant food probably affects people who have a compromised gut, often from poor diet and antibiotics. Fix the gut with probiotics and prebiotics and the lectins become a non-issue. Quercetin, marshmallow root, and glutamine can work wonders to heal a leaky gut.

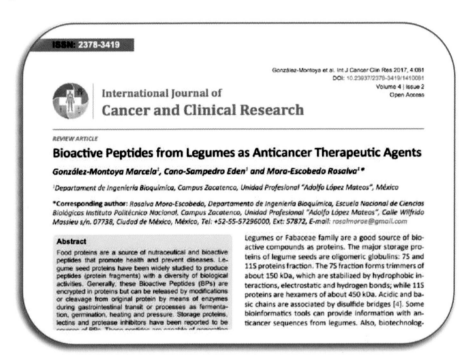

ISSN: 2378-3419

González-Montoya et al. Int J Cancer Clin Res 2017, 4:081
DOI: 10.23937/2378-3419/1410081
Volume 4 | Issue 2
Open Access

International Journal of
Cancer and Clinical Research

REVIEW ARTICLE

Bioactive Peptides from Legumes as Anticancer Therapeutic Agents

González-Montoya Marcela[1], Cano-Sampedro Eden[1] and Mora-Escobedo Rosalva[1]*

[1]*Departamento de Ingeniería Bioquímica, Campus Zacatenco, Unidad Profesional "Adolfo López Mateos", México*

*Corresponding author: Rosalva Mora-Escobedo, Departamento de Ingeniería Bioquímica, Escuela Nacional de Ciencias Biológicas Instituto Politécnico Nacional, Campus Zacatenco, Unidad Profesional "Adolfo López Mateos", Calle Wilfrido Massieu s/n. 07738, Ciudad de México, México, Tel: +52-55-57296000, Ext: 57872, E-mail: rosalmorae@gmail.com

Abstract

Food proteins are a source of nutraceutical and bioactive peptides that promote health and prevent diseases. Legume seed proteins have been widely studied to produce peptides (protein fragments) with a diversity of biological activities. Generally, these Bioactive Peptides (BPs) are encrypted in proteins but can be released by modifications or cleavage from original protein by means of enzymes during gastrointestinal transit or processes as fermentation, germination, heating and pressure. Storage proteins, lectins and protease inhibitors have been reported to be sources of BPs. These peptides are capable of preventing

Legumes or Fabaceae family are a good source of bioactive compounds as proteins. The major storage proteins of legume seeds are oligomeric globulins: 7S and 11S proteins fraction. The 7S fraction forms trimmers of about 150 kDa, which are stabilized by hydrophobic interactions, electrostatic and hydrogen bonds; while 11S proteins are hexamers of about 450 kDa. Acidic and basic chains are associated by disulfide bridges [4]. Some bioinformatics tools can provide information with anticancer sequences from legumes. Also, biotechnolog-

Legumes

Having a sack of beans in the house is like having a roof over your stomach. Beans are an incredible addition to your anti-cancer diet. Dried beans will store for a year on the shelf, or many years in a vacuum sealed can. Great way to have food saved for a rainy day. Soybeans are a staple in Asia. Soy is an interesting food. Many studies have shown soy to be a valuable part of your anti-cancer diet. However, GMO soy (most of soy in America) is of less value. Genetically modified, then soaked in glyphosate, GMO soy and other GMO products should be avoided by most people and all cancer patients. The Paleo and ketogenic advocates often eliminate beans from the diet, under the assumption that beans may cause an adverse reaction, such as an auto-immune disease. Indeed, some people have adverse reactions to various foods. But in most cases, it is the person's gut that needs healing, not elimination of wholesome foods. More on the gut in the chapter on "change the underlying causes".

The most scientifically examined and endorsed diet on earth, the Mediterranean diet, includes garbanzo beans often. Hummus is cooked garbanzo beans. In longevity studies, scientists find that the more beans people eat, the lower their risk for heart disease, cancer, diabetes, and nearly any other condition you can imagine. Beans are good for you.

Beans contain unique carbohydrates, stachyose and raffinose, that are of great interest to your gut bacteria, but must have a digestive enzyme in you to avoid gas and discomfort. To minimize flatulence from beans, soak them overnight, then discard the water, then pressure cook. Better yet, sprout the beans for 3-4 days, then pressure cook.

Beans contain <u>anti-cancer substances</u> [14] that have been researched and proven useful in your anti-cancer diet.

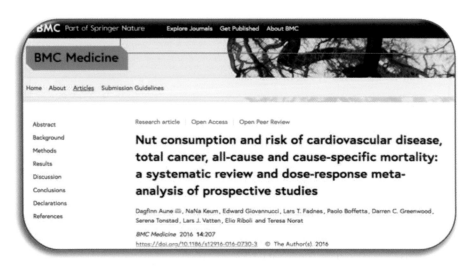

Nuts: Walnut, pecan, cashew, pine nut, Brazil nut, coconut

Consumption of nuts has consistently been shown to lower the risk for various diseases. For each 28 grams of nuts consumed (about a small handful) heart disease risk was lowered by 29%, <u>cancer by 15%</u>, death from lung problems 52%, infectious disease 75%, etc. The more nuts consumed, the better. Dose dependent response.[15] Raw nuts are high in lectins, which can be harsh on the gut if consumed to excess. Best if nuts are roasted or soaked overnight in water, then rinsed to reduce lectin content.

Seeds: Chia, hemp, papaya, poppy, sesame, pumpkin, watermelon, squash. Seeds have the source of life within. Eat these foods often.

Mar. Drugs **2014**, *12*(2), 851-870; https://doi.org/10.3390/md12020851

Open Access

Review

Fucoidan as a Marine Anticancer Agent in Preclinical Development

Jong-Young Kwak ✉

Department of Biochemistry, School of Medicine and Immune-Network Pioneer Research Center, Dong-A University, 32, Daesingongwon-ro, Seo-gu, Busan 602-714, Korea

Received: 15 November 2013; in revised form: 31 December 2013 / Accepted: 10 January 2014 / Published: 28 January 2014

Abstract: Fucoidan is a fucose-containing sulfated polysaccharide derived from brown seaweeds, crude extracts of which are commercially available as nutritional supplements. Recent studies have demonstrated antiproliferative, antiangiogenic, and anticancer properties of fucoidan *in vitro*. Accordingly, the anticancer effects of fucoidan have been shown to vary depending on its structure, while it can target multiple receptors or signaling molecules in various cell types, including tumor cells and immune cells. Low toxicity and the *in vitro* effects of fucoidan mentioned above make it a suitable agent for cancer prevention or treatment. However, preclinical development of natural marine products requires *in vivo* examination of purified compounds in animal tumor models. This review discusses the effects of systemic and local administration of fucoidan on tumor growth, angiogenesis, and immune reaction and whether *in vivo* and *in vitro* results are likely applicable to the development of fucoidan as a marine anticancer drug.

Seaweed: Kelp, kombu, wakame, nori, dulse, Irish moss

For much of human history, people living near the sea were a heartier group. There are many reasons for this advantage, including fish and kelp in the diet. There are hundreds of different land vegetables and hundreds of different sea vegetables (aka seaweed) categorized as either red, brown, or green. Green seaweed grows closer to the surface of the water, hence, the chlorophyll being used for photosynthesis. Red and brown seaweeds are found further below the water surface in deeper water.

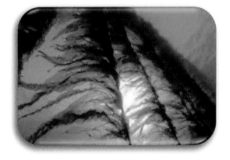

Over <u>2 billion people are deficient in iodine</u>, with half suffering blatant iodine deficiency.[16] Seaweed solves this problem with therapeutic doses of iodine. From 33-68% of people in England and Germany have measurable problems with thyroid function due to iodine deficiency.

Seaweed is a rich source of most of the trace minerals required by the human body but not added to the soil in agribusiness. Fucoidan in seaweed is a <u>powerful anti-cancer substance</u>. [17] Several studies have shown a reduced risk for breast cancer with seaweed consumption.[18] 99% of the seaweed on earth is consumed in southeast Asia. Western palates are adapting to the rich flavor of seaweed. Some people say that dried kelp tastes like green potato chips.

Mushrooms: Shiitake, oyster, white button, maitake, portobello, reishi, lion's mane

There are many therapeutic benefits of edible mushrooms. <u>Maitake</u>,[19] shiitake, reishi, lentinan, and other mushrooms have been used for <u>centuries in Chinese medicine</u>.[20] Some mushrooms are capable of enhancing immune function to thwart infections and cancer. Culinary mushrooms are tasty and healthy. Medicinal mushrooms will be front line medicine of the 21st century.

Medicinal Spices

Grandmother was practicing herbal medicine all day every day in the kitchen with her quiver of medicinal spices. Modern humans have substituted these powerful kitchen healers with salt, sugar, MSG, deep fried everything, and 2800 FDA approved food additives with questionable safety and no medicinal value. Columbus set sail over the edge of the earth in 1492 hoping to find a way to the "spice islands". In those days, food rotted quickly without the modern benefits of refrigeration or canning. Spices were used to 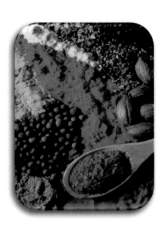 cover the flavors of food that wasn't yet dangerous, but was not very fresh either. Spices were treasured by royalty and hoarded by peasants. We now know why. Spices not only improve the flavor of food but have extraordinary healing capacity.

Scientists have proven beyond argument that medicinal spices could become front line therapies in the near future. Use these spices often liberally. For more details on the efficacy of these spices, see <u>HEALING SPICES</u> by Bharat B. Aggarwal, PhD.[21]

MEDICINAL SPICES

Ajowan	Coconut	Onion
Allspice	Coriander Cumin	Oregano
Almond	Curry leaf	Parsley
Amchur	Fennel seed	Pomegranate
Aniseed	Fenugreek seed	Pumpkin seed
Asafetida	Galangal	Rosemary
Basil	Garlic	Saffron
Bay leaf	Ginger	Safe
Black cumin seed	Horseradish	Sesame seed
Black pepper	Juniper berry	Star anise
Caraway	Kokum	Sun-dried tomato
Cardamom	Lemongrass	Tamarind
Celery seed	Marjoram	Thyme
Chile	Mint	Turmeric
Cinnamon	Mustard seed	Vanilla
Clove	Nutmeg	Wasabi
Cocoa		

Salt and Cancer

While Americans eat too much salt (sodium chloride), the public health measures to reduce sodium intake have gone overboard. About 10% of Americans are sodium retainers…they keep their salt and generate high blood pressure. However, for the remaining 90% of the population, broad sweeping recommendations to eat low sodium everything is unwise. Clear evidence shows that a low salt diet increases insulin resistance, which is bad for everyone.[22]

The 85 million Americans with high blood pressure have health issues that are far more complex than just excess sodium in the diet. The real issue is the ratio of electrolytes that fuels the battery of every cell in your body. Every cell in your body is bathed in a salt solution similar to the ocean. Blood, sweat, and tears are rich in sodium.

However… Americans eat too little magnesium, calcium, potassium, lithium, and too much sodium. It is this gross error and imbalance in the recipe for your electrolyte soup that can generate cancer, hypertension, and other problems. Fats in the diet dictate the permeability of the cell membrane, which has a major bearing on health and hypertension.

Most canned foods and many restaurants use excessive levels of salt. If you use reasonable amounts of sea salt or Himalayan salt on your healthy diet rich in plant foods (potassium) and insure that you get enough magnesium, then salt will not become a problem in your cancer recovery.

DRAGON-SLAYER SHAKE

Shakes can be a quick and easy meal substitute. Depending on your calorie requirements, use this shake in addition to or instead of the breakfast suggestions listed later. Many cancer patients have used this shake recipe to get them through the rigors of nausea from chemo.

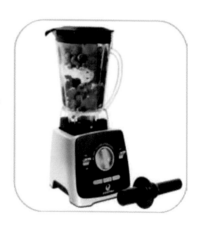

Take up to half of your pills with the "Dragon-Slayer shake" and save the remaining pills for later in the day. Taking supplements in small divided dosages helps to maintain sustained levels of nutrients in the bloodstream.

DRAGONSLAYER SHAKE: general combination of ingredients				
liquid 4-8 oz	protein1-4 T	Veg/Fruit	thicken 2T	other 1-3 T.
water	egg, soy, rice	raw or cook	froze banana	MCT
fruit juice	powder beef	carrots, beets	apple sauce	lecithin
vegetable juice	whey	broccoli	agar	powder greens
V8	bee pollen	cauliflower	carragenan	aloe
ice cubes	dry milk	cabbage	guar gum	vit/min powder
milk	wheat germ	tomato, fruit	gelatin	
soy milk	spirulina	asparagus	ice cubes	
rice milk	brewer yeast	spinach, kale	blueberries	
		collards	mango	

Ingredients:
- ♦ 4-8 ounces of liquid
- ♦ 10-15 grams (1-4 tablespoons) of powdered protein
- ♦ 1/4 to 1/2 cup veg/fruit, cooked or raw
- ♦ 1-3 tablespoons thickening agent
- ♦ 1-3 tablespoons of other ingredients, including your favorite powdered vitamin/mineral mix (i.e. ImmunoPower.com).

Directions: Using a powerful blender puree all ingredients.

Banana adds texture via pectin to make this shake have true milk shake viscosity. If the banana is frozen, it will give a thick "milkshake-like" texture to your drink.

For those who need to gain weight, add 2 tablespoons of MCT (medium chain triglyceride) oil from your health food store.

PUTTING IT TOGETHER

Picture your meal plate as a clock face. Choose quality protein foods for one third of your plate. Choose cooked wholesome plant foods for the next one third of your plate. Choose raw colorful fresh fruits and vegetables for the last one third of your plate. You can do this.

★★★★★ **AMAZON.COM**
TESTIMONIAL: Must read book. Wish I read it after first 'C' diagnosis.
The book gave us a lot of hope in fighting this cancer, whereas the doctors have applied a very negative view since we all have learnt there is a huge limitation of what chemo and RT can actually do on its own. We have taken the power back from the doctors and it feels good that we can now take charge by making sure the patient is being fed the food that the body needs. So far so good, even though we have been given the stage IV diagnosis, the doctors have not been able to explain why the tumors have shrunk (this was before treatment and just by changing the diet completely for three weeks before treatment could start)!!!
Everybody is different, but we know diet is making a huge difference.
It is must read book to allow you to have the power back and take away the feeling that the floor has been taken away from your feet.
Choose a doctor that supports your nutrition - it is critical. *John B.*

EAT OFTEN

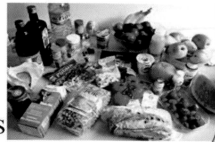

FRUITS
VEGETABLES
WHOLE GRAINS *avoid wheat, zonulin
LEGUMES
NUTS
SEEDS
SEA VEGETABLES
MUSHROOMS
MEDICINAL SPICES

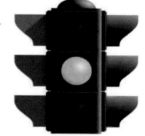

EAT OCCASIONALLY

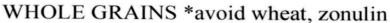

FISH
GRASS FED MEAT
EGGS
YOGURT
BUTTER

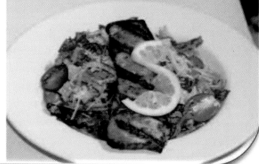

AVOID

FAKE FOODS
WHITES: SUGAR, FLOUR, RICE, POTATO
DEEP FRIED ANYTHING
HYDROGENATED OILS
HARD LIQUOR

LOOKING AT A HEALTHY MEAL PLATE

tomato,spinach,carrot,peppers,
fruit,broccoli,cabbage,onion,etc

fish, wild game, poultry,
Grass fed beef, eggs,
beans, dairy,spirulina,kelp

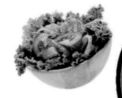

1/3
raw fr/veg

1/3
hi pro

1/3
cooked whole plant food

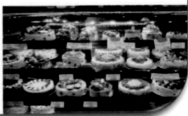

90% good
10% whatever

oatmeal,beans,rice,quinoa,tortilla,
yams,nuts,grains,legumes,cooked
vegetables, mushrooms, kelp

For more information about foods and their anti-cancer activity go to FoodisMedicine.com.

PATIENT PROFILE: SHRINKING LUNG CANCER

C.G. was diagnosed with non-small cell lung cancer stage 3. The tumor was about the size of a tennis ball. C.G. began using the principles in this book along with chemo and radiation. Originally, his doctor gave him 6 months to live. That was 2 years ago. The tumor is now the size of a small marble and shrinking with each chest X ray and CT scan. Doctor said "I don't know what you are doing, but keep doing it." C.G. says "Thank you for writing your book. So far, you have saved my life."

ENDNOTES

[1] http://www.euro.who.int/en/health-topics/disease-prevention/nutrition/news/news/2011/02/cancer-linked-with-poor-nutrition

[2] https://www.nap.edu/catalog/371/diet-nutrition-and-cancer

[3] https://www.aicr.org/cancer-prevention/food-facts/

[4] https://www.sciencedirect.com/science/article/abs/pii/S0309174005000422

[5] https://www.bmj.com/content/349/bmj.G4490.abstract

[6] https://link.springer.com/article/10.1007/s10549-013-2484-3

[7] http://cancerres.aacrjournals.org/content/58/3/442

[8] https://academic.oup.com/ije/article/35/2/307/694696

[9] https://www.bmj.com/content/347/bmj.f5001

[10] https://journals.physiology.org/doi/full/10.1152/physrev.00003.2008?view=long&pmid=21248165&

[11] https://onlinelibrary.wiley.com/doi/full/10.1111/j.1541-4337.2012.00189.x

[12] https://academic.oup.com/jn/article/133/11/3778S/4817990

[13] https://www.sciencedirect.com/science/article/pii/S0733521014000228

[14] https://www.tandfonline.com/doi/abs/10.1080/01635581.2015.1004729

[15] https://bmcmedicine.biomedcentral.com/articles/10.1186/s12916-016-0730-3

[16] https://www.ncbi.nlm.nih.gov/pmc/articles/PMC6284174/

[17] https://www.mdpi.com/1660-3397/12/2/851/htm

[18] https://www.ncbi.nlm.nih.gov/pmc/articles/PMC3651528/

[19] http://www.partnec.com/rd/rdgf/3/maitake_mxtract.pdf

[20] https://muse.jhu.edu/article/196008/summary

[21] https://www.amazon.com/Healing-Spices-Everyday-Exotic-Disease-ebook/dp/B0751NRF46

[22] https://www.sciencedirect.com/science/article/abs/pii/S002604951000329X

Chapter 13

RECIPES

Quick & Easy

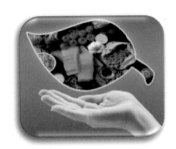

PLANNING YOUR MEALS

Eating should be both nourishing and fun. Of the hundreds of dietary programs that have been studied, none has been more thoroughly endorsed by the scientific community than the Mediterranean diet. This sample meal plan outlines the typical foods you eat under the Mediterranean diet. It covers the three main meals per day for a whole week. Keep in mind that this is just a rough guide to help you get started.

Some people have adverse food reactions. If you can't eat that food, then delete it. Feel free to add and remove items to fit your individual needs. While the scientific evidence overwhelmingly supports a

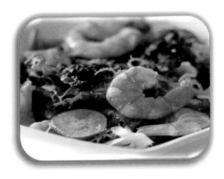

plant-based diet, there is mixed reviews on strict vegan diet. Two days here are vegan. Other days offer small servings of chicken, grass fed beef, fish, eggs, yogurt, and cheese.

This diet will be a dramatic improvement over the Standard American Diet (SAD). This diet offers you the taste, cost, convenience, nutrition, and health that you both like and deserve.

The serving portions are variable. This is to encourage you to adjust your servings and eating habits according to your own needs. It is up to you to make sure that you are not eating too much at any time.

This chapter contains a few useful recipes for anyone who wants to enjoy the benefits of the Mediterranean diet. There is no need to go to a fancy grocery store or restaurant to get a taste of these foods. The following recipes can easily be prepared in the comfort of your own home.

We have added some foods you may not be familiar with, however they are included to add some healthy alternatives. *Couscous* has fewer calories and carbohydrates than both brown and white rice, plus it higher in fiber than white rice. *Quinoa* is rich in protein, fiber, B vitamins and more dietary minerals per serving than many other grains.

Potatoes	Pigmented, purple, red, yams, sweet
Rice	Brown, Basmati, Jasmin, Wild, Black (avoid white)
Beverages	Teas, coffee, juices with pulp, homemade nut milk, coconut milk, filtered water, red wine at dinner
Grain Options	Brown rice, oatmeal, amaranth, buckwheat, berries, quinoa, millet, spelt, barley
Sweeteners	Honey, stevia, dates, other dried fruit
Meat & Butters	Grass fed, free range, wild caught
Medicinal Spices	Abundant use turmeric, cinnamon, pepper, ginger, rosemary, cumin, cardamom and others
Pressure cooker	As needed. Ideal for beetroot, grains, beans, potatoes

Day 1

- Breakfast: Spinach & Tomato on Toast. Orange and Kale Smoothie
- Lunch: Cauliflower with Lemon + Pumpkin Curry Soup
- Dinner: Fish with Lime & Cilantro
- Desert: Apple Crisp in Instant Pot

Day 2 - Lacto-Ovo-Vegetarian

- Breakfast: Avocado and Eggs on Toast.
  Banana Berry Blast Smoothie
- Lunch: Seasonal Vegetable Medley
- Dinner: Vegetable Burger
- Dessert: Chocolatey Chocolate Chip Muffins

Day 3

- Breakfast: Easy Vegetable Frittata. Creamy Matcha Smoothie
- Lunch: Garbanzo Bean Patty with Salad
- Snack: Lettuce Chicken Wraps
- Dinner: Cardamom Fudge with Lentils

Day 4

- Breakfast: Versatile Spicy Rice with Beans. Pear & Apple Juice
- Lunch: Rice Noodles with Vegetables
- Dinner: Instant Pot Tender Beef Stew
- Dessert: Peanut Butter Pudding

Day 5

- Breakfast: Tomato Toast w/ Ricotta. Orange & Ginger Smoothie
- Lunch: Asparagus & Rice Salad
- Dinner: Marinated Chicken with Honey
- Dessert: Multi Seed Superfood Balls

Day 6 – Lacto-Vegetarian

- Breakfast: Warm Breakfast Couscous. Tomato and Cucumber Juice
- Lunch: 4 Grain Salad with Cranberries
- Dinner: Garlic Mediterranean Vegetables
- Dessert: Ricotta with Honey and Almonds
-

Day 7

- Breakfast: Blueberry Delight. Ginger Turmeric Smoothie
- Lunch: Grilled Chicken or Seafood with Caprese Salad
- Dinner: Flatbread Pizza
- Dessert: Chocolate Avocado Pudding with Vanilla

Daily Snack Suggestions:

Organic popcorn
Avocado on gluten-free toast
Fresh pineapple chunks
Carrots with hummus tahini
Small seasonal fruit
Greek yogurt or cottage cheese
Slices of apple dipped in almond butter

Day 1

Breakfast

Spinach & Tomato on Toast
Servings – 4   Prep – 10 mins   Cook – 10 mins

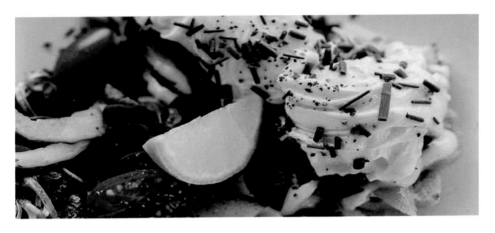

2 cups cherry tomatoes
2 cups spinach
2 tbsp fresh basil, chopped
 or 2 tsp of dried basil
2 tbsp of extra virgin olive oil

2 cups mashed potato
1 cucumber, sliced
½ tsp salt to taste
Toasted bread, roll, baguette
Lemon, quartered

Directions
1. Heat oil in a skillet, medium heat until the aroma is released (5 mins).
2. Add spinach, sliced tomatoes and herbs. Cook 5 mins. Stir often.
3. Serve on bread with spinach, cucumber, mashed potato, and lemon.

Orange and Kale Smoothie
Servings – 4   Prep – 10 mins   Cook – 0 mins

2-3 leaves of kale
1 ¼ cups fresh orange
2 celery stalks, juiced

2 apples, juiced
¼ cup flat-leaf parsley
¼ cup fresh mint

Directions
Place all ingredients in high speed blender until liquid. Serve over ice.

Lunch

Cauliflower with Lemon
Servings: 2   Prep: 10 mins   Cooking: 5 mins

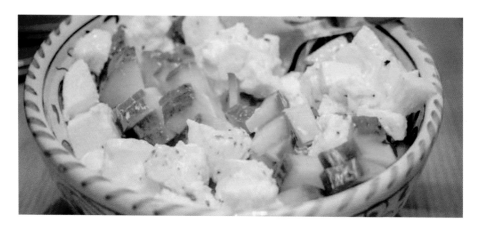

2 cups cauliflower
½ cup parsley, fresh
1/8 tsp sea salt

½ cucumber, chopped
½ lemon, juiced
¼ cup olive oil

Directions:
1. Finely chop and combine parsley and sea salt.
2. Transfer to a large mixing bowl, Add oil and lemon juice and mix.
3. Serve with fresh or blanched cauliflower.
4. Store remainder in refrigerator for up to 2 days

Pumpkin Curry Soup
Servings – 2   Prep – 15 mins   Cook – 10 mins

1 small pumpkin
¾ cup onion, chopped
2 cups vegetable broth
1 tbsp butter
2 tsp curry powder (turmeric,
  chili, coriander, cumin, ginger)
½ cup Greek yogurt
1 tsp lemon juice
Pinch pepper & salt

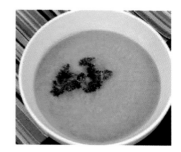

Directions
1. Place pumpkin in a saucepan with ½ vegetable broth.
2. Bring the broth to a boil, reduce heat, simmer until pumpkin is tender.
3. Blend mixture and puree until smooth.
4. Melt butter in pan and sauté onions. Add pepper, salt, curry and stir.
5. Cook mixture till lightly cooked, add remaining vegetable broth.
6. Increase heat. Continue to stir until mixture simmers.
7. Reduce heat and whisk yogurt to mixture. Add lemon juice.
8. Ladle into individual bowls. Garnish with parsley. Salt as needed.

Dinner

Fish with Lime & Cilantro
Servings – 4   Prep – 20 mins   Cook – 30 mins

4 pieces grilled or broiled salmon, salmon, cod, mahi, shrimp, or sardines	1 small bunch fresh cilantro (finely chopped)
2 limes, juiced	1 tbsp extra virgin olive oil
	Black pepper and sea salt to taste

Directions
1. Combine the cilantro, lime juice, pepper, salt, oil and spoon over fish.

Potatoes with Herbs
Servings – 2 to 4   Prep – 15 mins   Cook – 40 mins
Baby orange and purple potatoes hold their shape well.

Baby orange/ purple potatoes	1 tsp mustard seed
1 onion, diced	2 tbsp chives, chopped
1 cup spinach	2 tbsp parsley, chopped
1 tbsp sage, roughly chopped	1 ½ tbsp olive oil

Directions
1. Halve potatoes, then cook, preferably steamed. 30 mins. Drain.
2. In large skillet add olive oil, onion, spinach. Cook till tender.
3. Add potatoes and all herbs. Mix thoroughly.
4. Serve and sprinkle with bacon. Salt and pepper as needed.

Dessert

Apple Crisp in Instant Pot

Servings – 8   Prep – 30 mins   Cook – 5 mins

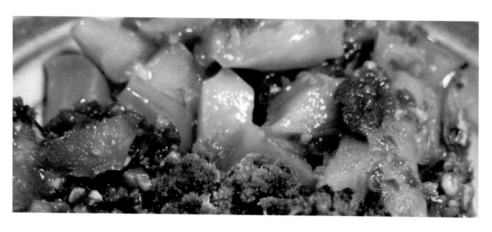

4 lbs apples (peeled, chopped)
1 ½ cups dates (pitted)
1 tsp cinnamon
1 tsp nutmeg
3 cloves
½ cup apple juice
2 tsp vanilla

1 cup oats
4 tbsp butter, softened

Topping:
1 cup heavy whipped cream
Nuts if desired

Directions

1. Place chopped apples and chopped dates in Instant Pot.
   Add ½ apple juice. Sprinkle with cinnamon, nutmeg, cloves.
2. In separate bowl mix oats, vanilla, butter, remaining apple juice.
3. Use spoon and drop/drizzle mixture over apples.
4. Secure and cook on high pressure 5 minutes.
5. Use natural release.
6. Allow mixture to cool. It will thicken.
7. Serve warm or cold with fresh cream and nuts if desired.

Day 2 – Lacto-Ovo-Vegetarian

Breakfast

Avocado & Spinach on Toast
Servings – 2   Prep – 5 mins   Cook – 0 mins

2 slices gluten free bread, toasted
2 avocados

1 tbsp chia seeds
1 cup spinach, chopped

Directions

1. Mash and spread avocado on toast
2. Sprinkle with chia seeds, then add spinach. Add salt or pepper.

Banana Berry Blast

Servings – 4   Prep – 10 mins   Cook – 0 mins

1 banana
¾ cup frozen blueberries
½ cup yogurt
½ - ¾ cup water, as needed
1 tsp Immunopower Gold

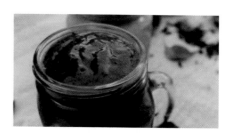

Directions

Place all ingredients in high speed blender until liquid. Serve.

Lunch

Seasonal Vegetable Medley

Servings – 4   Prep – 15 mins   Cook – 25 mins

1 tbsp olive oil
1 zucchini, sliced
2 carrots, sliced
2 cups green beans, chopped
1 cup peas

1 large onion, chopped
3 cloves garlic, minced
¼ cup fresh parsley
¼ cup fresh dill
1 cup toasted nuts (your choice)

Directions

1. Heat olive oil in a large saucepan over medium-high heat.
2. Add onion and garlic. Sauté 5 minutes. Add remaining vegetables.
3. Sir frequently until cooked.
4. Add toasted nuts.
5. Serve garnished with chopped parsley and dill.

Dinner

Vegetable Burger

Servings – 4 to 6   Prep – 20 mins   Cook – 25 mins

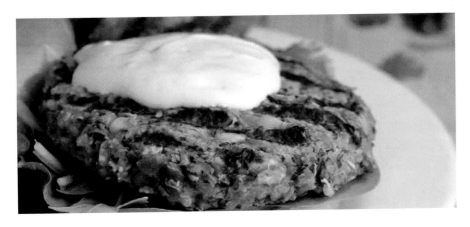

Patties:
2 tbsp olive oil
3 onions, finely chopped
2 cups seasonal vegetables (peas, cauliflower, beans, carrots)
2 small beetroot boiled, chopped
2 eggs

2 tbsp tomato paste
1 tbsp lemon juice
2 tbsp parsley, chopped
2 tbsp butter
Salt to taste
Serving Suggestions:
Top with sour cream or yogurt

Directions

1. In frypan add chopped mixed vegetables, tomato paste. Sauté.
2. Cover and cook on low heat. Stir every few minutes until half cooked.
3. Whisk eggs and add lemon juice, chopped parsley. Add to vegetables.
4. Shape the mixture into patties.
5. Heat griddle and add 1 tbsp butter. Place 4-5 patties on the griddle, and drizzle oil as needed while turning until golden brown.
6. Cook remaining patties.
7. Serve with quinoa or lentils, and broccoli and/or asparagus.
8. Top with sour cream or yogurt.

Dessert

Chocolatey Chocolate Chip Muffins
Servings – 12   Prep – 20 mins   Cook – 20 mins

3 cups rolled oats
1 cup cacao powder
2 cups dark chocolate chips
½ cup almonds, finely chopped
1 tbsp of baking powder

1 egg
1 ripe banana, mashed
1 cup applesauce, unsweetened
¼ cup honey (adjust to taste)
1 tbsp of vanilla

Directions

1. Preheat oven to 375 degrees.
2. Using a blender grind oats to flour. Pour into a large mixing bowl. Stir in baking powder.
3. Beat the egg in another bowl and add the cacao, chocolate chips, banana, apple sauce. Stir in vanilla and honey.
4. Spray 12 muffin cups with oil, fill with batter. Sprinkle with almonds.
5. Bake for 20 minutes or until the middle sets. Remove from oven and cool for 15 minutes before removing from tin. Cool before serving.

Day 3

Breakfast

Easy Vegetable Frittata
Servings – 4-6   Prep – 15 mins   Cook – 15 mins

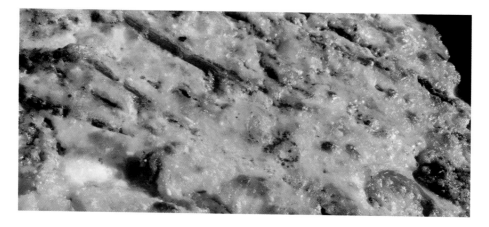

12 med-large organic eggs
1 medium red onion, chopped
10 oz spinach, finely chopped
6 asparagus, chopped
2 cloves garlic, crushed
1 bell pepper, chopped

1 tomato, sliced
2 tbsp Italian herbs
2 tbsp parsley
1 tsp salt and pepper to taste
1 tbsp olive oil
4 oz Parmesan cheese, grated

Directions

1. In a 10 inch oven safe frying pan (you will be baking later), sauté onion in olive oil to almost done. Remove onion and set aside.
2. On medium high heat toss in chopped peppers, spinach, asparagus and garlic. Add additional olive oil if needed.
3. In a separate bowl, use a fork to whisk the eggs.
4. Add remaining ingredients; tomato, herbs, salt and pepper.
5. Heat oven to 350 degrees.
6. Pour egg mixture into pan and stir. Sprinkle with parsley, parmesan.
7. Bake in oven 15 minutes.
8. Let cool for 10 minutes prior to serving.

Variation Suggestions – Step 4:
Artichoke and Goat Cheese: Add 1 cup artichoke and ½ cup goat cheese finely crumbled, mix with lemon zest and juice.
Mushroom and Romano Cheese: Add 1 pound mushrooms, stemmed and cut into ½ inch pieces. Add ¼ cup green scallions and ¼ cup Romano.

Creamy Matcha Smoothie
Servings – 2   Prep – 5 mins   Cook – 0 mins

1 cup favorite fruit, pureed
2 cups nut milk
2/3 cup spinach

½ tsp matcha powder
4 leaves mint, finely chopped

Directions
Place all ingredients in a high speed blender. Blend with ice if desired. Add honey if desired.

Lunch

Garbanzo Patty with Salad

Servings – 4 to 6   Prep – 20 mins   Cook – 30 mins

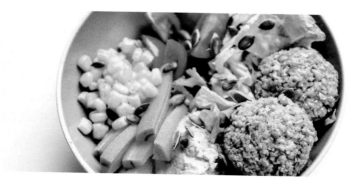

15-oz can garbanzo beans
2 cloves garlic, mined
1 medium onion, chopped
1 large egg, lightly beaten
1 tsp dried oregano

½ tsp ground cumin
1 tbsp lemon juice, fresh
Olive oil cooking spray
½ cup nuts, ground
Lettuce, carrot, corn

★★★★★ **AMAMAZON.COM**

<u>TESTIMONIAL:</u> **She also is now walking about six miles a day.**
I had gotten this book back in January of 2007, when my mother-in-law had colon cancer. I was the one taking care of her after her surgery and this book was very informative and very helpful. This book came in handy for me and I was able to change her diet completely.

The doctors wanted her to have chemo and radiation since her cancer markers were so high before the surgery and were still above the mark that they recommend for treatment, but my mother-in-law decided that since her lymph nodes and all the tissue around the tumor was negative of cancer, she opted out. With diet we were able to bring her markers under the mark that they recommend for treatment. The doctors are very impressed with her. *Ana Maria Olivas-Flores*

Directions
1. Process garbanzo beans, garlic, onion, egg, in food processor.
2. Add lemon juice, cumin, oregano, pepper and salt
3. Spread ground nuts on a plate. Make 16 round balls from bean mixture; roll in ground nuts for coating. Set balls on wax paper.
4. Spray a large skillet with your olive oil cooking spray. When the skillet is hot, add falafel balls to cook until browned, about 10 minutes.
5. Serve with salad of lettuce, carrot and corn.

Dinner

Chicken Lettuce Wraps
Servings – 4 to 6   Prep – 10 mins   Cook – 20 mins

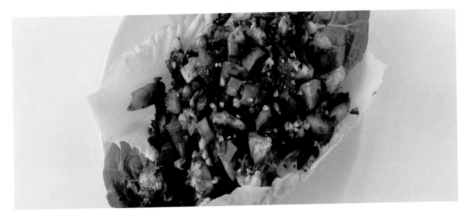

Chicken Recipe
3 lbs chicken thighs, diced
½ onion minced
1 cup red pepper diced
1 8-oz can water chestnuts, minced
1 tbsp extra virgin olive oil
2 tsp paprika
1 tbsp lemon grass, chopped
2 tbsp fresh parsley, chopped
1 tbsp cilantro, chopped

Sauce
3 tbsp soy sauce
3 tbsp hoison sauce
1 tbsp honey
¼ tsp ginger, powder

Serving Suggestion
Lettuce
Peanuts, crushed

Directions
1. Combine "Chicken Recipe" in saucepan and cook well. Stir often.
2. Mix sauce ingredients in bowl. No cooking needed.
3. Place lettuce leaves on platter and divide "Chicken Recipe".
4. Pour sauce over chicken. Repeat as necessary.
5. Chicken recipe suitable for freezing as needed.

Dessert

Cardamom Fudge with Lentils
Servings – 16-20 pieces   Prep – 45 mins   Cook – 20 mins

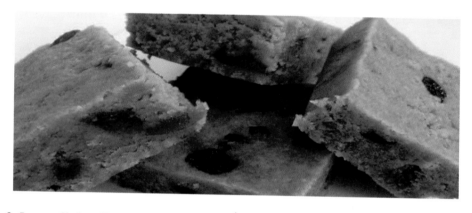

3.5 oz split lentils
16 oz water
2 cups nut milk
½ cup coconut flakes, unsweetened
10 almonds, chopped

2 tbsp cranberries
1 tsp cardamom powder
½ cup ghee
1/3 cup honey (more if needed)

Directions
1. Soak the lentils in water and set aside 2-3 hours. Strain lentils and cook in 1 cup milk till soft. Blend into a coarse paste.
2. Heat ghee in a saucepan, add the lentils and cook until light brown.
3. Blend honey into the mixture.
4. Add remaining milk. Cook till the mixture leaves the sides of the pan.
5. Add the coconut flakes, almonds, cranberries, cardamom. Mix well.
6. Remove from heat and spread onto a greased tray. Cool and slice.

Day 4

Breakfast

Versatile Spicy Rice with Beans

Servings – 2-4   Prep – 15 mins   Cook – 35 mins

1 cup rice, cooked
  (Jasmin, basmati, brown)
1½ cups black beans, cooked
3 tbsp olive oil
1 red pepper, diced
½ cup shallots

2 tsp turmeric
1 tbsp chili powder
1 tsp paprika
1 tsp cumin
Parsley or basil for garnish

Directions

1. In a large bowl, combine rice, beans, red pepper, shallots.
2. In a small bowl combine remaining ingredients. Drizzle over rice.
3. Stir fry with olive oil on high for a few minutes until rice is thoroughly heated and coated with spices.
4. Garnish with chopped fresh basil and/or parsley

Pear & Apple Juice

Servings – 2-4   Prep – 10 mins   Cook – 0 min

5 green apples, cored
2 pears, cored
1 orange, peeled
1 lemon, peeled
1 scoop ImmunoPower Gold

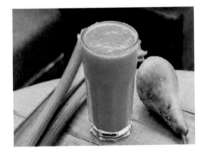

Directions

Place all ingredients in juicer or high speed blender. Serve immediately.

Lunch

Rice Noodles with Vegetables

Servings – 4   Prep – 20 mins   Cook – 15 mins

1 pack rice noodles
½ cup bell peppers, chopped
1 bunch asparagus
½ red onion, chopped
2 carrots (matchstick size)
1 cup spinach
2 cloves of garlic, minced

2 tbsp extra virgin olive oil
¼ tsp ground cumin
1 lemon, juiced
1 cup vegetable broth
1 tbsp ginger, minced
Dash of cayenne pepper

Directions

1. Cook rice noodles.
2. Sauté onion, carrots, garlic, cumin, ginger
3. In saucepan heat vegetable broth, then add noodles and vegetables.
4. Mix together with spinach.
5. Add lemon and cayenne as needed.

Dinner

Instant Pot Tender Beef Stew

Servings – 6   Prep – 10 mins   Cook – 30 mins
Made ahead of time and freeze

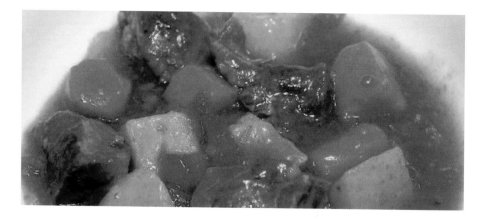

2 lbs grass fed beef, cubed
4 large garlic cloves, chopped
1 medium onion, finely chopped
2 tbsp olive oil, + extra to drizzle
6 oz tomato paste
1 carrot, chopped
1 celery stick, chopped

2 colored potatoes, chopped
4 cups beef broth
Pinch ground cloves
Fresh thyme sprigs
¼ cup parsley, chopped
2 tbsp ghee or butter
Salt and pepper to taste

Directions

1. Heat Instant Pot to Sauté. When warmed add ghee. Brown the beef for 7-8 mins. Add onions, garlic and keep stirring for 5 mins.
2. Add remaining ingredients and mix well.
3. Seal the pot. Set to stew or high pressure setting. Cook for 30 mins.
4. Carefully vent the pressure valve or allow manual release.
5. Serve with grains or seasonal vegetables.
6. Cover and refrigerate the stew for up to 5 days or freeze.
7. Reheat gently in a low oven or on the stovetop over low heat.

Dessert

Peanut Butter Pudding

Servings – 4   Prep – 15 mins   Cook – 0 mins

12 oz package tofu, soft
1/3 cup creamy peanut butter
1 tsp vanilla
2 tbsp coconut milk
½ cup toasted nuts

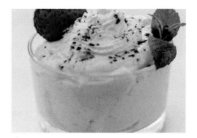

Directions

1. Puree tofu, peanut butter. Add honey, vanilla, coconut milk.
2. Blend well until smooth.
3. Divide among dishes. Cover and refrigerate 30+ mins.
4. Top with fresh whipped cream and toasted nuts.

Day 5

Breakfast

Tomato Toast with Macadamia Ricotta
Servings – 6   Prep – 15 mins   Cook – 15 mins

6 slices whole grain bread
½ pound tomatoes
½ cup ricotta
¼ tsp sea salt

Macadamia Spread
1 cup raw macadamia nuts
2 tsp fresh lemon juice
2 tsp white miso paste
2 cloves garlic

Directions
1. *Macadamia Spread.* Drain and rinse macadamia nuts and blend with lemon juice, miso, garlic and salt. Add water as needed to reach a creamy consistency. Refrigerate until ready to use.
2. *Toast.* Add Ricotta, sliced tomatoes, macadamia spread, salt.
3. Slice and serve.

Orange & Ginger Smoothie
Servings – 2-3   Prep – 10 mins   Cook – 0 min

2-3 leaves of chard
1 beet, finely chopped
1 orange
1 cup strawberries or other berry

1 lime, juiced
½ inch ginger root, grated
1 scoop ImmunoPower Gold
½ cup water, as needed

Directions
Place all ingredients in a high speed blender.

★★★★★ **AMAZON.COM**
TESTIMONIAL: I'm beating cancer now!
I am a biochemist newly diagnosed with breast cancer (DCIS stage 0) Sept. 2013. I have been looking for the most tissue-sparing treatment and for the best approach to boost my immune system to beat cancer. Having worked in a medical setting for about 30 years I do not expect our medical standard of care to be infallible.
PQ's scientifically well documented and common sense approach has led me to change my eating habits for the better, also adding supplements and greatly reducing common toxins and sugar from my diet. *Diane Mann, M.S.*

Lunch

Asparagus & Rice Salad

Servings – 4   Prep – 20 mins   Cook – 10 mins

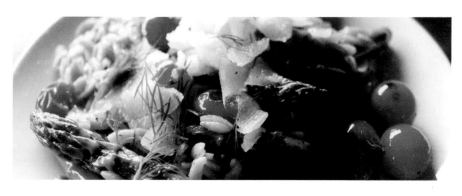

2 cups rice, cooked	½ cup dill
8 asparagus	1 cup parmesan cheese, sliced
2 cups cherry tomatoes	2 tbsp water as needed
2 scallions	1 lemon juiced
2 tbsp olive oil	1 tbsp garlic, minced
½ cup parsley	Salt and pepper

Directions

1. Sauté asparagus, tomatoes, garlic, parsley in olive oil.
2. In bowl add cooked rice, lemon juice, scallions. Warm on stove top.
3. Serve rice with sautéd medley. Garnish with dill, cheese, lemon juice.

Dinner

Marinated Chicken with Honey

Servings – 4   Prep – 30 mins   Cook – 50 mins

4 chicken breast halves, sliced	½ tbsp ginger, grated
Marinade:	1 tsp red pepper flakes
1/3 cup lemon juice	1 tbsp olive oil
1/3 cup balsamic vinegar	2 tbsp honey – add after cooked
3 tbsp soy sauce	*Garnish:* Lemon slices
1 tsp cumin and nutmeg	*Serve:* Fresh green vegetables

Directions

1. Combine chicken and ½ marinade mixture in bowl. Mix well.
2. Seal the bag and lay it on a baking pan. Turn it over several times making sure that the chicken is covered well.
3. Place in refrigerator and marinade for at least 2 hours or overnight.
4. When ready, remove chicken and marinade and cook in skillet on medium high heat until pink disappears.
5. Add other ½ marinade. Warm 5 mins.
6. Place chicken on platter along with fresh greens or vegetables.
7. Drizzle with marinade and garnish with lemon slices.

Dessert

Multi Seed Superfood Balls

Servings – 12   Prep – 15 mins   Cook – 0 mins

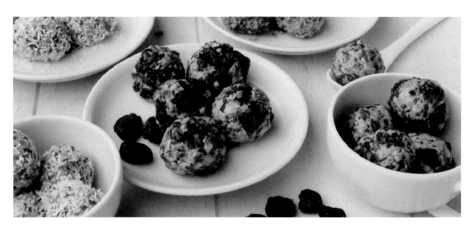

Balls:

1 cup pecans, toasted
¾ cup dates, finely chopped
¼ cup cacao
2 tbsp goji berries
2 tbsp cranberries

2 tbsp cacao nibs
2 tbsp flaxseeds
2 tbsp chia seeds
½ cup coconut flake

Toppings: Hemp seeds, coconut flakes (toasted optional), cacao nib

Directions
1. Place pecans in a food processor and gently process.
2. Add remaining ball ingredients
3. Blend until mixture sticks together.
4. Roll mixture into small balls and then roll around in desired toppings.
5. Store balls in an air-tight container in the refrigerator for up to 1 week.

Day 6 – Lacto-Vegetarian

Breakfast

Warm Breakfast Couscous
Servings – 4   Prep – 10 mins   Cook – 20 mins

Enjoy warm or cold

2 cups dry couscous
4 cups of water
½ cup dried cranberries
1 tsp each nutmeg, ginger, cinnamon and cumin

4 oz soft goat cheese, crumbled
Zest of small orange & lemon
3 tbsp olive oil
Honey if needed
Salt and black pepper

Directions
1. Bring 4 cups water to boil, add quinoa and cook till tender. Cool.
2. Cover cranberries with hot water and set aside until plump.
3. In small bowl add spices, zest, ½ cup water.
4. Heat 1 tbsp oil in skillet and add couscous and spice mixture. Stir until toasted and golden (about 3-4 mins).
5. Add cranberries, sprinkle with goat cheese, honey. Serve

Tomato & Cucumber Juice
Servings – 2   Prep – 10 mins   Cook Time – 0 mins

4 tomatoes
2 carrots
1 cucumber

2 limes, juiced
1 scoop ImmunoPower Gold
Salt and pepper

Directions
Place all ingredients in high speed blender. Serve over ice. Salt as needed.

Lunch

4 Grain Salad with Cranberries
Servings – 6   Prep – 10 mins   Cook – 10 mins

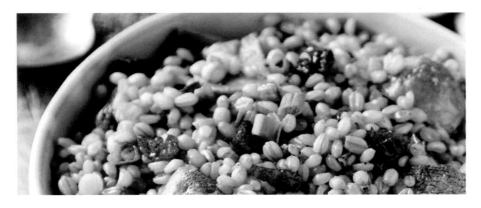

½ cup wheat berries, cooked
½ cup barley, cooked
½ cup bulger, cooked
½ cup quinoa, cooked
½ cup cranberries

2 green onion, chopped
½ cup onion, sliced
2 tbsp extra virgin olive oil
1 tsp cumin, turmeric each

Directions
1. Stir green onions, onions, spices in 1 tbsp oil till cooked and aromatic.
2. Soak cranberries in hot water until plump.
3. In large bowl add warmed grains, cranberries, then add mixture and blend with large spatula. Add additional olive oil if necessary.
4. Serve with seasonal salad or vegetables.

Dinner

Garlic Mediterranean Vegetables
Servings – 4 to 6   Prep – 20 mins   Cook – 40 mins

8 cups root vegetables, assorted, chopped. (Suggest yams, carrots, parsnips, potatoes - variety)
1 large red onion, sliced
1 red bell pepper, sliced
2 cloves garlic, minced

2 tsp ea. parsley, rosemary, basil
Salt and black pepper to taste
¼ cup of extra virgin olive oil
¼ cup balsamic vinegar
Serving Suggestion
1 cup lentils or bean

Directions
1. Toss the vegetables together with herbs, garlic, oil, salt and pepper. Place in a shallow pan.
2. Bake at 375 degrees in the oven for 40 minutes or until vegetables become tender. Stir once or twice during cooking.

Dessert

Ricotta with Honey and Almonds
Servings – 4 to 6   Prep – 20 mins   Cook – 30 mins

1 cup whole milk ricotta
½ cup almonds, sliced
1 tsp honey

Zest from an orange, optional
Fruit, optional

Directions
1. Combine ricotta, almonds, zest in a bowl. Stir well.
2. Spoon into large or individual serving bowls.
3. Sprinkle with sliced almonds. Drizzle with honey.
4. Serve with seasonal fruit.

Day 7

Breakfast

Blueberry Delight
Servings – 2 to 4   Prep – 10 mins   Cook – 10 mins

Fruit:
2 cups fresh or frozen blueberries
1/3 cup water
2 tsp lemon zest

Filling:
3 cups Greek yogurt
1 cup granola, toasted
3 tbsp honey

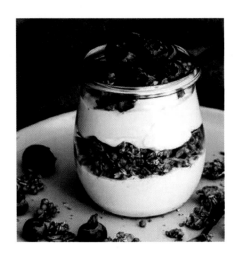

Directions
1. Combine blueberries, lemon, and water. Bring to boil 8-10 mins. Cool.
2. *Parfait*: Layer yogurt, blueberries, granola; alternating as desired.
3. Serve chilled.

Ginger Turmeric Smoothie
Servings – 2   Prep – 10 mins   Cook – 0 mins

1 large banana
1 cup nut milk
1 cup seasonal fruit

1 tbsp ginger root, grated
1 inch aloe vera, fresh
1 scoop ImmunoPower Gold

Directions
Place all ingredients in a high speed blender. Serve.

Lunch

Grilled Chicken with Caprese Salad
Servings – 4   Prep – 15 mins   Cook – 10 mins

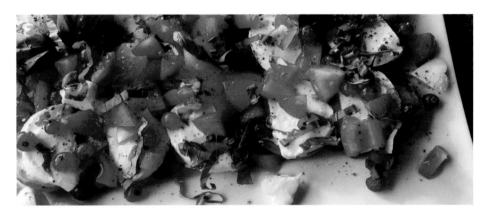

4 4-6 oz grilled chicken or seafood, cooked

Caprese Salad

1 lb fresh mozzarella
4-6 large ripe tomatoes, sliced
½ cup basil, chopped
1 tbsp parsley, minced
½ cup onions, sliced thinly

Dressing:
1 small clove garlic, minced
1 tbsp fresh lemon juice
½ tsp fresh oregano, minced
¼ cup of extra virgin olive oil

Directions:
1. On a large platter, layer alternatively with mozzarella and tomato slice.
2. Sprinkle with chopped tomato and fresh basil, parsley, onion.
3. *Dressing*: In small bowl add remaining ingredients and mix.
4. Drizzle dressing over salad, season as needed. Serve.

Dinner

Flatbread Pizza

Servings – 4   Prep – 15 mins   Cook – 15 mins

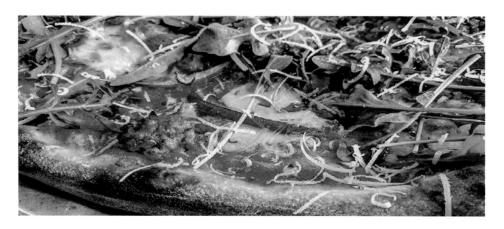

2-6 flatbreads
1 small can tomato paste
1 small red onion, finely chopped
1-2 tbsp extra virgin olive oil
2 tsp fresh oregano, chopped
2 tsp fresh thyme, chopped

3 cloves garlic, minced
¼ tsp chili powder
1 tsp turmeric
8 oz mozzarella cheese, shredded
Balsamic glaze
2 cups arugula

Directions

1. Sauté onion and garlic in 1 tbsp olive oil until slightly caramelized and well cooked.
2. Warm flatbread on skillet about 2 minutes each side with olive oil.
3. Combine onion mixture, herbs, spices, salt and pepper. Mix well.
4. Spread tomato paste over flatbread. Spread onion mixture, cheese.
5. Bake until melted, 15 mins. Drizzle with balsamic glaze and arugula.

Dessert

Chocolate Avocado Pudding

Servings – 4   Prep – 10 mins   Cook – 0 mins

Dairy-free, vegan and paleo. Delicious!

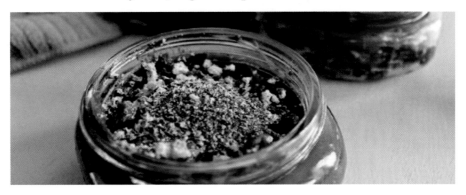

2 large avocados, chilled
½ cup full fat coconut milk
2-3 tbsp raw cacao powder

⅓ cup honey (or more)
1 tbsp vanilla extract
Sprinkle with sea salt and/or nuts

Directions

1. Scoop out the avocado flesh and put in a food processor.
2. Add the coconut milk, raw cacao powder, honey, vanilla extract, salt until blend until smooth and creamy.
3. Scoop chocolate avocado pudding into individual serving bowls.
4. Sprinkle with sea salt or other topping of your choice.

★★★★★ **AMAZON.COM**
TESTIMONIAL: If you only read one book on cancer & nutrition this is it!
This book might look like a lot of technical text when you first open it, but it is fantastic. I have stage IV cancer and this book was the turning point for me. I have read it cover to cover and then most of it again to my husband. Our family (kids included) has embraced the low sugar, and tons of veggies rule. Today I am strong and healthy and believe a huge part of that is due to the things I learned reading this book. *Julia*

Bonus Recipes

Smoothie Options

Berry Turmeric Smoothie
Servings – 4   Prep – 10 mins   Cook – 0 mins

2 cups beet greens	¼ tsp cinnamon
2 cups almond milk	1 scoop ImmunoPower Gold
2 cups berries	

Lemony Mint Smoothie
Servings – 4   Prep – 10 mins   Cook – 0 mins

4 cups spinach	6 leaves fresh mint
1 cucumber	1 lemon, juiced
2 apples	1 scoop ImmunoPower Gold

Ginger Limeade Smoothie
Servings – 4   Prep – 10 mins   Cook – 0 mins

1 lime, juice	1 apple
1 cucumber	½ tsp ginger, powder
½ red beet	1 scoop ImmunoPower Gold

Acai Berry with Hemp Smoothie
Servings – 4   Prep – 10 mins   Cook – 0 mins

1 cup acai berries	1 lemon, peeled
1 cup mixed berries	½ tsp maca powder
1 tbsp hemp heart seeds	Splash vanilla extract
1 cup liquid (nut milk or water)	

Directions for Each Recipe
Place all ingredients in high speed blender. Serve over ice.

Condiments/Dressings Options

Tomato-Cucumber Relish
Servings – 4   Prep – 20 mins   Cook – 0 mins

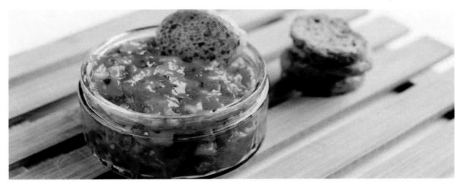

½ cup tomato, chopped
½ cup cucumber, chopped
¼ tsp dried mint, finely chopped

Fresh-ground black pepper and
salt to taste

Directions:
1. Combine all ingredients in a blender. Blend on low for 30 seconds.
2. Season with salt and pepper to taste.

Olive Oil Vinaigrette
Servings – 4-6 people   Prep – 10 mins   Cook – 0 mins

2 tbsp balsamic vinegar
2 tbsp red wine vinegar
1 tbsp fresh lemon juice
1 clove garlic, minced

1 tsp salt
½ cup of extra virgin olive oil
Dash ground black pepper

Directions
1. Combine vinegars, lemon juice, salt, garlic and pepper in a small bowl.
2. Whisk above with olive oil until well-blended. Serve with your salad of choice.

Dijon Lemon Mustard
Servings – 4   Prep – 10 mins   Cook – 0 mins

6 tbsp mustard seeds
4 tbsp lemon juice
3 tsp lemon zest
¼ cup extra virgin olive oil
¼ cup distilled white vinegar

¼ cup dry white wine (optional)
1 clove garlic, finely minced
½ tsp salt
¼ tsp black pepper
1 tbsp minced oregano

Directions
1. Blend all dry ingredients. Add remaining ingredients. Blend again.
2. Cover and refrigerate for 5+ hours. Can store for 3-4 weeks.

Dessert Option

Chocolate Truffles with Sweet Orange
Servings – 12   Prep – 50 mins   Cook – 0 mins

Truffle filling
1 cup cocoa powder, unsweetened
1 tbsp cup coconut cream
¼ cup orange juice
1 tbsp orange zest
2 tbsp honey
Chocolate coating
1 cup cacao powder

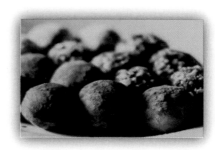

Directions
1. *Filling*: Combine all ingredients in a blender and blend well.
2. Place mixture in the freezer for about 45 mins. It needs to be firm enough to be scooped into balls. Adjust coconut cream as needed.
3. With a cookie or ice cream scoop, place balls on a lined baking sheet and place in the freezer for at least 30 minutes.
4. *Coating*: Roll balls in cocoa powder. Return to freezer for one hour.
5. Keep truffles in sealed container in freezer.

Chapter 14

SUPPLEMENTS AGAINST CANCER

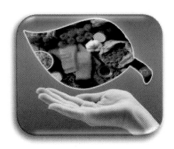

"It is not enough for a cancer patient to receive appropriate conventional therapy for his or her disease. To improve quality and quantity of life a regimen of good nutrition is essential."
Linus Pauling, PhD, twice Nobel laureate

WHAT'S AHEAD?

Cancer patients probably need more nutrients than can be obtained even from a healthy diet. No supplement is a magic bullet against cancer. While nutrition products need to be taken with professional guidance, the risk-to-benefit ratio heavily favors the use of supplements for most cancer patients. Supplements can:

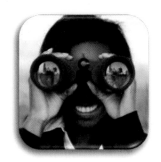

✓ stimulate immune function
✓ encourage "suicide" (apoptosis) in cancer cells
✓ improve cell-to-cell communication
✓ reduce the toxicity of chemo and radiation on the patient.

<u>77% of Americans take some nutrition supplement.</u>[1] <u>84% of those users express satisfaction</u> with the safety and efficacy of their supplements. The dietary supplement industry sells about $122 billion in products to Americans annually. The medical and pharmaceutical industries have made enormous efforts to discredit this health arena through lobbying to get supplements only available through prescription or media coverage of only negative issues with supplements.

92% of Americans DO NOT GET the Recommended Dietary Allowance (RDA, now called Reference Daily Intake, or RDI) for all listed essential nutrients. And there is compelling evidence that the RDA is a survival level for nutrient intake, not a level that allows for optimal health, nor recovery from cancer.

There are now over 50,000 scientific references that support the use of supplementing a good diet with vitamins, minerals, herbs, fatty acids, glandulars, probiotics, and food extracts in order to prevent or even reverse many common ailments.

For more information see:

Nutrition Therapy:
scientific, logical, inexpensive, non-toxic

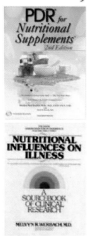 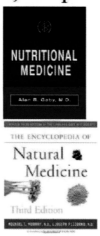 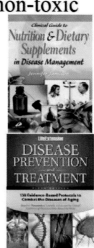

Notice the additional vitamins and minerals that are added to dog and cat food. Look at the amazing assortment of vitamins, minerals, herbs, etc; that are offered for horses. None of these products are sold due to the "placebo" effect, or simply because the animal believed in the product. Nutrients, like drugs, have a dose-dependent response curve. Meaning, the more you give, the greater the effect, until additional benefits taper off and toxicity becomes possible.

BEYOND DEFICIENCIES: META-NUTRIENT FUNCTIONS

For instance, at 20 milligrams of niacin per day, most adults have decent, normal health. At 100 mg/day of niacin, this B-vitamin becomes a powerful dilator of blood vessels and may improve circulation. At 2,000 mg/day, niacin becomes a potent agent at lowering cholesterol in the bloodstream of people with hypercholesterolemia.

Most adults can survive on 20-40 mg daily of vitamin C. The RDA is 65 mg, while studies show that women can lower their risk for cervical cancer by 50% simply by taking 90 mg of vitamin C daily. At 300 mg/day, vitamin C has been shown to add 6 years to the lifespan of male supplement users. People with virus infections or cancer have benefitted by taking 1,000 to 20,000 mg of vitamin C daily. Show me a drug that you can take 100 times the normal prescription dosage and not have some serious harmful effect. The point is: "While nutritional supplements are far from cure-alls, they do rate very favorably on the risk-to-benefit-to-cost scale when compared to prescription medications.

META NUTRIENT FUNCTIONS: BEYOND DEFICIENCY

VITAMIN D:
    400 iu prev. rickets
    2000-10,000 iu regulate 20% genome, prev.diseases
VITAMIN K:
    120 mcg/d prevent hemorrhaging
    500+ mcg/d improves bone health, cancer prev.

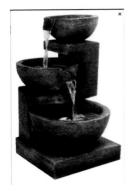

VITAMIN C: 60 mg/d prev.scurvy
90 mg/d lowers risk endom ca.
1000 mg/d enhances wound heal
FOLATE: 400 mcg/d avoid meg. anemia
10,000 mcg reverse dysplasia
30,000 mcg vasodilator, lo blood p.
NIACIN: 20 mg prev.pellagra
100 mg vasodilator
2000 mg lowers cholesterol

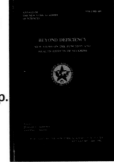

All substances consumed--from chemotherapy to allopathic drugs to vitamins, minerals, herbs, and even food--all have a "window of efficacy". Above that level is too much and may cause damage. Below that level is probably ineffective. With drugs, the window of efficacy is much narrower and, hence, great caution must be used in administering prescription medication. All nutrients have a wider window of efficacy than all drugs. Yet some nutrients are more likely to harm than others. Iron, copper, selenium, and vitamins A and D are the nutrients that must be used with discretion. Most other nutrients are unlikely to harm.

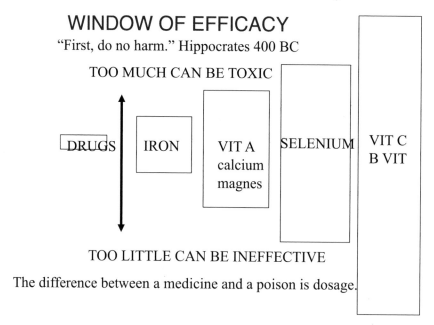

WINDOW OF EFFICACY
"First, do no harm." Hippocrates 400 BC

TOO MUCH CAN BE TOXIC

| DRUGS | IRON | VIT A calcium magnes | SELENIUM | VIT C B VIT |

TOO LITTLE CAN BE INEFFECTIVE

The difference between a medicine and a poison is dosage.

RISKS OF NUTRITION THERAPY
In an extensive review of the literature found in the New York Academy of Sciences textbook BEYOND DEFICIENCIES (vol.669, p.300, 1992), Dr. Adrienne Bendich found the following data on nutrient toxicity:

- ♦ B-6 can be used safely for years at up to 500 mg (250 times RDA)
- ♦ Niacin (as nicotinic acid) has been recommended by the National Institute of Health for lowering cholesterol at doses of 3,000-6,000 mg/day (150-300 times RDA). Time-release niacin is more suspect of causing toxicity as liver damage.

♦ Vitamin C was tested in 8 published studies using double-blind placebo-controlled design. At 10,000 mg/day for years, vitamin C produced no side effects.

♦ High doses of vitamin A (500,000 iu daily) can have acute reversible effects. Teratogenecity (birth defects) is a possible complication of high dose vitamin A intake.

♦ Vitamin E intake at up to 3,000 mg/day (300 times RDA) for prolonged periods has been shown safe.

♦ Beta-carotene has been administered for extended periods in humans at doses up to 180 mg (300,000 iu or 60 times RDA) with no side effects nor elevated serum vitamin A levels.

In MICRONUTRIENTS AND IMMUNE FUNCTION (NYAS, vol.587, p.257, 1990), John Hathcock, PhD, a Food and Drug Administration toxicologist, reported the following data on nutrient toxicity:

♦ Vitamin A toxicity may start as low as 25,000 iu/day (5 times RDA) in people with impaired liver function via drugs, hepatitis, or protein malnutrition. Otherwise, toxicity for A begins at several hundred thousand iu/day.

♦ Beta-carotene given at 180 mg/day (300,000 iu or 60 times RDA) for extended periods produced no toxicity, but mild carotenemia (orange pigmentation of skin).

♦ Vitamin E at 300 iu/day (30 times RDA) can trigger nausea, fatigue, and headaches in sensitive individuals. Otherwise, few side effects are seen at up to 3,200 iu/day (320 times RDA).

♦ B-6 may induce a reversible sensory neuropathy at doses of as low as 300 mg/day in some sensitive individuals. Toxic threshold usually begins at 2,000 mg for most individuals.

♦ Vitamin C may induce mild and transient gastro-intestinal distress in some sensitive individuals at doses of 1,000 mg (16 times RDA). Otherwise, toxicity is very rare at even high doses of vitamin C intake. More on vitamin C in the chapter on vitamins and the chapter on Rational Cancer Treatment.

♦ Zinc supplements at 300 mg (20 times RDA) have been found to impair immune functions and serum lipid profile.

♦ Iron intake at 100 mg/day (6 times RDA) will cause iron storage disease in 80% of population. The "window of efficacy" on iron is probably more narrow than with other nutrients.

♦ Selenium can be toxic at 1-5 mg/kg body weight intake. This would equate to 65 mg/day for the average adult, which is 812 times the RDA of 80 mcg. Some sensitive individuals may develop toxicity at 1,000 mcg/day.

CAUSES OF DEATH IN USA/YR

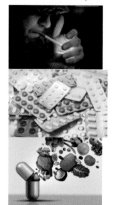

Heart disease 647,000
Tobacco 480,000
Alcohol 88,000
Prescription drugs 128,000
Illicit drug overdose 70,000
Car accidents 38,000
Skateboarding 40
Lawnmower accidents 69
Suicide 48,000
Drowning 3500
Heat stroke 1300
Foodborne illness 3000
Vitamin supplements 0
Source: https://aapcc.org/annual-reports/

CHOOSING YOUR VITAMIN SUPPLEMENTS

There are many vitamins, minerals, botanicals (herbs), fatty acids, food extracts, glandulars, and other nutrient compounds that can be of benefit to the cancer patient. You may take all of these "a la carte" at a cost of $1,500-$2,000 per month and 200+ pills per day, or you may consider using the ImmunoPower 7 supplement (ImmunoPower.com), which is a mixture of 70+ nutrition factors, in pill and powder form, that is much more convenient, complete, and cost-effective than the usual "life and death scavenger hunt" that cancer patients have embarked upon. ImmunoPower Gold may also be worth considering.

Vitamins can be expensive, especially since these are "out of pocket" expenses, meaning not reimbursable by insurance companies. Odd how insurance and Medicare will pay $3,000 per day for a cancer patient in intensive care, but neither will pay for nutrition supplements that might prevent the patient from developing malnutrition (cachexia) and ending up in the intensive care unit of a hospital. Choose the supplement regimen that best suits your ability to tolerate vitamins and your ability to pay for them.

PATIENT PROFILE

S.R. was diagnosed at age 48 with stage 4 non-Hodgkins B-cell lymphoma. Tumor was the size of a potato and choking off blood to the intestines. Underwent chemo regimen. S.R. used nutrition supplements in spite of oncologist's hostility to the subject. S.R. was able to work throughout chemo, travelling to trade shows, though he did lose his hair. Four years later S.R. was in complete remission and has learned the value of good nutrition, living more joyfully, and faith in God.

⭐⭐⭐⭐⭐ **AMAZON.COM**

TESTIMONIAL: **I read this book 18 years ago and still use it today!**
In 1996 I was diagnosed with stage 3 pancreatic cancer. I had developed an adenocarcinoma on the head of my pancreas. I was given the option of a Whipple (surgery), chemo and radiation. I did all three. After the surgery the "doctors" gave me no chance of survival as they discovered the cancer had migrated into my lymph system. During the chemo and radiation I was introduced to Patrick Quillin's book which became my food and nutrition bible then and as it is today. I completely changed my lifestyle. My outlook on life changed. I went through a rebirth. My doctors thought I was nuts and only grasping at straws until my 2-year survival date arrived. Once it appeared that the cancer was gone I asked each doctor who had attended me if they would take credit for the fact I was still alive? Each one answered with an emphatic NO! To this day I still follow the nutrition protocols I learned from Patrick Quillin's book! Believe me it is never too late to change your lifestyle and diet. *N.D.*

ENDNOTES

[1] https://www.crnusa.org/CRN-consumersurvey-archives/2015/

Chapter 15

HERBS

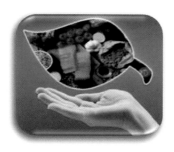

"Behold, I have given you every green plant, and it shall be food for you." Genesis 1:29

WHAT'S AHEAD?
Many herbs (botanicals) contain powerful healing ingredients for cancer patients. No herb is a magic bullet for all cancers. Herbs may help by:
- ✓ stimulating immune functions
- ✓ detoxifying the liver and body
- ✓ directly killing yeast and other cancer-causing microbes

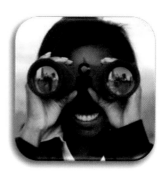

Until the late 20th century, the primary medicine available to keep the human species alive was botanical medicine, or herbs. Botanical medicine has been with us since before the dawn of time. Archeologists have found evidence of <u>herbal collections from 60,000 years</u> ago.

Of the 391,000 species of plants on earth, some are trees in your neighborhood, some are vegetables and fruit in your grocery store, and some become favorites of the apothecary. <u>40% of modern drugs</u> (OTC and prescription) are derived from plants or are a synthesized variation of plant extracts.

The beginning of all life on earth is photosynthesis. Plants harness the sun's energy and combine carbon dioxide in the air with water to yield sugar, glucose. From that humble beginning, add some nitrogen and trace minerals, and the plants become Merlin the Magician in creating a bewildering assortment of phytochemicals.

There are over 6000 known bioflavonoids in plants and another 600 known carotenoids. And this is just the beginning of the phytochemical soup produced by the plants of the earth. Some of these phytochemicals are so deadly that you not only cannot eat it, but cannot even cook your food over it, such as oleander. Yet oleander extracts are now being standardized and used to <u>treat advanced cancer patients</u>, with noteworthy success and minimal toxicity.[1] Remember: the difference between a medicine and a poison is dosage.

HERBAL MEDICINE

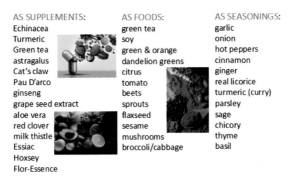

AS SUPPLEMENTS:	AS FOODS:	AS SEASONINGS:
Echinacea	green tea	garlic
Turmeric	soy	onion
Green tea	green & orange	hot peppers
astragalus	dandelion greens	cinnamon
Cat's claw	citrus	ginger
Pau D'arco	tomato	real licorice
ginseng	beets	turmeric (curry)
grape seed extract	sprouts	parsley
aloe vera	flaxseed	sage
red clover	sesame	chicory
milk thistle	mushrooms	thyme
Essiac	broccoli/cabbage	basil
Hoxsey		
Flor-Essence		

In Dr. Kelly Turner's brilliant book, <u>RADICAL REMISSION</u>, she interviewed people who were diagnosed with a stage 4 poor prognostic cancer and did not use traditional oncology and went into complete remission. Dr. Turner found 9 common strategies used by these cancer victors, including a plant-based diet and use of herbal medicines. The other 7 strategies were psycho-spiritual: community involvement, sense of purpose, hope, etc.

Our ancestors used to practice botanical medicine all day every day--in the kitchen. While we have a tendency to think of herbs as mysterious plant concoctions blended up for a very sick person by some eccentric older woman (the quintessential herbalist), in fact, our ancestors ate potent anti-cancer herbs in their diet and as seasonings each day. Columbus set sail in a mad suicidal adventure over the edge of the Earth in the unlikely event that he might find the Spice 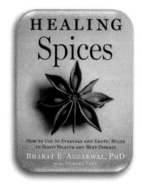 Islands, near India. Spices (a.k.a. seasonings, herbs, botanicals) have been used throughout history as a flavoring agent, preservative, and to cover the rotting stench of unrefrigerated food. As an unintentional by-product of using these seasoning agents our ancestors were able to keep the cancer incidence well below what we currently have. While this section pays homage to the scientific data using botanical extracts as anti-cancer medicines, you are encouraged to check out the brilliant book, HEALING SPICES.

The herbs listed below are by no means an exhaustive list, but the tip of the iceberg on herbs and cancer. This chapter alone could have been 1000 pages. We have spared you the onerous task of reading such a tome. Below are some of the best herbs for cancer. We encourage you to work with a trained herbalist for best results.

BOTANICAL (best form for absorption) suggested daily dosage
Primary functions in human body and anti-cancer activities

Oligomeric proanthocyanidins (OPC) 100-1000 mg
Potent antioxidant, supports vitamin C functions, penetrates the blood-brain barrier, reduces capillary fragility, enhances peripheral circulation, protects DNA from damage by radiation and chemotherapy.

Scurvy (deficiency of vitamin C) has played a huge role in human history. Humans roamed the oceans of the world throughout the 15th through the 19th centuries, often losing up to half of the people on board ship due to scurvy. The English physician, James Lind, discovered that limes cured scurvy in 1747 and began to wind down the death toll from scurvy, while also labeling the English sailors as "limeys".

BOTANICAL MEDICINE:
ready for prime time

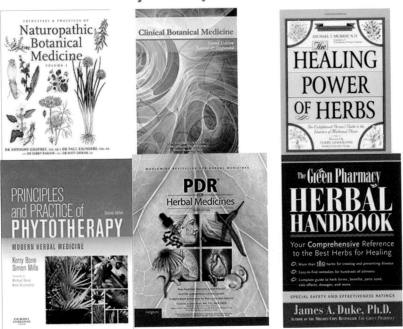

In 1930, Nobel prize winner, Albert Szent-Gyorgy, MD, PhD, isolated pure vitamin C. Ironically, the pure white crystalline vitamin C that Dr. Szent-Gyorgy isolated would not cure bleeding gums, whereas the crude brown mixture of citrus extract would. The difference between these two mixtures was "bioflavonoids", which include over 6,000 different chemical compounds that generally assist chlorophyll in photosynthesis and protect the plant from the harmful effects of the sun's radiation. The rainbow colors of fall foliage are Nature's art exhibit of bioflavonoids and carotenoids.

Some of the main categories of bioflavonoids include:

- anthocyanins; deep purple compounds found in black grapes, beets, red onions, and berries
- catechins and epigallocatechin, which are polyphenols found in apples and green tea

- ◆ ellagic acid, a true anti-cancer compound found in cranberries, raspberries, and other berries
- ◆ flavones, found in citrus fruit, red grapes, and green beans
- ◆ flavanols, such as quercetin, myricetin, found in kale, spinach, onions, apples, and black tea
- ◆ flavanones, such as hesperidin and naringen, found in citrus fruits of grapefruit, oranges, and lemons.

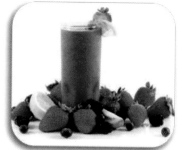

Some of the better-known bioflavonoids include rutin, which is defined in the DORLAND'S MEDICAL DICTIONARY as capable of "preventing capillary fragility." Hesperidin, quercetin, pycnogenol from pine bark, and proanthocyanidins are other popular bioflavonoids. While bioflavonoids are known to be essential in the diet of insects, bioflavonoids are not yet considered essential in the human diet.

As the science of nutrition matures, we are finding that some of the "star" nutrients of the past may be just "supporting actors" for the real star nutrients. For instance, tocotrienols and coenzyme Q may be more important than vitamin E in human health. Eicosapentaenoic acid (EPA from fish oil), though not considered essential, may be more important than alpha-linolenic acid (ALA from flax oil), which is considered essential. And bioflavonoids may be more important than vitamin C. OPC bound to phosphatidylcholine (lecithin) has been shown to improve absorption and cell access to OPC.

Animals with implanted tumors lived longer when given anthocyanin from grape rinds.[2] Flavonoids administered in the diet of rats helped to reduce DNA damage from benzopyrene carcinogens.[3] Bioflavonoids are potent chelators, helping to eliminate toxic minerals from the system.[4] Bioflavonoids in general help to reduce allergic reactions, which create an imbalanced immune attack against cancer and infections.

OPC traps lipid peroxides, hydroxyl radicals, delays the onset of lipid peroxidation, prevents iron-induced lipid peroxidation, and inhibits the enzymes that can degrade connective tissue (hyaluronidase, elastase, collagenase), which then helps to prevent cancer cells from "knocking down the walls" of surrounding tissue for metastasis. Bioflavonoids may inhibit tumor promotion.[5] Bioflavonoids enhance the activity of T-lymphocytes.[6] Various flavonoids have produced striking reductions in cancer incidence in animals, sometimes up to almost total inhibition of tumorogenesis.[7]

Silymarin (milk thistle) 100-500 mg
Stimulates liver detoxification and tissue regeneration, may also augment immune functions

---

Silybum marianum, or milk thistle, is a stout annual plant that grows in dry, rocky soils in parts of Europe and North America. Its seeds, fruit, and leaves are widely prescribed medication in Europe for most diseases affecting the liver. Silymarin has been shown to help regenerate liver tissue, protect the liver against toxic chemicals, and increase the production of glutathione (GSH), which is fundamental in the cell protecting itself against hydrogen peroxide that the cell produces.[8]

Since the liver is the primary detoxifying organ of the body and automatically becomes involved in the internal cancer battle, metastasis to the liver complicates cancer treatment. Among other functions, the liver also stores many vitamins and minerals, produces bile salts for fat digestion and absorption, and is generally one of the more versatile and essential organs in the body. For recovery from cancer to be possible, the liver must be healthy.

Echinacea (purpurea) 100-500 mg
Immune stimulant

Echinacea species consist primarily of E. angustifolia, E. purpurea, and E. pallida. Native American herbalists used echinacea more than any other plant for medicinal purposes. There are over 350 scientific articles worldwide on the immune-enhancing effects of echinacea, including the:
- activation of complement, which promotes chemotaxis of neutrophils, monocytes, and eosinophils; "gearing up" the immune cells
- solubilization of immune complexes
- neutralization of viruses.[9]

One of the components of echinacea, arabinogalactan, has shown promise as an anti-cancer agent in vitro.[10]

In patients with inoperable metastatic esophageal and colorectal cancers, supplements of echinacea (as Echinacin) provided modest improvements in immune functions, slowed the growth of some tumors, and increased survival time. [11] Outpatients with advanced colorectal cancers were given echinacea as part of therapy, with some patients experiencing stable disease, reduction in tumor markers, increases in survival time, and no toxicity reported. [12]

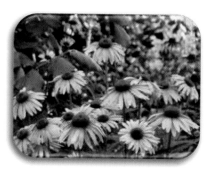

Curcumin (Curcuma longa) 500-5000 mg
Potent antioxidant, protector of DNA

Curry is an Indian spice mixture that includes turmeric as one of the flavoring agents. The active component in turmeric appears to be a bright yellow pigment, curcumin (a.k.a. Curcuma longa), which helps to enhance the immune system by protecting immune cells from their own poisons (pro-oxidants) used to kill cancer cells. Although common condiments like mustard are a good source of curcumin, curcumin is poorly absorbed unless 1% black pepper is added.

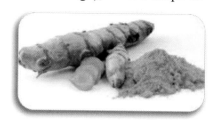

Curcumin appears to be a potent inhibitor of cancer. [13] In animal experiments, curcumin was shown to be directly toxic to tumor cells. [14] In a study with smokers, turmeric tablets were able to dramatically reduce the excretion of urinary mutagen levels (indicators of the possibility of cancer). [15] In patients with skin cancers (squamous cell carcinomas) who had failed therapy with chemo, radiation, and surgery, supplements or ointment of turmeric were able to provide significant reduction in the smell, size, itching, pain, and exudate of the lesions. [16]

Turmeric may be one of the more promising anti-cancer ingredients for 21st century oncology. [17] Researchers find:

"Results obtained from animal studies and other laboratory studies indicate that curcumin may have anti-inflammatory, antioxidant and anticancer properties, in particular."

A patented nanoparticle stabilized version of curcumin, C3 from Sabinsa, has been studied in <u>advanced colon cancer patients</u>.[18]

Ginkgo biloba (24% heteroside) 200-1000 mg
Improves circulation, augments the production of healthy prostaglandin PGE-1, immune stimulant, and adaptogen
(helps to regulate many cellular functions)

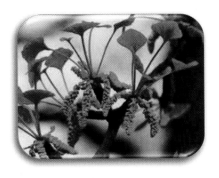

The ginkgo tree is one of the oldest living species on earth, having been around for over 200 million years. The ginkgo tree is an incredibly adaptable and tenacious plant. One ginkgo tree survived the near-ground zero nuclear blast in Hiroshima, Japan. Millions of these cone-shaped evergreen trees survive amidst air pollution, drought, and poor soil throughout the world. A ginkgo tree may live as long as 1,000 years. The leaves and berries contain a wide assortment of phytochemicals (collectively called "ginkgoflavonglycosides"), which have been a pivotal medicine in China for 5,000 years. There are now over 1,000 scientific studies published during the past 40 years demonstrating the medicinal value of ginkgo, with ginkgo extract becoming one of the more widely prescribed medications in Europe today. Annually over 100,000 physicians worldwide write over 10 million prescriptions for ginkgo.

There are several ways in which ginkgo may help the cancer patient:

◆ Vasodilator which expands the tiny capillaries that nourish 90% of the body's tissues, thus bringing oxygen and nutrients to the cells. In doing so, ginkgo improves depression[19] and general circulation to the organs.[20]

◆ Inhibits platelet aggregation, or the stickiness of cells. Stroke, heart attacks, and cancer metastasis are fueled by sticky cells that are generated by platelet activating factor (PAF). Ginkgo inhibits PAF.[21] By modifying PAF, ginkgo helps to reduce inflammation and allergic responses.[22]

- Antioxidant of exceptional efficiency.[23]   Slows down free radical destruction of healthy tissue, therefore protects immune cells in their semi-suicidal quest to kill cancer cells and also protects the favorable prostaglandin, PGE-1. This antioxidant activity also helps to stabilize membranes, where the lipid bi-layer is vulnerable to lipid peroxidation.
- This protection extends to the DNA, which is why Chernobyl workers were given ginkgo to protect them from further damage via radioactivity.

Astragalus (membranaceus) 100-500 mg
Adaptogen and immune stimulant

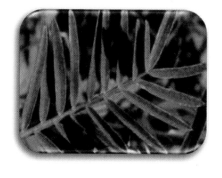

Adaptogens are a small and elite group of herbal compounds, including garlic and ginseng, which coordinate and regulate a broad spectrum of biochemical processes, including prostaglandins, cell membranes, blood sugar levels, etc. "Adaptogen" is the term coined in 1957 by the Russian pharmacologist I. Brekhman. Criteria for an adaptogen are that it must be:[24]

- innocuous, causing minimal harm in reasonable quantities
- non-specific in activity, that is, able to influence a wide range of physical, chemical, and biochemical pathways in the body
- a normalizer of functions, meaning that it will lower or raise a bodily measurement, depending on what needs to happen for improvement in overall health to occur, such as raising blood pressure in hypotensive individuals and lowering blood pressure in hypertensive individuals.[25]

Astragalus has also demonstrated anti-viral activity as it was able to shorten the duration and severity of the common cold in humans.[26] Researchers at M.D. Anderson Hospital in Houston found that astragalus was able to enhance the immune capacity using the cultured blood of 14 cancer patients,[27] as well as augment the anti-tumor ability of Interferon-2.[28] In a study of 176 patients undergoing chemotherapy for cancers of the gastrointestinal tract, astragalus and ginseng were able to prevent the normal immune depression and weight loss that occurs.[29] In a variety of human studies, astragalus has been shown to stimulate various parameters of the immune system, has anti-tumor activity, and inhibits the spreading (metastasis) of cancer.[30]

Panax ginseng (8%) 100-500 mg
Adaptogen, immune stimulant, anti-tumor activity, inhibits metastasis[31]

Ginseng is one of the oldest, most widely used, and scientifically studied of all the world's herbs. The original proponents of ginseng were Chinese physicians several thousand years ago, using it to treat nearly every conceivable ailment.   Given the known "adaptogenic" qualities of ginseng, the enthusiasm of these ancient Chinese doctors may have been well placed.   Ginseng is a plant species term (Panax), which is further subdivided into Panax quinquefolium (American ginseng), Panax japonicum (Japanese ginseng), Panax pseudoginseng (Himalayan ginseng), and Panax trifolium. [32]   Eleutherococcus senticosus, a relative newcomer to this category, contains some ginseng-like 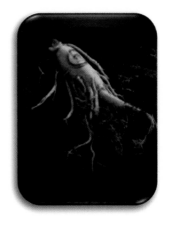 compounds (triterpenoid saponins), but is not considered true ginseng. Panax ginseng C.A. Meyer is the best studied in the scientific literature and is referred to in the followed studies.

The wide disparity in outcome of clinical studies using ginseng probably stems from the lack of active ingredients in many substandard ginseng products sold today. Ginseng's therapeutic value comes from the 13 different triterpenoid saponins, collectively known as ginsenosides, which are found in various concentrations in various types of ginseng grown on various soils and experiencing various drying and storage techniques.   While most ginseng is about 1-3% ginsenosides, better products will offer 8% concentration. In one study published in 1979, of the 54 ginseng products analyzed, 60% were worthless and 25% had no ginseng at all![33] It is the regularly-formed root from wild Panax ginseng that is most highly prized. Nearly 60,000 people are employed in Korea for the raising and processing of ginseng.

Ginseng may help cancer patients for the following reasons:

♦ **Adaptogenic qualities**. Ginseng is nearly unsurpassed in the plant kingdom for its ability to bring about biochemical adjustments in whatever direction is necessary.

♦ **Central nervous system stimulant**.[34] In various animal and human studies, ginseng provides both calming and stimulating effects simultaneously. It allows people to better adapt to stressful situations, including cancer. It also provides for energizing effects and improvement of moods and alertness.

♦ **Blood glucose regulator**. While ginseng will lower blood glucose levels in the diabetic individual or the one fed a high sugar diet, it will not lower blood glucose in the healthy individual fed a normal diet.[35] Since cancer is a sugar feeder, keeping blood glucose levels in check is a crucial job of ginseng.

♦ **Immune-stimulating effects**. Ginseng has been shown to stimulate the reticuloendothelial system, which means getting more macrophages ("big eaters") to gobble up (phagocytosis) cancer cells and cell debris.[36] In animals, ginseng was shown to prevent viral infections.[37] Ginseng can dramatically bolster host defense mechanisms in animals and humans.

♦ **Liver cleansing, protection, and stimulation**. Ginseng activates the macrophages in the liver, known as Kupffer cells, which are responsible for removing cellular debris from the body's most important detoxifying organ, the liver. Macrophages in the liver help to "take out the trash". Ginseng also helps to improve protein synthesis in the liver[38], reverse diet-induced fatty liver, and protect the liver from chemically-induced damage.[39]

♦ **Anti-clotting and metastatic**. Cancer spreads by adhering to blood vessel walls. Hence reducing the stickiness, or platelet aggregation, of cells is a major plus. Ginseng reduces platelet aggregation.[40]

♦ **Anti-cancer properties**. Ginseng is a potent inhibitor of cancer in animals[41] and humans.[42] Ginseng has the unique, paradoxical, and nearly miraculous ability to control cell growth, or hyperplasia. In healthy cells with adequate nourishment, ginseng encourages cell division. Yet under adverse conditions, ginseng helps to suppress abnormal cell division.[43] Ginseng helps to repair damaged DNA.[44]

In tumor-bearing mice, 8 days of ginseng administration brought about a 75% reduction in average tumor size.[45] Oral administration of ginseng in tumor-bearing mice inhibited the growth of liver cancer (solid ascites hepatoma), while inhibiting metastasis to the lungs.[46] Panax ginseng was able to enhance the uptake of mitomycin (an antibiotic and anti-cancer drug) into the cancer cells for increased tumor kill.[47] Ginseng was able to slow tumor growth and improve survival time in rats with chemically-induced liver cancer.[48]

SAFETY ISSUES
Ginseng and estrogen

Of the many supplements that may be useful for cancer patients, 2 of them contain estrogen-like compounds: soy and ginseng, which merit a special discussion. There is some controversy in the scientific community regarding the use of estrogen-like compounds in the treatment of breast or ovarian cancer patients.

Estrogen is an essential hormone produced by women throughout their menstruating years as part of fertility. Estrogen has 260 different functions in the human body, including antioxidant, maintenance of bone structure, and protection against cardiovascular diseases. If estrogen caused cancer, then every young healthy menstruating woman would be riddled with tumors. Estrogen does not cause breast or ovarian cancer, but it is a growth hormone and can accelerate the growth of anything, including hormone-dependent cancers.

There are 4 primary categories of estrogen-like compounds:

- **Estrogen**, which actually refers to a family of hormones, including estradiol, estriol, and estrone, manufactured in the female body for specific bodily functions.[49]

- **Phytoestrogens**, which are estrogen-like compounds in plants, which have about 0.05% (1/2000) the strength of estrogen and have demonstrated beneficial effects both pre- and post-cancer diagnosis. These compounds work like a mild version of Tamoxifen to compete with estrogen for binding to estrogen receptor sites.[50] Richest source of phytoestrogens is flax followed by soy.

- **Xenoestrogens**, which are estrogen-like compounds in herbicides, pesticides, and other commercial chlorinated hydrocarbons. These have been shown to have disastrous consequences of antagonizing all the negative aspects of estrogen.[51] Women with breast cancer have been found to have more chlorinated hydrocarbons, or xenoestrogens, in their bloodstream. These xenoestrogens are creating havoc in the wild, where male animals end up with dramatically deformed genitals, and females have reduced fertility and increases in birth defects.

♦ **Estrogen-receptors**, which are compounds that escort estrogen from the body, hopefully after it has performed its essential functions. The human body makes estrogen-receptors through the PGE-1 prostaglandin pathways when blood sugar levels are kept low and essential fatty acids (EPA, ALA, GLA, LA) are sufficient.

Tamoxifen is an estrogen binder that can be of value in short-term use to slow down breast cancer, but in long term use elevates the risk for heart attack, [52] eye, [53] and liver damage [54] and INCREASES the risk of endometrial cancer. [55]

Researchers, like Stephen Barnes, PhD at the University of Alabama, find that soy is able to inhibit the growth of hormone-dependent tumors, including breast and prostate. Soy and ginseng are Nature's "kinder, gentler" forms of Tamoxifen.

Adding all this complex biochemistry together and trying to make the recommendations simple, there are several reasons why the 4 above-mentioned categories of estrogen-like compounds are not equal. Soy products and ginseng have been used both to prevent and to reverse cancer. The macrobiotic diet, which uses soy as a pivotal source of protein, has not been shown to accelerate the course of breast or ovarian cancer. While soy and ginseng products can reduce the symptoms of menopause by working as phytoestrogens, they do not increase the risk for breast or ovarian cancer nor do they accelerate the disease once present.

However, that said, there probably are male and female specific foods, including these phytoestrogens found in highest amounts on soy and flax. Adult men probably need to be aware of the <u>testosterone-lowering effect of phytoestrogens</u>. [56]

Green tea polyphenols 100-2000 mg
Antioxidant, protector of DNA, immune stimulant

America was founded upon a tea revolt. The American colonists decided that, rather than pay the English King's taxes on tea without representation in the British Parliament, the colonist would rather go into caffeine "cold turkey" by throwing the tea into Boston harbor. While the

British have brought "high tea" into its revered limelight, tea was first introduced to England in the 17th century via trade with China, where it had been a favorite beverage for over 3,000 years. Of the 2.5 million tons of dried tea produced each year worldwide, most is grown and consumed in the Orient.

Tea comes from the plant Camellia sinensis, an evergreen shrub in which the young leaves can be either:

♦ lightly steamed to produce **green tea** or
♦ air dried and oxidized to produce **black tea**.

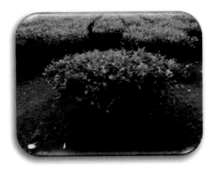

The potent polyphenols are maintained in green tea, since steaming denatures the enzymes that would normally convert the polyphenols to less beneficial ingredients. Green tea is healthier than black tea. While both forms of tea have caffeine, only 20% of tea produced annually comes as green tea.

Green tea contains a variety of polyphenolic compounds, including catechin, epicatechin, and the reputed chief active ingredient, epigallocatechin gallate. One cup of green tea contains 300 to 400 mg of polyphenols and 50 to 100 mg of caffeine. Green tea works as an antioxidant, perhaps even more potent than vitamins C or E.[57] In animals, green tea was able to induce major improvements in antioxidant and detoxifying enzymes in the body.[58] In human studies, green tea users have about half the cancer incidence of non-tea drinkers.[59] In test tube studies, green tea shut down the tumor promoters involved in breast cancer.[60] Green tea inhibits the formation of cancer-causing agents in the stomach, including nitrosamines.[61]

Green tea has been shown to <u>lower the risk for</u> cancer, heart disease, stroke, Alzheimer's and other common conditions associated with aging.[62]

The anti-cancer properties of green tea include:[63]

♦ Immune stimulant
♦ Inhibits platelet adhesion
♦ Antioxidant that protects immune cells for a higher tumor-kill rate, while protecting the valuable prostaglandin PGE-1
♦ Inhibits metastasis

- ◆ Inhibits the breakdown of connective tissue via collagenase, which is the primary mechanism for the spreading of cancer cells. [64]
- ◆ Green tea has recently been shown to <u>inhibit the replication</u> of the SARS/Coronavirus.[65]

Aloe powder 100-1000 mg
Immune stimulant, aids in cellular communication

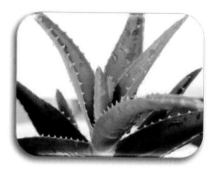

For 5,000 years, many cultures and herbalists around the world have been using aloe vera as a primary medicinal plant. King Solomon used it as his favorite laxative. Hippocrates, the father of modern medicine 2,400 years ago, used at least 14 different medicine formulas containing aloe. Alexander the Great conquered an island in order to have aloe for his soldiers.

Aloe thrives on neglect. All the plant needs is decent soil and a little water and sun, then you get to harvest one of Nature's most versatile and impressive healers. Fresh aloe gel applied topically may be the greatest skin cream on the planet earth. The yellow bitter part of the plant leaf is a proven laxative. And whole-leaf extracts have the ability to gear up the immune system, reduce swelling, improve healing, kill bacteria and viruses, and improve communication between cells (intercellular) and within the cell (intracellular). Aloe plants begin generating medicinally active mannans after 2 or 3 years. Younger plants are relatively ineffective.

Of the 300 species of aloe, it is aloe vera that has received the most attention. Aloe certainly typifies the complexity of understanding the healing properties of plants. There are over 200 biologically active ingredients in aloe vera, including prostaglandins, essential fatty acids (including GLA), vitamins, minerals, anthraquinones, and polysaccharides (longer chains of sugar-like molecules).[66]

In the movie, MEDICINE MAN, a doctor (Sean Connery) discovered a cure for cancer from a plant in the Amazon forest, which was rapidly being levelled by bulldozers and fire. But now he cannot reproduce his original concoction from the same plant. Spoiler alert: the active ingredient in his original cancer cure was from the spider feces that was found in the sugar used to dilute the herbal concoction. Moral of the story: We are still neophytes when it comes to understanding just what is the active ingredient(s) in medicinal plants, which is why using low-heat processing of the whole leaf aloe is crucial for preserving the active ingredient.

There are receptor sites on immune cells (macrophages) for D-mannose (one of the sugars in aloe) just like a key fitting a keyhole.[67]

Aloe may help the cancer patient in many ways.

◆ **Antibacterial & antifungal**. Aloe vera applied topically to burn regions of animals was superior to the common antibacterial medication used, silver sulfadiazine.[68]

◆ **Antiviral activity**. Feline leukemia is a form of cancer contracted by cats and caused by a virus. This disease is invariably fatal, with 70% of cats dying within 8 weeks of early symptoms. Most cats are euthanized as soon as the diagnosis is made. In one study, acemannan from aloe was injected weekly for 6 weeks into the cats, with a followup 6-week waiting period. After this 12 week study, 71% of the cats were alive and in good health. [69] Acemannan has also demonstrated a potent ability to fight the flu virus, measles, and the HIV virus, while also reducing the dosage required of the drug AZT.[70]

◆ **Anti-inflammatory**. Drugs, such as cortisone, that are effective at reducing inflammation also shut down wound recovery. Aloe has the ability to reduce swelling, while also enhancing wound recovery.

◆ **Immune stimulant**. Aloe has been shown to increase the activity of the immune system.[71] Aloe seems to provide neutrophils with more "bullets", or toxic substances to kill cancer and invading organisms.[72] Aloe (acemannan) increases the production of nitric oxide, a potent anti-cancer "napalm" used by immune cells.[73]

◆ **Anti-cancer activity**. Various fractions of aloe (mannans and glucans) have been found to have potent anti-neoplastic activity.[74]

◆ **Radio-protective**. Some forms of mannan are bone marrow stimulants and can protect mice against cobalt-60 radiation.[75] In my experience with cancer patients, those who took aloe before and during radiation therapy had minimal damage of healthy tissue while still getting an impressive anti-cancer effect from the radiation. Generalized radiation to the pelvic region for prostate or colon cancer can be particularly nasty in harming the bladder and gastrointestinal tract. One cancer patient used aloe throughout 40 rounds of pelvic radiation and suffered no burns and only mild GI distress.

♦ **Cell communication**. Many forms of carbohydrates, called glycoproteins, may play a key role in promoting healthy communication within the cell and between cells. Aloe may contribute an important carbohydrate (mannan) that becomes part of this crucial "telegraph system", which prevents or slows down cancer.[76] Given the 8 monosaccharides used in the body and the 18 configurations used to arrange these molecules, the possible number of "words" in this complex "telegraph" system works out to 18 to the 8th power, or over 11 billion "messages". No doubt, more important breakthroughs will come out of this new and exciting field of cell communication.

Cat's claw, 3:1 concentrate 200 mg
Immune stimulant, anti-inflammatory, DNA protector, antioxidant

---

Cat's claw, or Uncaria tomentosa, is a relative newcomer to Western botanical medicine. It has been used therapeutically for centuries by Native South Americans in the higher elevations of the Peruvian Amazon rain forest. Cat's claw is a woody vine that grows to 100 feet by wrapping around nearby trees. The root and inner bark are used to prepare herbal concoctions that have demonstrated some effectiveness at cleansing the gastrointestinal tract of parasites and re-establishing a favorable environment for healthy microflora bacteria.

Cat's claw may be able to:
♦ Inhibit free radicals[77]
♦ Stimulate the immune system[78]
♦ Cleanse and strengthen the intestinal tract
♦ Inhibit auto-immune diseases, such as Crohn's and rheumatoid arthritis
♦ Protect the DNA from damage[79]
♦ Slow down cancer growth[80]

Rhodiola rosea root extract, standardized to 4% Rosavins and 1% salidrosides; 200 mg
Adaptogen, cardio-protective, mood enhancer, energizer, hormonal regulator, immune enhancement

---

Rhodiola is an extremely tenacious herb that grows at high elevations in colder climates, such as Siberia. Rhodiola was a secret herb that was well researched by the Russians and used by Russian military and athletes in secrecy. At the end of the Cold War and the fall of the Berlin Wall, secrets from Russia began to trickle out to the rest of the world. 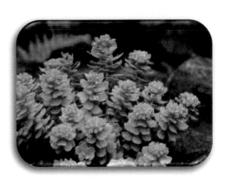 One of those valuable secrets was Rhodiola.

Rhodiola was first mentioned in the medical herb text DE MATERIA MEDICA by the Greek physician Dioscorides in 77 AD. Chinese emperors would regularly send expeditions to Siberia to retrieve the "golden root" Rhodiola for energy enhancement and libido.

Rhodiola has generated considerable enthusiasm among herbalist who find compelling scientific evidence that Rhodiola can act as an:

♦ adaptogen, enhancing many bodily functions in a non-specific fashion
♦ increase energy and improve moods[81]
♦ protect DNA from mutagens that can trigger cancer[82]
♦ protects the body from the damaging effects of certain chemo agents (cyclophosphamide)[83]
♦ increase endurance[84]
♦ elevate mental concentration and clarity[85]
♦ stress reliever, such as used by Russian cosmonauts in space
♦ cardioprotective effects during oxygen deprivation[86]
♦ anti-depressant, relieving depression in 64% of patients in a Russian study[87]
♦ hormone balancer, without triggering hormone-related cancers[88]

Rhodiola appears safe in doses up to 20,000 mg per day for adults. Recommended dosages range from 100 to 500 mg per day.[89]

OTHER BOTANICALS: Of the 114,000 plant extracts studied at the National Cancer Institute, only 26 were selected for secondary testing. There are literally thousands of botanical agents that hold promise in cancer treatment. The above list offers some of the better studied and more widely available herbal agents to help the cancer patients. Other herbs and herbal combinations worthy of consideration might include:

- Tianxian herbal concoction (tianxian.com).
- Hoxsey formula
- Essiac formula
- Goldenseal
- Licorice
- Pau D'Arco
- Burdock (Arctium lappa)
- Marigold (Calendula officinalis)
- Poke root (Phytolacca decandra)
- Sheep Sorrel (Rumex acetosella)
- Dandelion (Taraxacum officinale)
- Red clover flowers (Trifolium pretense)
- Nettle (Urtica dioica)

There are thousands of herbs commonly used in the Orient that are not widely available in the U.S., but possibly available through a trained herbalist.

SKIN CANCER

There are about 5.4 million basal cell and squamous cell carcinomas treated annually in the US. Surgical excision is about 90% effective as a long-term cure. Melanoma is a much more lethal and rare form of skin cancer that requires professional attention. For those people interested in treatment options for routine

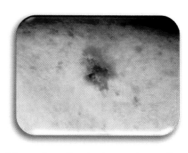

non-malignant skin cancer, you may consider the herbal escharotics (selectively burn away abnormal tissue when applied topically):
- ✓ PDQ herbal ointment[90]
- ✓ Cansema[91]
- ✓ Ecopolitan ointment[92]

For more information on how your body can fight cancer go to GettingHealthier.com.

PATIENT PROFILE: BEAT COLON CANCER

D.M. was 48 years of age when he was diagnosed with stage 4 colon cancer that had spread to the liver. His doctor used chemotherapy with little hope of any benefit from this therapy, much less a cure. D.M. began using the principles in this book including proper diet and nutrition supplements to reverse his cancer. Within 6 months he was disease-free and has remained so for 2 years. D.M. writes, "I really believe your book helped to save my life."

ENDNOTES

[1] https://cancerres.aacrjournals.org/content/74/19_Supplement/4658

[2] . Koide, T., et al., Cancer Biotherapy & Radiopharmaceuticals, vol.11, p.273, Aug.1996

[3] . LeBon, AM, et al., Chem.Biol.Interactions, vol.83, p.65, 1992

[4] . Havsteen, B, Biochem Pharmacol., vol.32, p.1141, 1983

[5] . Fujiki, H., in Plant Flavonoids in Biology and Medicine, vol.1, p.429, Liss Publ., NY, 1986

[6] . Berg, P, in Plant Flavonoids in Biology and Medicine, vol.2, p.157, Liss Publ., NY, 1988

[7] . Wattenberg, L., et al., Cancer Research, vol.30, p.1922, 1970

[8] . Werbach, M., et al., BOTANICAL INFLUENCES ON ILLNESS, p.30, Third Line, Tarzana, CA, 1994

[9] . Werbach, M., IBID, p.189

[10] . Luettig, B., et al., J. Natl.Cancer Inst., vol.81, p.669, 1989

[11] . Lersch, C., et al., Tumordiagen Ther., vol.13, p.115, 1992

[12] . Lersch, C., et al., Cancer Invest., vol.10, p.343, 1992

[13] . Nagabhushan, M., et al., J. Am.Coll. Nutr., vol.11, p.192, 1992

[14] . Kuttan, R., et al., Cancer Lett., vol.29, p.197, 1985

[15] . Polasa, K., Mutagen, vol.7, p.107, 1992

[16] . Kuttan, R., et al., Tumori, vol.73, p.29, 1987

[17] https://jbuon.com/archive/21-5-1050.pdf

[18] https://link.springer.com/article/10.1186/s13063-015-0641-1

[19] . Schubert, H., et al., Geriatr Forsch, vol.3, p.45, 1993

[20] . Kleijnen, J., et al., Br. J. Clin.Pharmacol. vol.34, p.352, 1992

[21] . Kleijnen, J., et al., Lancet, vol.340, p.1136, 1992

[22] . Koltai, M., et al., Drugs, vol.42, p.9, 1991

[23] . Pincemail, J., et al., Experientia, vol.45, p.708, 1989

[24] . Shibata, S., et al., Econ.Med.Plant Res., vol.1, p.217, 1985

[25] . Siegel, RK, JAMA, vol.243, p.32, 1980

[26] . Chang, HM, et al., Pharmacology and Applications of Chinese Materia Medica, vol. 2, World Scientific Publ., Teaneck, NJ, p.1041, 1987

[27] . Sun, Y, J. Biol Response Modifiers, vol.2, p.227, 1983

[28] . Chu, DT, et al., J. Clin.Lab.Immunol., vol.26, p.183, 1988

[29] . Li, NQ, et al., Chung Kuo Chung Hsi I Chieh Ho Tsa Chih, vol.12, p.588, 1992

[30] . Boik, J., CANCER AND NATURAL MEDICINE, p.177, Oregon Medical, Princeton, MN, 1995

[31] . Boik, J. CANCER AND NATURAL MEDICINE, p.180 Oregon Medical, Princeton, MN, 1995

[32] . Murray, MT, HEALING POWER OF HERBS, p.265, Prima Publ., Rocklin, CA 1995

[33]. Ziglar, W., Whole Foods, vol.2, p.48, 1979

[34]. Samira, MMH, et al., J.Int.Med.Res., vol.13, p.342, 1985

[35]. Ng, TB, et al., Gen.Pharmacol., vol.6, p.549, 1985; see also Yamato, M., et al., Proceedings of the 3rd Intl Ginseng Symp, p.115, 1980

[36]. Jie, YH, et al., Agents Actions, vol.15, p.386, 1984; see also Gupta, S., et al., Clin.Res., vol.28, p.504A, 1980

[37]. Singh, VK, et al., Planta Medica, vol.51, p.462, 1984

[38]. Oura, H., et al., Chem.Pharm.Bull., vol.20, p.980, 1972

[39]. Hikino, H., et al., Planta Medica, vol.52, p.62, 1985; see also Oh, JS, et al., Korean J.Pharmacol., vol.4, p.27, 1968

[40]. Yamamoto, M., et al., Am.J.Chin.Med., vol.11, p.84, 1983

[41]. Yun, TK, et al., Cancer Detect.Prev., vol.6, p.515, 1983

[42]. Yun, TK, et al., Int.J.Epidemiol., vol.19, p.871, 1990

[43]. Lee, KD, Jpn.J.Pharmacol., vol.21, p.299, 1971; Fulder, SJ, Exp.Ger., vol.12, p.125, 1977

[44]. Rhee, YH, et al., Planta Medica, vol.57, p.125, 1991

[45]. Hau, DM, et al., Int. J. of Oriental Med., vol.15, p.10, 1990

[46]. Yang, G., et al., J. of Trad. Chin. Med., vol.8, p.135, 1988

[47]. Kubo, M., et al., Planta Med, vol.58, p.424, 1992

[48]. Li, X., et al., J. Tongji Med Univ., vol.11, p.73, 1991

[49]. Murray, RK, et al., HARPER'S BIOCHEMISTRY, 24th ed, p.550, Lange, Stamford, CT 1996

[50]. Boik, J., CANCER AND NATURAL MEDICINE, p.44, Oregon Medical, Princeton, MN 1995

[51]. Davis, DL, et al., Environmental Health Perspectives, vol.101, p.372, Oct.1993

[52]. Nakagawa, T., et al., Angiology, vol.45, p.333, May 1994

[53]. Pavlidis, NA, et al., Cancer, vol.69, p.2961, 1992

[54]. Catherino, WH, et al., Drug Safety, vol.8, p.381, 1993

[55]. Seoud, MAF, et al., Obstetrics & Gynecology, vol.82, p.165, Aug.1993

[56] https://www.ncbi.nlm.nih.gov/pmc/articles/PMC3074428/

[57]. Ho, C., et al., Prev.Med., vol.21, p.520, 1992

[58]. Khan, SG, et al., Cancer Res., vol.52, p.4050, 1992

[59]. Yang, CS, et al., J. Natl., Cancer Inst., vol.85, p.1038, 1993

[60]. Komori, A., et al., Jpn.J.Clin.Oncol., vol.23, p.186, 1993

[61]. Stich, HF, Prev.Med., vol.21, p.377, 1992

[62] https://www.sciencedirect.com/science/article/abs/pii/S0024320505012415

[63]. Boik, J., CANCER AND NATURAL MEDICINE, p.178, Oregon Medical, Princeton, MN 1995

[64]. Beretz, A, et al., Plant Flavonoids in Biology and Medicine II, p.187, Liss Publ., 1988

[65] https://www.tandfonline.com/doi/full/10.1080/07391102.2020.1779818

[66]. Haller, JS, Bull.NY Acad.Sci., vol.66, p.647, 1990

[67]. Lee, YC, Adv.Exp.Med.Biol., vol.228, p.103, 1984

[68]. Robson, MC, et al., J.Burn.Care Rehab., vol.3, p.157, 1982

[69]. Sheets, MA, et al., Mol.Biother., vol.3, p.41, 1991

[70]. Kahlon, JB, et al., Mol.Biother., vol.3, p.214, 1991

[71]. t'Hart, LA, et al., Planta.Med., vol.55, p.509, 1989

[72]. t'Hart, LA, et al., Int.J.Immunopharmacol., vol.12, p.427, 1990

[73]. Karaca, K., et al., Int.J.Immunopharmacol., vol.17, p.183, 1995

[74]. Kamasuka, T., et al., Gann, vol.59, p.443, 1968

[75]. Tizard, IR, et al., Mol.Biother., vol.1, p.290, 1989

[76]. Murray, RK, et al., HARPER'S BIOCHEMISTRY, p.648, Lange Medical, Stamford, CT 1996

[77]. McBrien, DC, et al., LIPID PEROXIDATION AND CANCER, Academy Press, NY 1982

[78]. Wagner, H., et al., Planta Medica, vol.12, p.34, 1985

[79]. Rizzi, R., et al., J. Ethnopharmacol., vol.38, p.63, 1993

[80] . DeOlivera, MM, et al., Anals Acad.Brasil Ciencias, vol.44, p.41, 1972

[81] . Spasov, AA, Phytomedicine, vol.7, no.2, p.85, 2000

[82] . Saratikov, AS, Stimulative Properties of Rhodiola Rosea, in RHODIOLA ROSEA IS A VALUABLE MEDICINAL PLANT, Tomsk, Russia, Izdatelstvo Tomskogo Univ., 1987

[83] . Udintsev, SN, European J.Cancer, vol.27, no.9, p.1182, 1991

[84] . Seifulla, RD, Sports Pharmacology Source Book, Moscow, Mosovskaya Prauda, 1999

[85] . Shevtsov, VA, Phytomedicine, vol.10, no.2-3, p.95, 2003

[86] . Afanasev, SA, Biokhimiia, vol.61, no.10, p.1779, 1996

[87] . Krasik, ED, New data on the therapy of asthenic conditions: clinical prospects for the use of golden root extract, Kemerov, Riussia, Russian Academy of Medicinal Sciences, p.298, 1970

[88] . Eagon, PK, abstract from American Association of Cancer Research meeting, 2003

[89] . Brown, RP, THE RHODIOLA REVOLUTION, Rodale Press, 2004

[90] http://pdqherbals.com/6594.html

[91] https://www.alphaomegalabs.com/cansemar-black-topical-salve-22g.html

[92] http://www.ecopolitan.com/doctor-t

Chapter 16

GLANDULARS

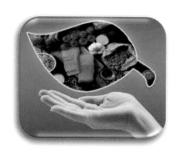

"Health begins on the farm, not the pharmacy."
Alan Gaby, MD author of Nutritional Medicine

WHAT'S AHEAD
- ✓ The thymus gland and spleen are valuable parts of the immune system that can sometimes be "worn out.
- ✓ Taking thymus and spleen glandular concentrates sometimes improves immune functions.
- ✓ Melatonin is a valuable antioxidant and anti-cancer agent.

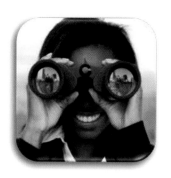

Glandular therapy has been practiced, at least inadvertently, since the dawn of mankind. A gland is an organ in the body that secretes or excretes something, all part of the endocrine system. For instance, the pineal gland in the brain secretes melatonin, which acts as an antioxidant, regulator of our biological clock, anti-aging hormone, and works to prevent and slow cancer. Essentially, as we age or are exposed to toxins, stress, and malnutrition, our glands do not perform their jobs ideally. This is where glandular therapy can be of benefit.

One of the more commonly practiced forms of glandular therapy is the use of natural desiccated thyroid extract to treat people with underactive thyroid glands. We are merely replacing what Nature is not making. Glandular therapy can be a rate-limiting step in the cancer patient getting well and oftentimes requires professional assistance in determining which gland is not working up to par and how to fix the problem.

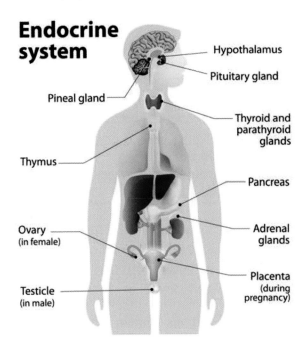

In the seminal book, NUTRITION AND PHYSICAL DEGENERATION, Weston Price, DDS, relates that Native Americans in the cold regions of northern Canada avoided scurvy in the winter by first eating the raw adrenal gland from any animal captured. Adrenal glands provide the most concentrated depot of vitamin C in the body. Our hunter-gatherer ancestors would offer the liver and heart of the captured animal to the slayer. Liver and heart are among the organs that are rich in CoQ, carnitine, lipoic acid, trace minerals, and a variety of nutrients that are missing in our diets.

At least 5 million Americans take synthetic thyroid (levothyroxine) to maintain normal thyroxin levels in the blood. This is glandular therapy. We now use gelatin extracts (which are from connective tissue of hooves and hides) of glucosamine sulfate and chondroitin sulfate to improve connective tissue diseases, such as osteo and rheumatoid arthritis. There are peptides in each gland that are specific to that gland, such as thymus and spleen, which will be targeted to that gland once consumed.

As we mature, many of our glandular functions deteriorate. [1] Although our biochemistry textbooks would have us believe that polypeptides, such as those found in glandular extracts, are all hydrolyzed (broken down) in the digestive processes of the gut, in fact, many peptides survive this chemical gauntlet. How else do we explain the passage of Immunoglobulin A from mother's milk to bolster the newborn infant's immune system, or the food proteins that pass directly into the bloodstream and trigger allergic responses? Glandular replacement therapy, such as thymus and spleen, may be useful for many people who are struggling with life-threatening diseases.

Thymic concentrate 500 mg
Bolsters functions of thymus gland, which is crucial to the maturation of immune cells into T-cells

---

In 1930 an article appeared in the Journal of the American Medical Association by a physician using <u>thymus extract to treat cancer</u>.[2] Since then there have been <u>numerous efforts to assess the effectiveness</u> of thymus extracts in cancer patients, with the likelihood of reducing infections in chemo and radiation patients.[3]

The thymus gland in humans usually atrophies with aging. Anyone over 30 years of age probably has a thymus gland that is well below optimal in size and functional capacity. There are thymus-derived factors with hormone-like activity, called thymosins, that have long been recognized for their potential at stimulating immune functions.[4] An extract of thymus, thymosin 5, was able to stimulate immune functions in mice with induced tumors.[5] Thymus extract is more of an immune regulator than an immune stimulant. In human lung cancer patients receiving chemotherapy, thymus supplements provided for longer survival time.[6] Thymus extract (TP-1) was able to increase lymphocyte counts in incurable gastrointestinal cancer patients treated with chemotherapy.[7]

Researchers followed over 1,000 patients who had been treated with thymus extract (TFX) over the course of 15 years and found the thymus to be extremely helpful in normalizing immune panels and improving outcome in a wide variety of immune suppressive disorders.[8] Researchers at the University of California isolated a fraction of thymus (thymic protein A), which improved immune parameters in mice.[9] Probably a wide variety of subsets of peptides and glycoproteins in thymus work to improve differentiation of bone marrow (B-cells) lymphocytes into active T-cells that can recognize and destroy cancer cells.

Spleen concentrate 500 mg
Bolsters functions of the spleen gland, a storage and filtering organ for the blood and immune system

---

The human spleen oftentimes atrophies with aging. Supplements of spleen extract have been used in conjunction with ginseng as a clinically tested immune stimulant for cancer and AIDS patients in Europe.

Adrenal supplements: DHEA, pregnenolone, cortisol
The primary substrates (raw materials to make) many hormones in the human body. May induce more optimal functioning for immune protection and hormonal balance

---

We hit our prime around age 20 for many biological measurements, including production of the above hormones from the adrenal glands (just above the kidneys). As we age, our internal production of these hormones drops predictably, with a 90 year old person having lost 90% of their original DHEA.

Since DHEA is a natural substance, it cannot be patented, hence research on this subject is sketchy. Without NIH or Big Pharma funding, there is no grant funding for these promising therapies. Cholesterol, pregnenolone, and DHEA are the beginning steps for manufacturing most of the sex hormones in the body.

Supplements of DHEA are usually made from wild yam and taken in doses of 5-100 mg/day. Supplements of DHEA have shown possible benefits for <u>mild depression</u>.[10] While the above adrenal supplements have been touted for many anti-aging benefits, it should be noted that most college and professional organizations ban the use of DHEA in athletes, which probably means that they do have an effect on athletic performance.

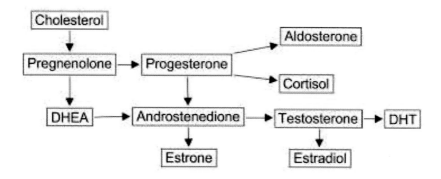

As always, the difference between a medicine and a poison is dosage. While these supplements can provide mild to major improvements in some individuals, they can also exacerbate some health problems. You can have your hormone levels tested through a health care professional, which then allows a more targeted use of these potentially beneficial supplements.

Melatonin 3-20 mg at bedtime
Regulates circadian rhythm, enhances immune system (IL-2) against tumor, antioxidant, stimulates thymus (immune enhancement), inhibits several different tumor lines, reduces toxicity (myelodysplasia) from chemo and radiation, may reduce lean tissue wasting (cachexia), stimulates immune system to become more toxic against tumors

---

There is a pea-sized gland in the center of the human brain called the pineal gland. This gland has been the source of intense research and interest since it was first called "the third eye" by scientists two centuries ago. Actually, ancient mystics placed great emphasis on development of this region of the brain nearly 2000 years ago.

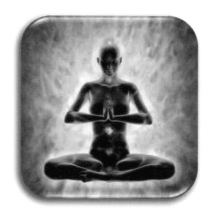

There is evidence that our toxic world full of light at night, alcohol, and an invisible sea of electrical emissions all dampen down the normal effectiveness of the pineal gland. Studies in other creatures find that melatonin is the

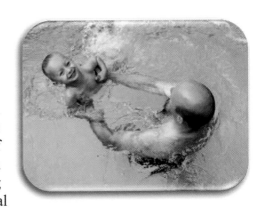

"juvenile" hormone, which is directly responsible for the effects of aging. Melatonin may be one of the master hormones in the human body, coordinating and regulating growth and aging, and very essential for optimal health.

Melatonin is now being used around the world as part of <u>comprehensive cancer treatment</u>, with reduced side effects of chemo as a common benefit.[11] Only side effects noted from melatonin supplements are drowsiness upon awakening. If so, reduce or discontinue dosage. Do not use melatonin in conjunction with other psychotropic drugs, such as Prozac, Lithium, or monoamine oxidase inhibitors.

- ♦ Tumor regressions were found in 36% (5 out of 14) patients studied with liver (hepatocellular carcinoma).[12]
- ♦ Melatonin was effective as sole therapy in refractory cancer patients (have not responded to other conventional therapies), with improvement in quality of life and control of cancer growth.[13]
- ♦ Melatonin was effective against metastatic lung cancer (non-small cell) in patients who had failed first-line therapy (cisplatin).[14]
- ♦ Melatonin prevented the common side effect from IL-2 therapy of thrombocytopenia (low platelet numbers in the blood).[15]
- ♦ Melatonin was shown effective in patients with relapsed melanoma.[16]
- ♦ In cancer patients who had failed all other cancer therapies, melatonin provided a 39% response rate (stopped tumor progression) with no side effects, and nearly all patients reported an improved sense of well-being.[17]
- ♦ Melatonin along with Tamoxifen produced better results in metastatic breast cancer patients than Tamoxifen treatment alone.[18]

PATIENT PROFILE: A LIFE WELL LIVED

"Cancer is the best thing that ever happened to me." V.G. was at the podium speaking to a hundred people at a Celebrate Life Reunion of cancer victors. V.G. had come to our hospital with stage 4 breast cancer, in great pain, and expecting imminent death. She went through our medical program while following the principles in BEATING CANCER WITH NUTRITION. V.G. had dramatic shrinkage of her tumors and went on to write THERE'S NO PLACE LIKE HOPE, which provided inspiration to thousands of her readers. V.G. lived another 14 years beyond her death sentence with relatively good quality of life before passing away. V.G. found her values and attitudes dramatically changed by her experience with cancer. Cancer is a life-threatening disease that presents to you the opportunity of turning your life into a masterpiece...just like V.G.

For more information on how your body can fight cancer go to GettingHealthier.com.

ENDNOTES

[1] . Klatz, R., et al., STOPPING THE CLOCK, Keats, New Canaan, CT, 1996

[2] https://jamanetwork.com/journals/jama/article-abstract/233614

[3] https://www.cochranelibrary.com/cdsr/doi/10.1002/14651858.CD003993.pub3/abstract

[4] . Oats, KK, et al., TIPS, p.347, Elsevier Press, Aug.1984

[5] . Wada, A., et al., J.Nat.Cancer Institute, vol.74, no.3, p.659, Mar.1985

[6] . Chretien, PB, et al., NY Acad Sci, vol.332, p.135, 1979

[7] . Shoham, J., et al., Cancer Immunol. Immunother., vol.9, p.173, 1980

[8] . Skotnicki, AB, Med. Oncol. & Tumor Pharmacother., Vol.6, no.1, p.31, 1989

[9] . Hays, EF, et al., Clin Immun. & Immunopath., vol.33, p.381, 1984

[10] https://www.ncbi.nlm.nih.gov/pubmed/25039497

[11] http://ar.iiarjournals.org/content/32/7/2747.short

[12] . European J.Ca., vol.30A, p.167, 1994

[13] . Oncology, vol,48, p.448, 1991

[14] . Oncology, vol.49, p.336, 1992

[15] . J.Biol.Regul.Homeostat.Agents, vol.9, no.2, p.52, 1995

[16] . J. Pineal. Research, vol.21, p.239, 1996

[17] . Anticancer Research, vol.18, p.1329, 1998

[18] . British J.Cancer, vol.71, p.854, 1995

Chapter 17

LIPIDS (FATS)

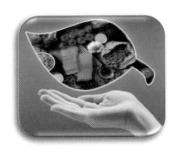

Science advances one funeral at a time.
Max Planck, PhD, Nobel prize in physics 1918

WHAT'S AHEAD
- ✓ Human health is highly dependent on the quality and quantity of our fat intake.
- ✓ Dietary fats form cell membranes and prostaglandins, playing a vital role in immune surveillance of cancer.
- ✓ Therapeutic fats, such as fish oil, borage oil, CLA, and shark oil can stimulate immune functions and help to slow cancer.

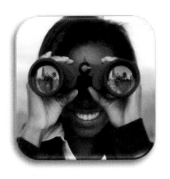

Fat is both essential for human health and potentially toxic. Most Americans eat too much fat, the wrong kind of fat, AND do not get enough of the essential fatty acids.

DIETARY FATS		
THERAPEUTIC	GOOD	BAD
fish, primrose, borage, MCT, lecithin, hemp, sesame, CLA, shark oil, rice bran, wheat germ, black currant	olive, safflower, soy, walnut, almond, pecan, avocado, cashew, coconut, palm, butter, pumpkin, canola	hydrogenated (trans), or oxidized (from fast food deep fryers), or not enough vitamin E, olestra

Dietary fats are another example of "it's not nice to fool with mother nature." Trans fats (aka hydrogenated fats) were created as a "superior" substitute for butter and lard. Turns out that trans fats, due to the slightly different 3-dimensional structure, are extremely toxic in the human system. Every 2% of kcal from trans fats yields a 20% increase in the risk of heart disease. Overcooking fats also corrupts the normal structure of fats. This chapter is not meant to dazzle or confuse you, but rather impress the reader with the inherent wisdom of eating your indigenous diet.

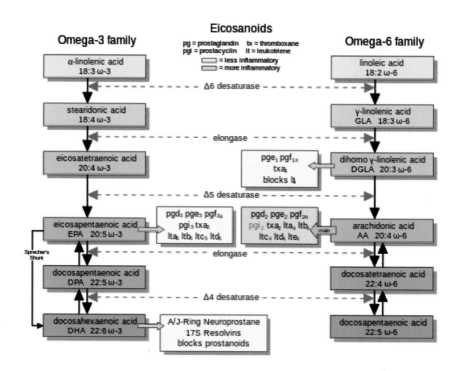

Dietary fats provide calories, help absorb fat soluble vitamins (A,D,E,K), and the required omega 6 oil (linoleic acid) and omega 3 oil (linolenic acid). Fats in the diet play an important role in cancer and health, because the fats in your diet become the fats in your cell membranes. Most importantly, fats in the diet provide precursors (raw materials to make) the prostaglandins, or eicosanoids.

In 1935 a researcher isolated a substance from seminal fluid from sperm and the prostate gland and coined it "prostaglandin". Later, researchers found that most animal cells make some prostaglandins. By 1971 researchers finally cracked the code on explaining how aspirin works through inhibiting certain prostaglandins. In 1982 a group of researchers earned the Nobel Prize in medicine for their work on prostaglandins. Prostaglandins, leukotrienes, and thromboxanes comprise the group of potent fatty acids known as eicosanoids. These are incredibly powerful bioregulators in the control of cancer.

CELLULAR ABNORMALITIES
THAT MAY GENERATE CANCER

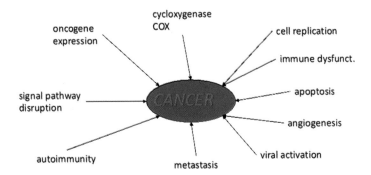

ALL ARE CONTROLLED BY EICOSANOIDS

Lieb, J, Prostaglandins Leukotriennes Essential Fatty Acids, vol.65, no.5, p.233, Nov.2001

Think of driving your car down a winding mountain road. At times you need to steer to the left. At other times you need to steer to the right to keep on the road. Same with eicosanoids, which become "bad" when your body steers the wrong direction.

Eicosanoids control inflammation, vasodilation, immune response, making of blood vessels (angiogenesis), cell replication, and the expression of cancer genes (oncogenes). Hence, "steering" your eicosanoids properly through diet becomes crucial for health and controlling cancer.

In general, the best way to "steer" your eicosanoids is by having well controlled blood glucose (because insulin affects this system), consuming reasonable amount of therapeutic fats (EPA, GLA, CLA, DHA) in the diet or as supplements, and limiting intake of omega 6 oils from corn, soy, safflower, etc. Avoid trans fats, aka hydrogenated fats. This field of eicosanoids dovetails with the field of cannabis research because we generate our own <u>cannabinoids when our eicosanoids</u> are properly regulated.[1]

Fish and krill oil 1-6 grams, including Vitamin A & Vitamin D
Augments immune system, improves production of favorable prostaglandin PGE-1, prevents metastasis of cancer cells by changing the stickiness of cells, improves cell membrane dynamics to augment nutrient absorption and toxin elimination

---

When the Senate Diet Goals were released by a blue-ribbon panel of nutrition experts in 1977, they included the recommendation to decrease fat intake from 40% of calories to 30%. Yet, experts then looked at the Greenland Eskimos, who get 60% of their calories from fat and practically no dietary fiber, yet mysteriously had little cancer or heart disease. Three factors saved these people from an otherwise disastrous diet:

1) genetic adaption, at least 40,000 years to adjust to this uniquely skewed diet

2) fish oil, which contains a very special and highly unsaturated fat, eicosapentaenoic acid (EPA)

3) no sugar in the diet, which helps the body make PGE-1, a healthy prostaglandin

EPA is, essentially, Nature's anti-freeze. In the Arctic regions of the world, the ocean temperature drops to below freezing, yet water-based life will explode at that temperature, like leaving out a water balloon on a sub-freezing night. So Nature provides the algae in the ocean with this special fat, EPA, which prevents freezing and bursting at low temperatures. Smaller fish eat the algae, and bigger fish eat

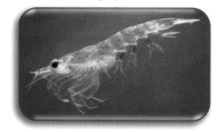

the smaller fish, until we have major concentrations of EPA in cold water fish, like cod, salmon, mackerel, tuna, krill and sardines. Krill is a small shrimp like creature that lives in the Antarctic Ocean and feeds on phytoplankton (small plants). During feeding season, one whale can eat up to 8000 pounds of krill daily. Krill oil has shown <u>impressive benefits in human</u> ailments, including cancer.[2]

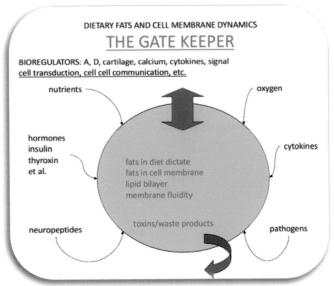

DIETARY FATS AND CELL MEMBRANE DYNAMICS

THE GATE KEEPER

BIOREGULATORS: A, D, cartilage, calcium, cytokines, signal cell transduction, cell cell communication, etc.

nutrients — oxygen

hormones insulin thyroxin et al.

cytokines

fats in diet dictate fats in cell membrane lipid bilayer membrane fluidity

toxins/waste products

neuropeptides

pathogens

IS FISH OIL AN ESSENTIAL NUTRIENT?

Convincing evidence that fish oil and fish can reduce[3]:

♦ heart disease
♦ sudden heart attack
♦ infant development abnormalities
♦ autoimmune disorders (i.e. lupus and multiple sclerosis)
♦ Crohn's disease
♦ cancer of breast, prostate, colon
♦ hypertension
♦ rheumatoid arthritis

EPA may help the cancer patient:

♦ Changes membrane fluidity. Cell membranes contain fats that are a direct reflection of our diet, including the unnatural hydrogenated fats found in Crisco and Pop Tarts. When we are talking about dietary fats, the old saying is literally true, "you are what you eat." Cell membranes that are fluid and flexible and allow the proper nutrients to pass into the cell will improve overall wellness, thus discouraging abnormal cell growths, like cancer. Cells that are flexible with EPA can squeeze down narrow capillaries to feed the distant tissue. Cells that are rigid with too much saturated or hydrogenated fat or having been "tanned" from too much sugar in the blood will not be able to move down narrow capillaries, like a car trying to get down a hotel hallway.

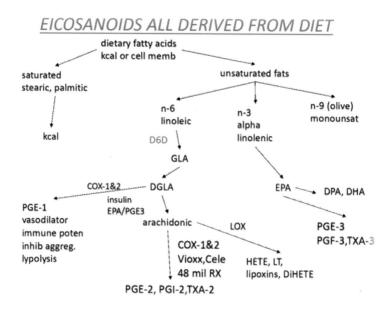

EICOSANOIDS ALL DERIVED FROM DIET

- ♦ Increase prostaglandin E-1, (PGE-1), which favors reducing the stickiness of cells for less risk of metastasis.[4] PGE-1 also bolsters immune functions, dilates blood vessels, elevates production of estrogen receptors, and provides other benefits for the cancer patient.
- ♦ Slows tumor growth in animals.[5] Slows tumor growth by altering protein synthesis and breakdown.[6]
- ♦ Augments medical therapies. EPA improves tumor kill in hyperthermia and chemotherapy by altering cancer cell membranes for increased vulnerability.[7] Increases the ability of adriamycin to kill cultured leukemia cells.[8] Tumors in EPA-fed animals are more responsive to Mitomycin C and doxorubicin (chemotherapy drugs).[9]

EPA and GLA were selectively toxic to human tumor cell lines while also enhancing the cytotoxic effects of chemotherapy.[10]

♦ **Reduces initiation, promotion, and progression of hormonally driven cancers**, such as breast, prostate, and ovarian. An EPA-rich diet significantly lowered the levels of estradiol, a marker for breast cancer, in the 25 women studied who were at risk for breast cancer.[11] Modulates estrogen metabolism for reduced risk and spreading of breast cancer.[12]

Fish oil may be as effective as any cancer treatment available. In a study examining end-stage refractory cancer patients who have exhausted all chemo and radiation options, fish oil supplements provided a substantial improvement in length of life and immune functions compared to placebo.

DOES FISH OIL SUPPLEMENTATION AS SOLE THERAPY IMPROVE OUTCOME IN PATIENTS WITH SOLID TUMORS?

"...consider alternative, less toxic treatment approaches..."

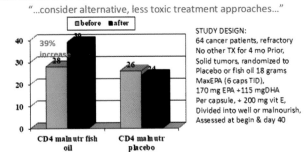

STUDY DESIGN:
64 cancer patients, refractory
No other TX for 4 mo Prior,
Solid tumors, randomized to
Placebo or fish oil 18 grams
MaxEPA (6 caps TID),
170 mg EPA +115 mgDHA
Per capsule, + 200 mg vit E,
Divided into well or malnourish,
Assessed at begin & day 40

"Omega 3 prolonged survival of all patients...resulted in significant ($p<0.025$) increase in survival for all patients compared with placebo"
Gogos, et al., Cancer, vol.82, p.395, 1998

CAN FISH OIL IMPROVE OUTCOME IN CANCER TREATMENT?

♦ anti-cachectic; prevents and reverses wasting syndrome[13]
♦ induces apoptosis (suicide) in cancer cells[14]
♦ upregulates immune function[15]
♦ reduces stickiness of cells to slow metastasis[16]
♦ improves insulin sensitivity, lowers blood glucose, impairs tumor angiogenesis (making of blood vessels)[17]

Flax oil is rich in alpha-linolenic acid (ALA), which is a precursor to EPA. While flax oil is cheaper and more palatable than fish oil, it requires enzyme conversion steps in the body to turn flax oil (ALA) into fish oil (EPA). ALA converts to EPA at about 4% the efficiency of giving fish oil. ALA <u>converts very poorly to EPA</u> if the diet has any meaningful amount (3% kcal) of polyunsaturated fats (e.g. soy, corn, safflower).[18] One study found that the more flax meal was fed to lab animals, the fewer and smaller were the metastatic tumors spreading from the implanted melanoma cancer.[19]

Borage or Evening primrose oil 1-6 grams (of which 9-20% is GLA)
Improves production of PGE-1, selectively toxic to tumor cells.

Our ancestors consumed a diet of range-fed animals who grazed on wild grain, nuts, and seeds. In these foods is a wide assortment of valuable fatty acids, including gamma linolenic acid (GLA), which is richly concentrated in the evening primrose and borage plants. Intake of GLA in modern Americans has dropped off substantially with the consumption of corn-fed beef, which is rich in linoleic acid that generates the tumor-promoting eicosanoids. The reason why range-fed lean buffalo was good for Native Americans, yet corn-fed high fat beef is not so good for modern Americans, is primarily the quality and quantity of fats in these two animals. A ratio of approximately 4:1 of EPA to GLA is very favorable for host defense mechanisms to fight off cancer.

> D6D (delta 6 desaturase): rate limiting step in arachidonic
> <u>MAKING THE CASE FOR GLA SUPPLEMENTATION</u>
>
> PRODUCTION OF GLA VIA D6D REDUCED VIA:
> ' aging
> ' stress (catecholamines)
> ' insulin resistance
> ' diabetes
> ' high glycemic diet
> ' alcohol
> ' viral & other infections
> ' trans fatty acids (partially hydrogenated oils)
>
> supplementation with GLA (borage, primrose) may be warranted in arthritis, CAD, cancer, autoimmune diseases, mental illness
>
> *Horrobin, DF, Prog.Lip.Res., vol.31, p.163, 1992*

We are able to make less GLA internally as we age, are exposed to stress and toxins, become compromised by disease, and eat hydrogenated fats--which describes millions of Americans. GLA in the diet helps to drive PGE-1, mentioned above, while also being selectively toxic to tumor cells.[20] GLA was selectively toxic to cultured human breast cancer cells.[21] In 21 human cancer patients with refractory (failed medical treatment) and untreatable malignancies, GLA was able to provide measurable benefits, including weight gain and reduction in tumor mass based on radiological evidence.[22]   When healthy and cancer cells are cultured with EPA and GLA, the healthy cells begin to outgrow the cancerous cells.[23]

One study found that when GLA was given to women with breast cancer in conjunction with Tamoxifen therapy, there was a 400% increase in the number of women who achieved complete response when compared to women just receiving Tamoxifen.

CAN GAMMA LINOLENIC ACID IMPROVE OUTCOME IN BREAST CANCER TREATMENT?

Kenny, FS, et al., Int.J.Cancer, vol.85, p.643, 2000
"Phase 2 study suggests high dose oral GLA to be a valuable new agent in tx ER/PR br.ca."

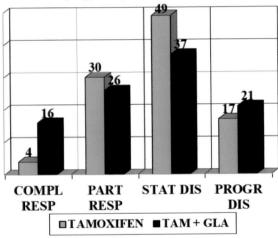

STUDY DESIGN:
47 elderly endocrine sensitive br.ca. patients received tamoxifen as 1st line tx (controls) compared to 38 matched patients receiving tamoxifen (20 mg od) + gamma linolenic acid 2.8 g/d. No drop outs & no side effects in 42% exper. group. Results at 6 mo. after beginning tx.
"Phase 2 study suggests high dose oral GLA to be a valuable new agent in tx ER/PR br.ca."

Shark oil 1-6 grams (20% alkylglycerols)
Improves the production of white (immune) and red (erythrocyte) cells from the bone marrow. Protects against the damaging effects of radiation therapy.

While it may be true that "sharks don't get cancer", it is more than cartilage that works in the shark's favor. Shark liver oil is rich in a compound called "alkoxyglycerols" or "alkylglycerols". The highest concentration of alkoxyglycerols in Nature are found in mother's milk, bone marrow, and shark liver oil, which is an

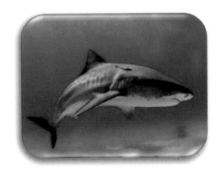

indication of the importance of this fatty compound. Bone marrow seems to derive the greatest benefit from alkoxyglycerol administration by nourishing the "cradle of all blood cells". Bone marrow is responsible for manufacturing red blood cells (hemopoiesis, or hematopoiesis) and white blood cells for the immune system.

Shark oil may help cancer patients

♦ Reversing anemia. Many cancer patients become anemic, or deficient in red blood cells, which leads to weakness and increased risk for infections. Shark liver oil encourages normal production of red blood cells, which is a much better strategy than giving high dose iron supplements.

♦ Protecting healthy tissue from radiation damage. In cancer patients given shark oil capsules before, during, and after radiation therapy, there was a 67% reduction in radiation-induced injuries. [24] Administration of shark oil capsules prior to radiation provided a 47% reduction in both severe (such as fistulas) and less harmful injuries from radiation therapy for cervical/uterine cancer. [25]

♦ May slow cancer growth. Shark oil was able to reduce cancer mortality in a human clinical trial. [26] Patients with uterine cancer who were given alkylglycerols throughout their cancer treatment had regression of tumor growth. [27]

Conjugated linoleic acid (CLA) 1-3 grams
Improves cellular communication to prevent and reverse cancer, stabilizes blood glucose, antioxidant and immune regulator.

"Close" is not good enough in either computer cables or fatty acid requirements in the human body. Americans often consume fats that are unhealthy, like hydrogenated fats, and are deficient in valuable fats, like CLA. A tiny difference in molecular structure, just like computer cables, can make a huge difference in whether this fat will help or hinder your cellular machinery.

CLA is a collection of unique "18 pin" fatty acids found primarily in the meat and milk of grazing animals, like beef and dairy. CLA is one of the more exciting recent developments in anti-carcinogenic fats. There is 300-400% more CLA in spring and summer milk and most Australian dairy products due to the availability of fresh green pasture land, which augments CLA content in the milk and fat of grazing animals.[28]

CONJUGATED LINOLEIC ACID (CLA)
a promising anti-cancer nutrient

☞ isomers of linoleic acid produced by bacteria in gut of ruminants
☞ only dietary sources are milk and meat of ruminants
☞ anticarcinogenesis (50%⇓ br.ca. animals), ⇑apoptosis
☞ immunomodulation: ⇓cachexia, ⇑cell mediated response
☞ body composition alteration: ⇑lean mass, ⇓fat mass
☞ antiatherosclerosis
☞ normalizes impaired glucose tolerance in diabetic rats
☞ antioxidant? reduced malondialdehyde, lipid peroxides
☞ ⇑vitamin A status

Whigham, LD, Pharmacological Research, vol.42, 6, p.503, 2000
Kelly, GS, Alternative Medicine Review, vol.6, no.4, p.367, 2001
Kritchevsky, D, British Journal Nutrition, vol.83, p.459, 2000
McDonald, HB, J.American College Nutrition, vol.19, no.2, p.111S, 2000

CLA is just another example of my first axiom of nutrition: "Nature knows best." Scientific studies in the past have come up with some conflicting results regarding diet and cancer. While most studies find that a high fat diet increases the risk for cancer, one recent study found that milk fat may protect women against breast cancer.[29] While most nutritionists argue that beef, in general, increases the risk for cancer, one prospective epidemiological study found that people consuming meat along with green or yellow vegetables on a daily basis had up to a 75% reduction in colon cancer incidence compared to those who consumed either meat or vegetables alone.[30]

CLA makes a good argument for humans consuming an omnivorous diet, since there is far more CLA, carnitine, EPA, taurine, and lipoic acid in animal foods than in plant foods. Dr. Weston Price was a dentist and, in my humble opinion, one of the more important nutritionists in history. He toured the world in the 1930s with his nurse-wife visiting numerous cultures and found many different diets. But he never found a group of people who were complete vegans...all of our ancestors ate some animal food. Maybe CLA is one of the nutrients that we need from a healthy mixed diet.

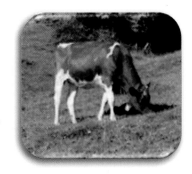

CLA is a unique fat, derived from linoleic acid, which is one of the two essential fatty acids in human nutrition, along with alpha-linolenic acid. CLA has unsaturated bonds in either the 9 & 11 position or the 10 & 12 carbon position. It comes in both "cis" (looks like a horseshoe) and "trans" (looks like a lightning bolt) isomers. Bacteria in the gut of ruminants, like cows, sheep, deer, and buffalo, can produce CLA. Yet there is more CLA in grilled beef than raw beef, so the cooking process also enhances CLA content.[31] Of all the nutrition factors studied, CLA is one of the more impressive at arresting cancer cells in animal and test tube studies.[32]

CLA may be able to help the cancer patient through:

◆ Cellular communication. Healthy cells know when to grow and when to stop growing and when to die. Cancer cells lose this crucial "knowledge". There is evidence that CLA assists in "signal transduction" pathways that tell cancer cells to commit suicide (apoptosis).

◆ Protection from toxins. CLA provided major cancer protection against toxins (like DMBA) in animal studies.[33] CLA may protect us from cancer by encouraging detoxification pathways.[34]

◆ Antioxidant. There is a large and growing list of non-essential dietary antioxidants, including CLA, ellagic acid, curcumin, quercetin, and epicatechin, which have shown remarkable abilities to slow down the oxidative damage, or the "rusting" that occurs constantly in all human beings.[35] Antioxidants can provide immune cells with a protective shield as they dowse the cancer cells with potent free radicals. Antioxidants can protect the healthy tissue of the patient, while the chemotherapy and radiation become more selective at destroying tumor tissue that does not absorb antioxidants as effectively as do healthy cells. However, other researchers found that if CLA is an antioxidant, then it does not protect cells in the usual antioxidant fashion, as shown by protection of cell membranes in culture.[36]

◆ Inhibitor of the cancer cascade. Cancer results from a series of deterioration steps in the cells. Cancer results after the stages of initiation, promotion, and progression have occurred. Hyperplasia (rapid cell growth) can worsen into metaplasia (above normal cell growth), can further deteriorate into dysplasia (abnormal cell growth), which can become neoplasia (new form of cell growth, or cancer). There are numerous pre-cancerous conditions, including fibrocystic breast disease, diverticulosis (colon), oral leukoplakia (mouth), cervical dysplasia (cervix), and benign prostatic hypertrophy (prostate), which all need more attention from both patient and physician. CLA seems to prevent this cancer cascade or avalanche from occurring. CLA also reverses cancer in animals even when they possess a genetic predisposition for cancer.[37]

♦ Neutralizing the potential damage from other fats. Animals fed varying levels of fat (10-20% by weight, similar to American diet) in the diet and different types of fat (corn oil vs lard) were protected against breast cancer when fed only 1% of the diet as CLA.[38]

♦ Generating unknown but valuable fatty acid by-products from the liver. In animal studies, CLA in the diet generated a unique collection of fats in the liver and outside of the liver.[39] Maybe CLA also provides the raw ingredient for the liver to make something very valuable in the body.

♦ Shuts down abnormal cell growth. CLA in test tube studies (in vitro) has shown a remarkable ability as a cytotoxic (kills cancer cells) and cytostatic (stops or slows cancer growth) agent in a wide variety of human cancers, including melanoma, colorectal, prostate, ovarian, glioblastoma (brain), mesothelioma, leukemia, and breast.[40]

♦ Some studies have found that CLA enhances immune functions[41] while another study showed no effect on the immune system while feeding the animals a diet that was 50% sucrose.[42] A high sugar diet is a much more powerful "vector" than micronutrients like CLA.

♦ Improve glucose and insulin levels. CLA manages to also make cells more sensitive to insulin, thus lowering insulin requirements and blood glucose levels. Researchers from Penn State and Purdue boldly state: "CLA may prove to be an important therapy for the prevention and treatment of non-insulin dependent diabetes mellitus." [43] Controlling blood glucose can provide the cancer patient with major assistance in slowing cancer growth.

♦ Timing is crucial. Studies with animals show that when CLA is fed to animals from post-weaning through puberty, it can prevent breast cancer from occurring even when a potent carcinogen is injected in the animals. However, if animals are deprived of CLA until the breast cancer occurs, then CLA must be fed to the animal for the remainder of its life in order to prevent a recurrence of cancer.[44] Apparently, CLA in young animals helps to ensure proper maturation of the mammary glands and to prevent the initiation and promotion phases of cancer.

For more information on how your body can fight cancer go to <u>GettingHealthier.com.</u>

PATIENT PROFILE

G.V. was originally diagnosed with breast cancer over 20 years ago. Then, at 58 G.V. was diagnosed with Stage 4 ovarian cancer. G.V. met with PQ after having been given a poor diagnosis by her oncologist. "I was not in a good place at that time." Deciding she was going to take a different route, G.V. decided to change her lifestyle and diet. She had always been reasonably healthy but made many small changes. G.V. started seeing a Functional Medicine doctor. Dietary changes included eating mostly organic produce, eating grass fed beef (about 3oz daily), juicing, bone broth, <u>ImmunoPower</u> and other supplements. Other lifestyle changes include adding daily healing prayer, reducing stress, simplifying her life, and intermittent fasting, usually 16 hours a day. Breakfast is often coffee with cinnamon and MCT oil. Her day often starts with a workout at the gym. Many of the minor health issues, noticed by PQ, have since disappeared including a persistent cough. G.V. is a grandmother with 5 grandchildren who keep her busy. She has started a non-profit to teach children and teens the benefits of sustainable gardening. PQ helped her change her life for the better and was very encouraging from the outset. G.V. is now in remission and is feeling better than she has in 20 years.

★★★★★ **AMAZON.COM**

<u>TESTIMONIAL:</u> **If you've been diagnosed with cancer, you owe it to yourself to pick up a copy today.**

"As an oncology nutritionist, I use the nutritional approaches described in Dr. Quillin's book on a daily basis. Science tells us they work. My patients' results show me they work." *Kim Dalzell, PhD, RD, LD*

★★★★★ **AMAZON.COM**

<u>TESTIMONIAL:</u> **Excellent resource and empowering.**

As an RD for 20 years , a former Oncology Nutritionist and a breast cancer survivor, I have bought so many copies of this book and given them away, I can't even count. Excellent resource, and empowering....it is another tool that I use to stay healthy. *Maureen Yorke*

ENDNOTES

1 https://www.sciencedirect.com/science/article/abs/pii/S0090698002000606

2 https://onlinelibrary.wiley.com/doi/full/10.1111/1541-4337.12427

3 . Connor, W., Am.J.Clin.Nutr., vol.71, no.1, p.171S, Jan.2000

4 . Gorlin, R., Archives Intern. Med., vol.148, p.2043, Sept.1988

5 . Karmali, RA, J. Nat. Cancer Inst., vol.73, p.457, 1984

6 . Wan, JM, et al., Fed. Amer Soc Exper Biol., vol.A350, p.21, 1988

7 . Burns, CP, et al., Nutrition Reviews, vol.48, p.233, June 1990

8 . Guffy, MM, et al., Cancer Research, vol.44, p.1863, 1984

9 . Cannizzo, F., et al., Cancer Research, vol.49, p.3961, 1981

10 . Begin, ME, et al., J.Nat.Cancer Inst., vol.77, p.1053, 1986

11 . Karmali, RA, J.Internal Med. suppl, vol.225, p.197, 1989

12 . Osborne, MP, et al., Cancer Investigation, vol.6, p.629, 1988

13 . Ross, JA, Curr.Opin.Coin.Nutr.Metab.Care, vol.2, no.3, p.219, May 1999

14 . Hardman, WE, J.Nutr., vol.132, no.11 supp, p.3508S, Nov.2002

15 . Kelley, DS, Nutrition, vol.17, no.7, p.669, Jul.2001

16 . Woutersen, RA, Mutat.Res, vol.443, no.1, p.111, Jul.1999

17 . Rose, DP, Nutr.Cancer, vol.37, no.2, p.119, 2000

18 https://www.sciencedirect.com/science/article/abs/pii/S0952327812000580

19 . Lin,Y., Cancer Letters, vol.124, pl.181, 1998

20 . Begin, ME, et al., Prostaglandins, Leukotriennes, and Medicine, vol.19, p.177, Aug.1985; see also Begin, ME, Anticancer Research, vol.6, p291, 1986

21 . Takeda, S., et al., Anticancer Research, vol.12, p.329, 1992

22 . Vander Merwe, CF, et al., British J.Clin.Practice, vol.41, p.907, 1987

23 . Begin, ME, et al., Prostaglandins, Leukotrienes & Medicine, vol.19, p.177, 1985

24 . Brohult, A., et al., Acta.Obstet.Gynecol.Scand., vol.56, p.441, 1977

25 . Brohult, A., et al., Acta.Obstet. Gynecol.Scand., vol.58, p.203, 1979

26 . Brohult, A., et al., Acta. Chem.Scand., vol.24, p.730, 1970

27 . Brohult, A., et al., Acta Obstet.Gynecol.Scand., vol.65, p.779, 1986; see also Acta.Obstet.Gynecol.Scand., vol.57, p.79, 1978

28 . Riel, RR, J.Dairy Sci., vol.46, p.102, 1963

29 . Knekt, P., et al., Br.J.Cancer, vol.73, p.687, 1996

30 . Hirayama, T., in DIET AND HUMAN CARCINOGENESIS, Joosens, JV , p.191, Elsevier, NY

31 . Sebedio, JL, et al., Biochimica et Biophysica Acta, vol.1345, p.5, 1997

32 . Ip, C., et al., Nutrition & Cancer, vol.27, no.2, p.131, 1997

33 . Ip, C., et al., Cancer Research, vol.54, p.1212, 1994

34 . Liew,C., et al., Carcinogenesis, vol.16, no.12, p.3037, 1995

35 . Decker, EA, Nutrition Reviews, vol.53, no.3, p.49, Mar.1995

36 . van den Berg,JJM, et al., Lipids, vol.30, no.7, p.599, 1995

37 . Ip, C., et al., Carcinogenesis, vol.18, no.4, p.755, 1997

38 . Ip, C., et al., Carcinogenesis, vol.17, no.5, p.1045, 1996

39 . Belury, MA, et al., Lipids, vol.32, no.2, p.199, 1997

40 . Shultz, TD, et al., Cancer Letters, vol.63, p.125, 1992; see also Visonneau, S., et al., J.Fed.Amer.Society Experimental Biology, vol.10, p.A182, 1996

41 . Cook, ME, et al., Poultry Science, vol.72, p.1301, 1993; see also Miller, CC, et al., Biochem.Biophys.Res.Commun., vol.198, p.1107, 1994

42 . Wong, MW, et al., Anticancer Research, vol.17, p.987, 1997

43 . Houseknecht, KL, et al., Biochem. Biophys.Res.Commun., vol.244, p.678, 1998

44 . Ip, C., et al., Nutrition & Cancer, vol.24, p.241, 1995

Chapter 18

MINERALS

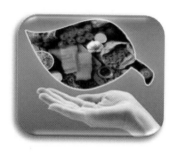

Look deep into nature, and then you will understand everything better.
Albert Einstein, PhD, Nobel laureate 1921

WHAT'S AHEAD

Minerals are inorganic substances that provide structure and enzyme activity in the human body.

✓ Since modern agriculture does not add trace minerals back to the soil, our food is becoming increasingly devoid of essential trace minerals.

✓ Selenium, zinc, chromium, boron and magnesium assist in cancer prevention and reversal.

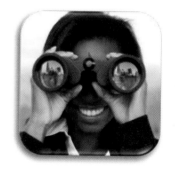

Minerals are the inorganic substances left over in ashes. Organic matter (based on carbon) can be burned. Minerals cannot be burned, although they will melt or vaporize at very high temperatures. Minerals in the human body work in many different arenas, from the structure provided by calcium in the bones and teeth, to the regulatory effect in enzymes provided by zinc, to the detoxifying effect from molybdenum and selenium. The body is a giant electrical battery, with minerals and water providing the conduction of electricity that keeps us healthy.

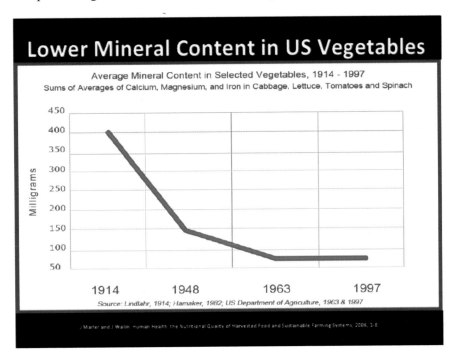

Of the 118 elements in the periodic table that form the building blocks for the entire planet earth, 83 are considered possibly useful or essential in human nutrition. Of which 16 have been classified as essential for humans, yet only 3 elements are added to the soil in modern agribusiness: NPK.

The remaining 86 minerals that are found in the human body are not added to the soil, thus are found in ever-diminishing amounts in our diet and bodies. This is not good. There are some crucial minerals involved in cancer prevention and reversal (such as selenium, zinc, chromium, boron, magnesium). Iron is a unique mineral, since it is the rate-limiting mineral in new growth, from red blood cells to spurring cancer growth. It is crucial that iron levels in your body and diet are ideal to recover from cancer and do not favor the growth of cancer.

ELEMENTS REQUIRED FOR HUMAN HEALTH

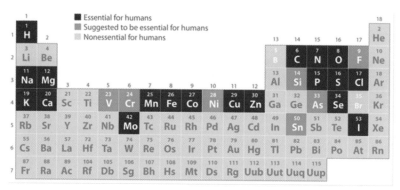

83 elements possibly involved in human and plant health
MAJOR ELEMENTS: H, C, O
major elements in agriculture: N, P, K
minor elements in agriculture: Mg, Ca, S, Na, Cl
trace elements in agriculture: B, Cu, Mn, Mb, Zn, I, Co, Se
64 elements remaining unimportant?

MINERAL (best form for absorption) suggested daily dosage
Primary functions in human body, anti-cancer activities

Calcium (glycinate, ascorbate) 100-500 mg
Electrolyte balance and cellular communication

Calcium is the most abundant mineral in the human body. While 99% of the body's calcium is bound up in the bones, the remaining 1% that is circulating is crucial for nerve and muscle function as well as regulating cell metabolism. There are calcium receptor sites on most cell membranes that help to control the flow of nutrients into and out of the cell as well as cell proliferation.

More than 5% of hospitalized cancer patients have elevated levels of calcium in the blood (hypercalcemia).[1] Abnormalities in calcium metabolism are common and usually caused by a <u>deficiency of vitamin D3 and/or K2</u>.[2] Hypercalcemia is not because the patient is eating too much calcium, but sometimes caused by either a parathyroid hormone substance secreted by the tumor or tumors cause the release of bone calcium to correct acidic conditions from the tumor. While some experts have argued that <u>too much calcium</u> increases the risk for health ailments[3], 1200 mg/d of calcium supplements for 4 years offered no risk and <u>some protection against prostate cancer</u>.[4] Actually, vitamins D3 and K2 play crucial roles in regulating calcium metabolism.

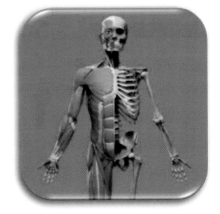

Best food sources of calcium include dairy products, dark green leafy vegetables (like kale and spinach), and cooked bones (like canned salmon). While the RDA of calcium is 800-1,200 milligrams daily, most Americans fall well short of this mark. Best supplemental sources of calcium are soluble forms of aspartate, citrate, lactate, orotate, etc. Calcium works with magnesium, sodium, potassium, and some ultra-trace minerals to regulate the "battery of life", or cell membrane potential that is crucial. Calcium also works with magnesium, phosphorus, protein, zinc, vitamin C, B-6, boron, and other nutrients to maintain proper mineralization of the skeleton, while dumping just the right amount of calcium into the bloodstream to keep the heart pumping merrily. Calcium metabolism is truly a delicate balancing act. <u>Calcium and magnesium levels in drinking</u> water are inversely associated with cancer risk.[5]

A low calcium intake increases the risk for colon cancer.[6] This effect may be due to calcium binding to bile acids in the colon to prevent carcinogenic by-products from forming, or due to the role calcium may play in regulating new cell growth. In human cancer patients, supplemental calcium increased the efficacy of radiation therapy to the bones and vulva.[7] Half of the patients with colon polyps (pre-cancerous growth) who were given supplements of calcium (1,250 mg as carbonate) had a significant decrease in cell proliferation. Calcium seems to tame the beast of hyperproliferative growth, like pre-cancerous growths.[8] Patients at high risk for developing colon cancer all showed a decrease in colon cell proliferation with calcium supplements.[9]

Magnesium (aspartate, glycinate) 400-800 mg
Essential for energy metabolism, low intake can spontaneously induce lymphoma

---

Magnesium is essential in at least 300 different enzyme reactions in the human body, including the pervasive conversion of ATP for energy. Think of magnesium as the essential "blasting cap" that allows the "dynamite" of ATP to release the essential energy for all of our metabolic needs. In animals, magnesium deficiency can spontaneously generate bone tumors and lymphomas. [10] Numerous studies show that a diet low in magnesium will increase the risk for various forms of cancer. Magnesium not only works with other electrolytes to maintain the sodium-potassium pump,

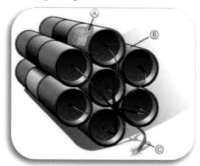

but also has a central role in regulating DNA synthesis and the cell cycle. Advanced patients of Covid appear to have common magnesium deficiencies with magnesium supplementation offering <u>improved clinical outcome</u>. [11]

The RDA for magnesium has been lowered from 400 mg daily to 350 mg, not because the evidence warranted this change but because few Americans came even close to consuming the RDA. The average American intake is 143-266 mg/day, which explains why low magnesium intake has been linked to an increase in the incidence of hypertension, heart disease, depression, migraines, fatigue, immune suppression, fibromyalgia, glaucoma, and much more. Best food sources of magnesium are kelp, whole grains, nuts, and molasses. Magnesium aspartate is the best absorbed form of magnesium supplements. Since magnesium is rarely added to soil in fertilizers, there are ever diminishing levels of magnesium in our soil and foods grown on that soil.

Symptoms of magnesium deficiency include depression, excess sweating, fatigue, frequent infections, and high blood pressure, which are all common in cancer patients. Many drugs, including diuretics, and alcohol cause a loss of magnesium from the system.

Potassium (citrate) 300-1000 mg
Essential ingredient for "electrolyte soup" that dictates healthy cell membrane

---

Potassium is the primary cation (positively charged ion) inside the human cell. Potassium is found primarily in plant foods, with the richest sources being avocado, banana, tomato, and potato. Meats and fish can provide a significant amount of potassium to the diet. Many studies show that a diet high in sodium (or salt) and low in potassium (found in plant food) increases the risk for heart disease and cancer, among other diseases.[12] Cells only exist due to the sodium/potassium pump which provides the voltage for the cell and life.

SODIUM POTASSIUM PUMP AND CANCER

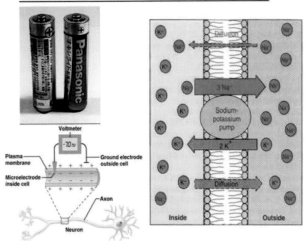

Excess sodium and deficient potassium change that voltage which lowers the amount of oxygen in the tissue to force healthy cells to become anaerobic (without oxygen) which then becomes a neoplasm--cancer. Potassium is crucial for nerve and muscle function and the conversion of glucose into glycogen for storage. The first symptom of potassium deficiency is usually weakness and fatigue.

SODIUM POTASSIUM PUMP AND CANCER

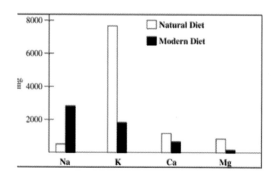

The FDA has set an upper limit of 99 mg allowed of potassium in tablet form due to the concerns that people with poorly functioning kidneys (less than 1% of the population) might suffer potassium overload. Meanwhile, 90% of the population do not get optimal amounts of potassium in the diet, especially in the right ratio with the other crucial electrolytes of sodium, calcium, and magnesium.

The range of potassium intake that is recommended by the RDA board is 1.9 to 5.6 grams daily. Up to 3 grams daily can be lost in perspiration and through the use of diuretics, like anti-hypertensive medication, alcohol, and coffee. While many American health authorities have crusaded against the use of salt (sodium) at the table, actually a deficiency of potassium, magnesium, and calcium are much more likely to be at fault in hypertension, heart disease, and various forms of cancer.

ICU physicians are finding that patients with advanced Covid are suffering from a deficiency of potassium and that replenishing that potassium improves outcome in the patient.[13] One of the basic guidelines for the Dr. Gerson anti-cancer diet was to increase potassium (through more plant food) and decrease sodium intake.

Zinc (yeast bound, picolinate, or chelate) 10-20 mg
Potent immune stimulant, essential in over 200 enzyme reactions in the body, including immune cell production and cell replication.

Zinc is the most multi-talented mineral in the body, participating in everything from sexual development, to immunity, to maintenance of nerve tissue, to the zinc-dependent antioxidant enzyme SOD (superoxide dismutase). Apoptosis, or programmed cell death, which is missing in cancer cells, may be regulated by zinc.[14] The average American consumes about 10 milligrams of zinc daily, which is well shy of the 15 mg RDA. Best food sources of zinc include shellfish, organ meats, meat, fish, pumpkin seeds, ginger root, nuts, and seeds.

Zinc is a crucial mineral for optimal immune functioning. Low zinc status will lower T-cell counts, reduce thymic hormone levels, and reduce reactions to pathogens and cancer. Reduced zinc levels and cancer are both common in the elderly. Zinc supplements of only 20 mg/day improved immune functions via jump starting the thymus gland in institutionalized elderly subjects.[15] Loss of appetite is one of the first symptoms of zinc deficiency. Zinc supplements usually restore appetite, which is a common problem in cancer patients. A low intake of zinc increases the risk for cancers of the esophagus[16], lung[17], and prostate.[18] Cadmium from tobacco and pollution will readily replace zinc in the prostate and may lead to benign prostatic hypertrophy (enlarged prostate) and prostate cancer.[19] <u>Zinc supplements have shown promise</u> at improving clinical outcome in Covid patients.[20] Doses were up to 220 mg/d.

Iron (yeast bound or chelate) 2-20 mg
Essential for red blood cell synthesis (hematopoiesis) to properly oxygenate tissues, essential for energy metabolism and immune cell production.

Iron has the narrowest "window of efficacy" of all nutrients. Too much or too little will create a health problem. Iron is one of the most commonly deficient nutrients in America and around the world.[21] When iron is bound to proteins, such as hemoglobin, there is no problem. But when unbound, iron causes free radical damage.

Iron can be hoarded by infecting bacteria and cancer cells to further invade healthy tissue. Iron deficiency can lead to suppressed immune function.[22] Therefore, iron supplements must be provided:
♦ in conservative doses: 5-25 mg/day
♦ in the most bioavailable chelated form
♦ in conjunction with multiple antioxidants to protect against the potential free radical damage from iron.

Iron is involved in:

♦ hemoglobin production for transporting oxygen to the cells
♦ myoglobin in the muscles
♦ oxidative burst as immune cells kill cancer cells
♦ one of the ways to induce cancer death through chemo drugs
♦ cytochromes for energy metabolism
♦ other iron-containing enzymes like NADH.

Symptoms of deficiency include anemia, lethargy, behavioral problems, poor body temperature regulation, reduced immunity and others. Since the RDA for iron is 10-15 mg and most Americans do not consume this amount, the right form (chelated) of iron supplements may be extremely valuable for people who also get adequate antioxidants at the same time to prevent the metabolic wrecking-ball effect from iron as a free radical.

SAFETY ISSUES

Many cancer patients are found to be anemic, which can precipitate the "knee jerk" response for recommending high doses of iron supplements, such as ferrous sulphate. This is a very bad idea. As mentioned above, iron supplements should be taken in conservative doses and in chelated versions, such as the heme form found in the blood. However, there is a prevailing opinion among scientists that iron can be harmful and even carcinogenic.[23] Some scientists are using an iron-binding drug, Deferoxamine, to treat cancer patients[24], as if we haven't learned our lesson after 30 years of trying to "starve the cancer out of the patient" with anti-metabolites, such as leucovorin.

Iron is an essential mineral for ALL OF LIFE, including humans and tumors. Unbound iron, which is caused by acidosis, is a serious issue that needs to be addressed by the health care practitioner. Iron can generate free radicals that can increase the risk for cancer. Donating blood often, especially among adult males, provides a win-win situation where the donor lowers their risk for cancer.[25]

Actually, iron is a rate-limiting growth nutrient for almost all forms of life, from a growing infant, to a tumor cell, to your lawn grass. The innate wisdom of the human body recognizes that iron can be a wrecking ball by generating free radicals and can also help the "enemy within" of any bacteria, yeast, or tumor cell to grow. That is why 99% of the iron in the human body is bound to hemoglobin or transferrin. It is

UNBOUND iron that creates the problem for humans. And why does the iron become detached from its normal escort?

The answer is: reduction in pH, or acidification of the body tissues, probably from fungal or cancer metabolites. Yeast give off a host of organic acids that reduce the pH in the human body and create problems, one of which is unbinding the iron. This effect is not unlike unhitching your prize stallion that normally does yeoman's work when attached to the plow or family wagon. But allowed to run amuck, the stallion (or iron) can do great damage. The key here is not to throw the baby out with the bathwater. We need adequate iron to extract energy from food (cytochrome system) and conduct aerobic metabolism (hemoglobin bringing oxygen to the cells). We also use iron as part of our immune system in killing invaders, such as cancer, with an oxidative burst.

Copper (chelate) 1-4 mg
Involved in several important enzyme reactions, including cytochromes for energy and superoxide dismutase for free radical protection.

Copper is important for the construction of tough connective tissues, which is how the body tries to envelop a tumor. Copper is crucial for energy metabolism via cytochrome c. Copper supplements have slowed tumor growth in animals.[26] Copper, via ceruloplasmin, helps to prevent the oxidation of fatty acids that can destroy DNA and cell membranes. The RDA of copper is 1.5-3 mg/day. Best sources of copper in the diet include organ meats, shellfish, and legumes.

Iodine (yeast bound, or kelp, or potassium iodide) 50-5000 mcg
Assists the thyroid gland in regulating basal metabolism, which is often low in cancer patients, is a selective toxin for disease-causing microorganisms in the gut.

Iodine is primarily involved in the thyroid hormone, thyroxin, which regulates basal metabolism throughout the body. Additionally, iodine seems to modify the effects of estrogen on breast tissue, thus reducing fibrocystic breast disease, which doubles the risk for developing breast cancer.[27] Low thyroid output is a fundamental insult in many women with breast cancer.[28]

There is an intriguing link between <u>iodine in the diet, thyroid function, and breast cancer</u>.[29] Breast tissue is a sponge for iodine. Larger breasts require more iodine to maintain health. <u>Many Americans are deficient in iodine, which is both essential for thyroid function</u> and is a powerful anti-microbial agent.[30] In primitive exploration times, adventurers would fill a helmet with soupy water from a river, then drop in iodine pills, which kill the parasites and bacteria but not the human who drinks this water. Iodine is an <u>amazing mineral in human metabolism and an unsung hero in the war on breast cancer</u>.[31]

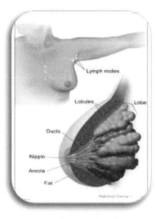

Seafood, especially kelp, provides the best sources of iodine. The fortification of salt with iodine (iodized salt) has been a classic example of public health measures that significantly reduced the incidence of goiter, or iodine deficiency expressed as clinical hypothyroidism. Yet, for various reasons, subclinical hypothyroidism is still rampant in the U.S. Iodine is also a selective toxin for microorganisms in the gut, helping to kill parasites and intestinal infections.

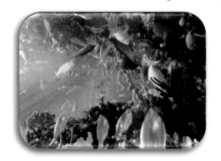

NOTE. If basal temperature is below 97.8 F, then medical assistance may be needed in the form of prescription thyroxin supplements to bolster basal metabolism.

Manganese (yeast bound or chelate) 1-2 mg
Essential mineral cofactor in various enzyme reactions, including an important antioxidant system of SOD (superoxide dismutase)

Manganese-deficient animals develop low insulin output and problems with the connective tissue and processing of fats. Recommended intake is 2-5 milligrams daily for adults, with over half the female population consuming less than adequate amounts of manganese.[32] Best food sources of manganese are whole grains, nuts, and fruits grown on manganese-rich (properly fertilized) soil. There are at least 3 different minerals, including manganese, copper, and zinc, that play a role in variations of the critical antioxidant enzyme system SOD.

Chromium (yeast bound, picolinate, GTF niacinate) 200-600 mcg
Essential mineral for proper energy metabolism, especially related to controlling blood sugar levels and preventing lean tissue wasting.

All of your 37 trillion body cells need energy all of the time. A primary source of energy is glucose/sugar. However, in order for glucose to enter the cell to be burned, there needs to be a healthy cell membrane, plus adequate insulin, plus GTF (glucose tolerance factor) which contains chromium. GTF could be the golden key that unlocks the cell membrane allowing glucose inside. Without adequate GTF in the body, insulin levels are raised, which can be disastrous. Glucose-dependent tissues, like the brain, lens of the eye, kidney, and lungs, suffer the most when blood sugar levels are abnormal.

Without proper burning of glucose in the cells, the body resorts to the backup energy substrates of protein (which causes lean tissue wasting, a.k.a. cachexia) and fat (which elevates levels of fats in the blood for increased risk of heart disease). GTF is also critical for immune functions and may even play a role in regulating cell growth.[33] Deficiencies of chromium in humans typically lead to impaired glucose metabolism, elevated blood fats, and peripheral neuropathy (tingling numbness in extremities).

An estimated 90% of the American population do not consume the minimum recommended intake of 50 micrograms daily. Researchers at the United States Department of Agriculture have estimated that up to 25% of heart disease in America could be prevented merely by consuming adequate quantities of chromium. Human subjects who took 400 micrograms daily of chromium supplements lost more fat and gained more lean tissue than those who took 200 mcg. Another study found that 600 mcg of chromium provided significant 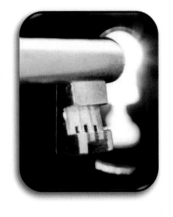 drops in fasting blood glucose in diabetics.[34] Several studies have shown that chromium supplements lower fasting blood glucose levels in normal healthy individuals.[35] Remember, a crucial strategy in fighting cancer is to starve the cancer of its favorite fuel, which is sugar.

Chromium is concentrated in whole grains and beans grown on chromium-rich soil, which is rare since chromium is not typically used in fertilizer. Brewer's yeast, liver, black pepper and molasses are decent sources of chromium. Chromium is stripped out of most food refining processes, including the milling of wheat to white flour and cane sugar to refined white sugar. 86% of Americans consume white bread rather than whole grain bread. The average American consumes 150 pounds per year of refined sugar, which increases the need for chromium while increasing the EXCRETION of chromium. The most bioavailable forms of chromium supplements are GTF, chromium picolinate, and chromium polynicotinate; the least bioavailable are the chromium salts like chromium chloride.

Selenium (yeast bound or selenomethionine) 200-600 mcg
Immune stimulant, detoxifying agent via glutathione peroxidase, may selectively control the growth of abnormal tissue

---

Selenium presents a fascinating story for the cancer patient. Until the 1960s, selenium was considered a toxic mineral by the FDA. An abundance of information beginning to appear in the 1960s showed that selenium may be one of our greatest allies in the war on cancer. Selenium is found in widely varying amounts in the diet, due to huge differences of selenium found in the soil. In places like South Dakota and Montana, there is so much selenium in the soil that animals grazing on the grass can develop selenium toxicity, or "blind staggers", which involves nerve and behavior problems. Some historians claim that General Custer's horses bolted on him in the Battle of Little 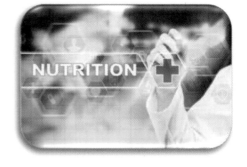 Bighorn because the horses were suffering from selenium toxicity. In Finland, where the selenium-deficient soil leads to a high incidence of cancer and heart disease, wheat flour is enriched with selenium just like we add iron to our white flour. About 70 million Chinese are affected by <u>low selenium in their soil and diet</u> with Keshan (heart disease), osteoarthritis, cancer and other health problems in abundance as a result.[36]

Wheat germ, seafood, and Brazil nuts are the best sources of selenium. The RDA is 70 micrograms, while the average intake is just over 100 micrograms. When lining up maps showing selenium content in the soil with cancer incidence, there is a strong link between low selenium intake and higher cancer risk.[37] In a recent prospective double-blind human intervention study, supplements providing 200 mcg of selenium were able to reduce the incidence of various cancers by up to 60%.[38] Selenium is a potent immune stimulator.[39]

Selenium-deficient animals have more heart damage from the chemo drug, adriamycin.[40] Supplements of selenium and vitamin E in humans did not reduce the efficacy of the chemo drugs against ovarian and cervical cancer.[41] Animals with implanted tumors were then treated with selenium and cis-platin (chemo drug) and showed a reduced toxicity to the drug with no change in anti-cancer activity.[42] Selenium supplements helped repair DNA damage from a carcinogen in animals.[43] Selenium was selectively toxic to human leukemia cells in culture.[44]

Garlic grown on selenium-enriched soil develops a unique anti-cancer activity. Selenium in a biological envelope, such as yeast-bound or selenomethionine, is the best absorbed and safest form of selenium.

SAFETY ISSUES

Selenium toxicity may begin as low as 1,000 mcg/day in some people, but toxicity is more common at about 65,000 micrograms (65 mg) for the average healthy adult.[45]

Molybdenum (yeast bound or chelate) 100-200 mcg
Essential mineral for detoxification pathways

Molybdenum functions as a mineral cofactor in hydroxylation enzyme reactions, such as uric acid and sulfite processing. When sulfites build up in the human system, cysteine metabolism is affected, which is crucial for detoxification. Most diets supply

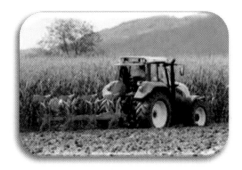

only around 50-100 micrograms daily of molybdenum and do not meet the safe and adequate levels of 75-250 mcg recommended by the Food and Nutrition Board. There is no RDA for molybdenum.

Large-scale farming does not add molybdenum to the soil as part of broad-spectrum fertilization, which further compounds the problems of common molybdenum deficiencies. It is found in vegetables that are grown on molybdenum-rich soil. Beans and organ meats are the best sources of molybdenum. This is an extremely non-toxic mineral, with animal studies showing that an intake of 100-5,000 milligrams per kilogram of diet is necessary to produce toxicity symptoms.[46]

Vanadium (vanadyl sulfate)20-60 mcg
Crucial mineral for controlling blood glucose

Vanadium is not added back to the soil in agri-business, and hence may be missing from the American diet, which typically contains 10-60 micrograms daily of vanadium.[47] When non-insulin dependent diabetics were supplemented with 100 milligrams daily (100,000 micrograms) of vanadyl sulfate, blood glucose levels dropped by 14%.[48] Vanadium in the form of vanadyl sulfate has shown promise in helping to control rises in blood glucose in human diabetics.[49] Toxicity may begin at 13 milligrams (13,000 micrograms) of vanadium daily. Best food sources of vanadium include mushrooms, shellfish, dill, parsley, and black pepper.

Boron (boric acid) 3-20 mg
Crucial for bone development, immune function, wound healing, hormone regulation, magnesium uptake, and more.[50]

Boron is a trace mineral found in small amounts in some soils around the world, but unpredictable in the food supply. While there is no RDA or estimated average requirement for boron, the scientific data says we are missing something in human nutrition. Gardeners, like myself, know the value of simply dissolving a tablespoon of borax in a 5 gallon bucket of water and distributing it around the garden can do wonders for plant growth. Human diets low in fruits and vegetables are nearly guaranteed to be deficient of boron. Borax/boron has been useful in the treatment of arthritis, due to its key role in magnesium metabolism.[51]

Boron shows promise as a powerful anti-cancer agent, with experts considering <u>boron a potential chemotherapeutic agent</u>.[52]

For more information on how your body can fight cancer go to <u>GettingHealthier.com</u>

PATIENT PROFILE: BEAT LUNG CANCER
E.M. was a 52-year old female with advanced lung cancer when she was admitted to our hospital. Her doctor back home had told her to "get her affairs in order." She began chemo and nutrition with excellent compliance in her new healthy diet. A year later, she was in complete remission. We planted a tree at our Celebrate Life Reunion in honor of her 5-year survival, the official definition of a cure by the American Cancer Society.

ENDNOTES

[1] . Heath, DA, Br., Med.J., vol.298, p.1468, 1989

[2] https://www.sciencedirect.com/science/article/abs/pii/S037851222030284X

[3] https://cebp.aacrjournals.org/content/11/8/719.short

[4] https://cebp.aacrjournals.org/content/14/3/586.short

[5] https://www.tandfonline.com/doi/abs/10.1080/00984100050027798

[6] . Sorenson, AW, et al., Nutr.Cancer, vol.11, p.135, 1988

[7] . Iakovkeva, SS, Arkh.Patol., vol.42, p.93, 1980

[8] . Wargovich, MJ, J.Am.Coll.Nutr., vol.7, p.295, 1988

[9] . Buset, M., et al., Cancer Res., vol.46, p.5426, 1986

[10] . Seelig, MS, in ADJUVANT NUTRITION IN CANCER TREATMENT, p.284, Quillin, P (eds), Cancer Treatment Research Foundation, Arlington Heights, IL 1994

[11] https://www.tandfonline.com/doi/full/10.1080/07315724.2020.1785971

[12] . Jansson, B., Cancer Detect.Prevent., vol.14, p.563, 1991

[13] https://journals.sagepub.com/doi/full/10.1177/0004563220922255

[14] . Cousins, RJ, in PRESENT KNOWLEDGE IN NUTRITION, p.293, ILSI, Washington, 1996

[15] . Boukaiba, N, et al., Am.J.Clin.Nutr., vol.57, p.566, 1993

[16] . Barch, DH, J.Am.Coll.Nutr., vol.8, p.99, 1989

[17] . Allen, JI, et al., Am.J.Med., vol.79, p.209, 1985

[18] . Whelen, P., et al., Br.J.Urol., vol.55, p.525, 1983

[19] . Feustel, A., et al., Urol.Res., vol.12, p.253, 1984

[20] https://www.sciencedirect.com/science/article/pii/S0306987720309695

[21] . Yip, R., et al., in PRESENT KNOWLEDGE IN NUTRITION, p.277, ILSI, Washington, 1996

[22] . Dallman, PR, Am.J.Clin.Nutr., vol.46, p.329, 1987

[23] . Reizenstein, P., Med.Oncol. & Tumor Pharmacother., vol.8, no.1, p.229, 1991

[24] . Donfrancesco, A, et al., Acta Haematol., vol.95, p.66, 1996

[25] https://academic.oup.com/jnci/article/100/14/996/917996

[26] . Sorenson, RJ, in TRACE SUBSTANCES IN ENVIRONMENTAL HEALTH XVI, U.Missouri 1982

[27] . Ghent, WR, et al., Can.J.Surg., vol.36,p.453, 1993

[28] . Callebout, E., in THE DEFINITIVE GUIDE TO CANCER, Diamond, J. (eds), p.116, Future Medicine, Tiburon, 1997

[29] https://breast-cancer-research.biomedcentral.com/articles/10.1186/bcr638

[30] http://www.svhi.com/newsletters/2006/slf-012006.pdf

[31] https://www.optimox.com/pdfs/IOD02.pdf

[32] . Keen, CL, et al., in PRESENT KNOWLEDGE IN NUTRITION, p.339, ILSI, Washington, 1996

[33] . Stoecker, BJ, in PRESENT KNOWLEDGE IN NUTRITION, p.347, ILSI, Washington, 1996

[34] Mossop, RT, Central African J.Med., vol.29, p.80, 1983

[35] Anderson, RA, et al., Metabolism, vol.32, p.894, 1983

[36] https://www.ncbi.nlm.nih.gov/pmc/articles/PMC3967180/

[37] . Schrauzer, GN, in VITAMINS, NUTRITION, AND CANCER, p.240, Karger, Basel, 1984

[38] . Clark, LC, et al., J.Amer.Med.Assoc., vol.276, p.1957, 1996

[39] . Kiremidjian-Schumacher, L., et al., Environmental Res., vol.42, p.277, 1987

[40] . Coudray, C., et al., Basic Res.Cardiol., vol.87, p.173, 1992

[41] . Sundstrom, H., et al., Carcinogenesis, vol.10, p.273, 1989

[42] . Ohkawa, K., et al., Br.J.Cancer, vol.58, p.38, 1988

[43] . Lawson, T., et al.,Chem.Biol.Interactions, vol.45, p.95, 1983

[44] . Milner, JA, et al., Cancer Research, vol.41, p.1652, 1981

[45] . Hathcock, JN, in MICRONUTRIENTS AND IMMUNE FUNCTIONS, vol.587, p.257, NY Acad.Sci., 1990

[46] . Nielsen, FH, in PRESENT KNOWLEDGE IN NUTRITION, p.359, ILSI, Washington, 1996

[47] Harland, BF, et al., J.Am.Diet.Assoc., vol.94, p.891, 1994

[48] Cohen, N., et al., J.Clin.Invest., vol.95, p.2501, 1995

[49] Brichard, SM, et al., Trends Pharmacol.Sci., vol.16, p.265, 1995

[50] https://www.ncbi.nlm.nih.gov/pmc/articles/PMC4712861/#:~:text=As%20the%20current%20article%20shows,magnesium%20absorption%3B%20(5)%20reduces

[51] https://journals.sagepub.com/doi/abs/10.1177/026010600401700403?journalCode=naha

[52] https://www.ncbi.nlm.nih.gov/pmc/articles/PMC3967180/

Chapter 19

ENZYMES

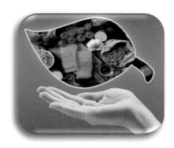

Americans are digging their graves with spoons, knives and forks.

WHAT'S AHEAD

Enzymes are organic catalysts that either tear apart molecules or put them together. Life would be impossible without enzymes.

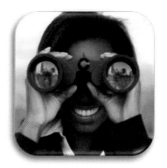

✓ Taking enzyme supplements with your meal can help to better digest and absorb food

✓ Taking enzyme supplements in between meals can help to dissolve the coating around the cancer that makes it invisible to the immune system.

Enzymes are organic catalysts that speed up the rate of a chemical reaction. In simple terms, enzymes in the body either "glue" stuff together (called conjugase) or tear stuff apart (called hydrolase). Without enzymes, life on earth could not exist. Enzymes wear out and are still a great source of mystery to leading researchers.

In the 1920s, scientists in Germany found that cancer patients seemed to lack a factor in the blood. They began injecting animal tumors with pineapple juice extract, which contains the proteolytic enzyme bromelain, and watched a measurable shrinkage or disappearance of many cancers in animals.

Nick Gonzalez, MD was instructed to find the flaws in the protocol advocated by Donald Kelly, DDS for treating cancer using proteolytic enzymes. Dr. Gonzalez not only was unable to find flaws, but became so enthused about the Kelly Protocol that Gonzalez used it

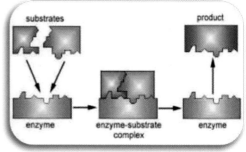

for decades to treat pancreatic cancer patients, who are considered poor prognostic. [1]   Given the extremely poor results from conventional oncologists using chemo and radiation for pancreatic cancer, it is noteworthy the many successes achieved by Dr. Gonzalez using enzymes and other non-toxic therapies. [2]   As expected, the pharmaceutically edited Wikipedia lists Dr. Gonzalez as "quack and fraud" and erroneously cites poor results from Dr. Gonzalez patients. Dr. Gonzalez died mysteriously at age 67 in otherwise good health in 2015.

Certain enzymes when taken orally as pills can reduce the toxicity of chemo and radiation, while extending the quality and quantity of life for most cancer patients. The German FDA has approved the use of injectable forms of enzymes, which are 100 times more potent than taking oral enzymes which must pass through the gut into the bloodstream.

To make the field of enzymes in cancer treatment even more interesting, tumors generate their own enzymes to invade the body's tissues. Oncologists find that tracking proteolytic enzymes (cysteine, serine, aspartic, metalloproteinases) can help monitor the extent of the cancer.

> **Enzymes (especially protease) 50,000 USP units or 200-1000 mg**
> Break up circulating immune complexes to improve efficiency of immune system, erode protective coating on tumor, break down toxic by-products of tumor metabolism that create weight loss and depression in cancer patients.

There are approximately 1,300 different enzymes produced in most human cells. With about 100,000 chemical reactions occurring per second in each 37 trillion cells in the adult human body, the importance of enzymes cannot be overstated. Without hydrolase enzymes in your gut, the digestion of food could not occur. Our body makes digestive enzymes to break down large food particles into usable molecules:

◆ proteins are digested into amino acids by the action of proteases, including trypsin and chymotrypsin
◆ starches are digested into simple sugars by the action of amylase
◆ fats are digested into fatty acids and glycerol by the action of lipase.

Our ancestors ate a diet high in uncooked foods. Cooking food denatures enzymes, like changing the white on an egg from waxy to white when it is cooked. It makes no difference whether you cook the food over a fire, on the barbeque, in the microwave oven, or fry it on the stovetop...all forms of heat denature enzymes. All living tissue contains an abundance of hydrolase enzymes as part of the lysosomes, or "suicide bags", which are there to mop up cellular debris and destroy invading organisms. When our ancestors ate this diet high in uncooked food, they were receiving a regular infusion of "enzyme therapy" as a lucky by-product. These hydrolytic enzymes would help to digest the food, and about 10% of the unused enzymes would end up crossing through the intestinal wall into the blood stream.

Undernutrition without malnutrition <u>extends lifespan</u> in primates and probably in humans.[3] Why this occurs is less obvious. Many good European studies support the use of digestive enzymes as a critical component of cancer treatment. Your mouth, stomach, and intestines will make a certain amount of enzymes to digest your food into smaller molecules for absorption through the intestinal wall into the bloodstream. Enzymes absorbed into the bloodstream help to break up immune complexes, expose tumors to immune attack, and assist in cell differentiation. People who eat less food may live longer because they are able to absorb a certain percentage of their unused digestive enzymes, which then have many therapeutic benefits. Indeed, as far back as 1934, an Austrian researcher, Dr. E. Freund, found that cancer patients do not have the "solubilizing" tumor-destroying enzymes in their blood that normal healthy people have.

The vast majority of cancer patients are older people, who have demonstrated a reduced output of digestive enzymes. Raw foods, which are high in hydrolytic enzymes, may sometimes help cancer patients.

There are 30 years of good research from Europe showing that enzyme therapy may help cancer patients. Digestive enzymes can:

- reduce tumor growth and metastasis in experimental animals [4]
- prevent radon-induced lung cancer in miners [5]
- improve 5-year survival in breast cancer patients. Stage I at 91%, stage II at 75%, and stage III at 50% [6]
- bromelain (enzyme from pineapple) inhibited leukemic cell growth and induced human leukemia cells in culture to revert back to normal (cytodifferentiation) [7]
- reduce the complications of cancer, such as cachexia (weight loss), pain in joints, and depression
- reduced the secondary infections from certain chemo and radiation methods, especially bleomycin-induced pneumo-toxicity.[8]

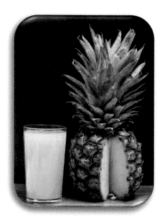

Proteolytic enzymes (proteases), such as bromelain from pineapple, seem to dissolve the "stealth" coating that keeps tumors invisible from the cancer patient's "radar". Proteases also break up "circulating immune complexes", which makes the immune system more efficient against cancer. Proteases have recently been found to be part of the body's complex regulation and communication system, possibly helping to induce apoptosis (suicide) in cancer cells.[9] Best food sources of these proteolytic enzymes are raw pineapple, papaya, mango, and kiwi.

Wobenzym is a unique clinically-tested product from Germany with a proprietary blend of various plant and animal-derived digestive enzymes, coupled with rutin (a bioflavonoid) all packaged in an enterically coated pill to survive the acid bath of the stomach and move into the intestines for absorption.

Serrapeptase (technically Serrato Peptidase) is a proteolytic enzyme produced by bacteria in the gut of silkworms. Serrapeptase has been studied and used extensively in Europe and Asia for over a quarter century, and seems to reduce swelling and digest unnecessary fibrin in the body. In one study, 70 women with fibrocystic breast disease were randomly divided into either treatment with serrapeptase or placebo group. The serrapeptase group had a greater reduction in breast swelling and pain than the placebo group.[10]

Enzymes are measured in USP (United States Pharmacopeia) comparison to pancreatic extract. One of the functions of the pancreas is to make digestive enzymes. A 4x label on your enzymes means "4 times the potency of pancreatin USP". Therefore, 500 mg of 4X pancreatin is equal in digestive capacity to 2,000 mg of pancreatin USP. 50,000 USP units is a good target for any given meal or in between meal dosage.

Enzymes taken with a meal will help to digest the food, but will not be absorbed into the bloodstream to help fight the cancer. About 10% of enzymes taken on an empty stomach will be absorbed into the bloodstream to help fight the cancer. Enzymes are one of the more fragile molecules in nature, easily denatured (change in 3 D shape) by temperatures above 108 F.

PATIENT PROFILE

MAC was initially diagnosed with 2B breast cancer in 2009. PQ had a phone consultation with MAC in May 2015 at a time when she was very weak. Though she is not feeling 100% and experiences nausea and dizziness due to her medication, she is leading a more normal life. She is currently taking many supplements including selenium, 8000 IU Vitamin D, maitake mushroom, NAC, olive leaf extract, alpha lipoic acid, CO10 and a pea-based protein drink daily. She believes her daily juicing contributed significantly to her recovery. She is currently in remission.

For more information on how your body can fight cancer go to GettingHealthier.com

ENDNOTES

[1] https://www.tandfonline.com/doi/abs/10.1207/s15327914nc330201

[2] http://www.alternative-therapies.com/at/web_pdfs/gonzalez1.pdf

[3] https://europepmc.org/article/med/10885801

[4]. Ransberger, K, et al., Medizinische Enzymforschungsgesellschaft, International Cancer Congress, Houston 1970

[5]. Miraslav, H., et al., Advances in Antimicrobial and Antineoplastic Chemotherapy, proceedings from 7th international congress of chemotherapy, Urban & Schwarzenberg, Munchen, 1972

[6]. Rokitansky, O., Dr. Med., no.1, vol.80, p.16ff, Austria

[7]. Maurer, HR, et al., Planta Medica, vol.54, no.5, p.377, 1988

[8]. Schedler, M., et al., 15th International Cancer Congress, Hamburg, Germany, Aug.1990

[9]. Mynott, TL, et al., J. Immunology, vol.163, no.5, p.2568, Sept.1, 1999

[10]. Kee, WH, Singapore Med.J., vol.30, no.1, p.48, 1989

Chapter 20

VITAMINS

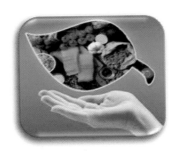

Natural forces within us are the true healers.
Hippocrates, father of modern medicine, circa 370 BC

<u>WHAT'S AHEAD</u>
Many vitamins are essential in the human diet, but are deficient in the typical American diet. Vitamins in therapeutic levels can take on meta-vitamin functions.
- ✓ Some vitamins, such as vitamin E succinate and K, may help to destroy tumor cells directly
- ✓ Some vitamins, such as C and E succinate, can become selectively toxic to tumors
- ✓ Some vitamins, such as D, A, E, K2, and B6, improve immune functions to help the body recognize and destroy cancer cells.

> **Vitamin A, retinol**
> Down-regulates cancer at genetic level, immune stimulant, improves cell differentiation process, helps with cell-to-cell communication.

Along with iron and iodine, vitamin A is one of the most common micronutrient deficiencies in the world. Around the world, an estimated 500,000 people each year go permanently blind because of clinical vitamin A deficiency. Vitamin A was the first micronutrient to be recognized for its role in preventing cancer. Vitamin A is one of the most multi-talented of all substances in human nutrition and plays a key role in preventing and reversing cancer. While vitamin A and beta-carotene are considered interchangeable, more recent evidence shows that these two nutrients have some overlapping functions and some distinctly different functions. A drug analog of vitamin A (all trans retinoic acid) has become a near cure all for acute promyelocytic leukemia, with one study showing a 96% cure rate.[1] Some companies use an emulsified vitamin A so that it stays in the blood stream longer, which may be important for extremely high doses of A (>100,000 iu/day) in cancer patients.

All of the known functions of vitamin A relate either directly or indirectly to the cancer patient:[2]

♦ **Cell division.** Billions of times each day, cells divide in the precarious process of cell division, i.e. proliferation or hyperplasia. Without vitamin A, this fragile process can easily turn into cancer, or neoplasia. Vitamin A is crucial for cancer prevention.[3] Vitamin A deficiency may be one of the primary insults leading to lung cancer.[4] There are probably binding sites on the human DNA for vitamin A. Researchers found that one of the most common cancers in Third World countries, cervical cancer, was linked to Human Papilloma Virus, which was then linked to shutting off the cancer-protective gene, called p53, which was then linked to a low intake of vitamin A. Essentially, vitamin A keeps the p53 active and protecting our DNA against cancer, even from viral attack.

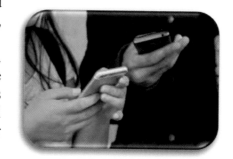

♦ **Cell-to-cell communication,** a.k.a. gap junction. Cells communicate via a text message system of ions floating in and out of cell membrane pores. This intercellular communication helps to maintain cooperation and coordination of cell functions. Without vitamin A, the communication system becomes distorted, and cancer can arise.

♦ Maintenance of epithelial tissue, or skin. The vast majority of cancers, including lung, breast, colon, and prostate, all arise from the epithelial tissue and are called carcinomas. Other categories of cancers include: leukemia (cancer of the bone marrow that produces red & white cells), lymphoma (cancer of the lymph cells and glands), and sarcomas (cancers of the structural tissue).[5] When the body is deprived of vitamin A, skin (epithelial) cancer is more likely to result. Giving therapeutic doses of vitamin A has been shown to slow down and reverse some forms of cancer.

♦ Immune stimulant.[6] Vitamin A deficiency brings changes in the mucosal membranes, changes in lymphocyte sub-populations, and altered T- and B-cell functions.[7] There are many studies linking vitamin A supplements to the curing of measles.[8] Vitamin A supplements brought a 19% reduction in respiratory infections in children.[9] HIV-positive pregnant women with the lowest quartile of serum vitamin A had a 400% increase in the risk of transmitting their HIV virus to their unborn infant.[10]

♦ Anti-cancer activity. Vitamin A supplements as sole therapy in patients with unresectable (cannot be surgically removed) lung cancer measurably improved immune functions and tumor response.[11] Vitamin A, and not beta-carotene, improved lymphocyte levels and reduced complications after surgery in lung cancer patients.[12] In

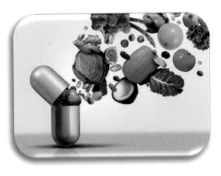

patients treated for bladder cancer, the incidence of recurrence was 180% higher in patients who consumed the lowest quartile of vitamin A in the diet.[13] High doses of vitamin A (200,000 iu/week) were able to reduce damaged and potentially cancerous mouth cells by 96%.[14] Vitamin A and its synthetic analogues have been shown to improve cancer treatment in oral leukoplakia, laryngeal papillomatosis, superficial bladder carcinoma, cervical dysplasia, bronchial metaplasia, and preleukemia.[15] Vitamin A supplements of 300,000 iu per day were provided in a placebo-controlled trial with 307 patients with stage I non-small-cell lung cancer. 37% of the treated group experienced a recurrence, while 48% of the non-treated group had a recurrence, thus bringing a 25% reduction in tumor recurrence, when used as the sole therapy.[16]

SAFETY ISSUE

Up to 1 million iu of vitamin A per day has been given for 5 years without side effects in European cancer clinics.[17] One study found that women taking as little as 10,000 iu/day during pregnancy had a slightly elevated risk for having a child with birth defects (teratogenicity).[18] Another study from the National Institutes of Health found no increase in birth defects in women taking 25,000 iu/day of vitamin A. An FDA biochemist, John Hathcock, PhD, states that toxicity with vitamin A at these low levels mainly involves people with confounding medical conditions, including compromised liver function.[19]

Cancer clinics in Europe often administer up to 2.5 million iu/day of vitamin A in emulsified form for several months under medical supervision. While these doses are not recommended without medical supervision, it shows the relative safety of vitamin A in the general population. Giving at least 300,000 iu per day of retinol palmitate in 138 lung cancer patients for at least 12 months created self-terminating unremarkable symptoms in less than 10% of these patients and only caused interruption of treatment in 3% due to symptoms that were potentially related to vitamin A excess. Upset stomach (dyspepsia), headache, nosebleeds, and mild hair loss were the most common and self-limiting symptoms.

Since primitive meat-eating populations would usually eat the liver of the animal first, which is the most concentrated source of pre-formed vitamin A, descendants of carnivorous people probably have a much greater tolerance and need for higher doses of A. By increasing the intake of vitamin E, many people will be able to avoid toxicity from high doses of vitamin A, since it is the lipid peroxide products from A that can cause damage to the liver. Vitamin E prevents lipid peroxidation.

**PREGNANT WOMEN SHOULD NOT USE
HIGH DOSES OF VITAMIN A**

Beta-carotene 15 mg (=25,000 iu) as mixed natural carotenoids
Immune stimulant, helps with cell-to-cell communication

It is easy to appreciate the beauty of carotenoids on a crisp, fall day with the autumn foliage at its peak. Carotenoids are usually pigmented substances produced by plants to assist in photosynthesis and to protect the plant from the damaging effects of the sun's radiation. Of the 800 or so carotenoids that have been isolated, the most famous are beta-carotene, alpha-carotene, lutein, zeaxanthin, lycopene, and beta-cryptoxanthin. Most carotenoids are pigmented molecules that are red, yellow, or orange in color. A few carotenoids, such as phytoene and phytofluene, are colorless.

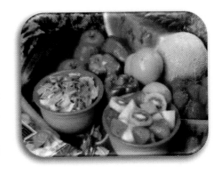

Over 200 epidemiological studies[20] show that a diet rich in fruit and vegetables will lower the risk for a variety of cancers. Of the 15% of annual lung cancer patients who are not smokers, which totals over 22,000 deaths per year, fruits and vegetables can provide major protection against lung cancer.[21]

Beta-carotene and other carotenoids have been thoroughly reviewed regarding their role in cancer and it has been found: "...carotenoids exert an important influence in modulating the actions of carcinogens."[22] Beta-carotene has been shown to play a major role in the "telegraph"-like communication between cells that prevents or reverses abnormal growths. This "gap junction communication" is one of many reasons why beta-carotene protects us from cancer.[23] Beta-carotene selectively inhibited the growth of human squamous cancer cells in culture.[24] Beta-carotene and canthaxanthin provided significant protection in animals against the cancer-causing effects of radiation.[25]

Carotenoids may partially compensate for the "sins" of our unhealthy lifestyles. In one study, researchers from the National Cancer Institute and Harvard tracked over 47,000 healthy individuals and found that lycopenes, even from pizza sauce, were protective against prostate cancer.[26] Other studies have found that beta-carotene supplements can reverse the pre-cancerous condition (oral leukoplakia) brought about by chewing betel nut,[27] which is a Third World version of chewing tobacco.

Beta-carotene affects the cancer process in a variety of ways:

♦ alters the adenylate cyclase activity in melanoma cells in culture, which affects cell differentiation and, thus, whether a cell will turn cancerous or not[28]

♦ potent anti-oxidant, [29] which spares immune cells in the microscopic "war on cancer" and protects the healthy prostaglandins

♦ provides a certain level of tumor immunity in mice inoculated with cancer cells[30]

♦ protects the DNA against the damaging effects of carcinogens[31]

♦ according to studies by Food and Drug Administration researchers, beta-carotene protects against the cancer-causing effects of a choline deficient diet in animals

♦ once cancer has been initiated, either chemically or physically, beta-carotene inhibits the next step in the cancer process of neoplastic transformation[32]

♦ there is a synergistic benefit of using vitamin A with carotenoids in patients who have been first treated with chemo, radiation, and surgery for common malignancies[33]

♦ beta-carotene and vitamin A together provided a significant improvement in outcome in animals treated with radiation for induced cancers[34]

♦ carotenoids (from Spirulina and Dunaliella algae) plus vitamin E and canthaxanthin were injected in animal tumors, with the result being complete regression, as mediated by an increase in Tumor Necrosis Factor (TNF) in macrophages in the tumor region[35]

♦ in 20 patients with mouth cancer who were given high doses of radiation and chemo, beta-carotene provided significant protection against mouth sores (oral mucositis) induced by medical therapy, although there was no significant difference in survival rates[36]

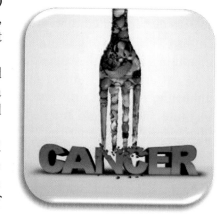

♦ in animals, beta-carotene provided cancer protection against a carcinogenic virus, which would normally damage the DNA[37]

Betatene is a special, mixed carotenoid extract from Dunaliella algae that has been shown in scientific studies to potently inhibit the development of breast tumors in animals.[38] Betatene consists of a rich mixture of various carotenoids, primarily naturally-occurring beta-carotene, along with smaller amounts of lycopene, alpha-carotene, zeaxanthin, cryptoxanthin, and lutein.

BETA-CAROTENE CAUSES LUNG CANCER?

SAFETY ISSUES

There is virtually no toxicity to beta-carotene at any dosage, other than the mild pigmentation (carotenemia) that occurs in the skin region.[39] With our primitive analytical tools, scientists isolated the most likely champion of the carotenoids, beta-carotene, and conducted several human intervention trials funded by the National Cancer Institute to examine whether beta-carotene would reduce the incidence of lung cancer in heavy smokers. It didn't.[40] And in two studies, the beta-carotene supplemented groups had slightly elevated incidences of lung cancer. The press loved this huge controversy and made sure that everyone knew about it. Unfortunately, only a small portion of the story was told.

Issues not covered by the press included:

♦ Those individuals who had the highest SERUM beta-carotene at the start of these two studies had a lower incidence of lung cancer. Beta-carotene ABSORBED does indeed reduce the risk of suicidal lifestyles, such as smoking.

♦ Prominent researchers in nutrition and cancer have published papers showing that antioxidants, like beta-carotene, can become pro-oxidants in the wrong biochemical environment, such as the combat zone of free radicals generated by heavy tobacco use.[41] Nowhere in Nature do we find a food with just beta-carotene. All foods contain a rich and dazzling array of anti-oxidants.

♦ After 35 years of heavy smoking, the damage is done. The damaging effects of tobacco cannot be neutralized by one "magic bullet" pill of synthetic beta-carotene, with coal tar-based food dyes added to ensure a homogenous color in the beta-carotene capsules.

♦ It is the synergism of multiple carotenoids that protects people. If beta-carotene truly provoked lung cancer, then what about the 200 studies showing that a diet rich in fruit and vegetables (best sources of beta-carotene) significantly lowers the incidence of cancer?

♦ One nutrient alone may be ineffective or counterproductive for cancer patients, while a host of compatible nutrients in the proper ratio can be extremely effective at slowing or reversing cancer.

> **D-3 (cholecalciferol) 2000-50,000 iu**
> Helps to squelch cancer at genetic level, reducing the production of gene fragments (episomes) by working with calcium receptors

Late spring and early winter are known as the "killing season" among epidemiologists. People have been inside for months. Anyone sick can easily spread that germ to others. No exercise, fresh air, or sunlight all add up to the highest morbidity and mortality occurring around February through April in the northern hemisphere. <u>Low vitamin D is considered a crucial factor</u> in this high-risk season, since sunshine exposure generates vitamin D in the skin.[42] The Covid epidemic of 2020 rode in on the coattails of winter and diminished with the summer. Covid clinicians are finding <u>vitamin D supplements valuable in preventing</u> and curing a wide range of viral infections, including flu and Covid.[43]

As the fledgling science of nutrition grows in knowledge and analytical tools, we keep discovering more nutrients and more functions of the nutrients that we thought we already understood. Such is true for vitamin D, which actually is not a real vitamin in the sense of needing it in the diet.[44] We can manufacture vitamin D in the body by the action of sunlight on the skin converting cholesterol to D.

As a simple metaphor, think of most human cells containing a "switch" that can activate cancer, called the oncogene. Vitamin D puts a protective plate over that oncogene "switch" to prevent cancer from starting or spreading.

Nature always seems to provide. In areas of the world where sunshine is unpredictable at best, indigenous people had traditional diets that were rich in fish liver, which is the most concentrated food source of vitamin D. Cloudy regions of the world, those above the Tropic of CANCER, have had notoriously higher rates of tuberculosis; cancers of the breast [45], ovaries [46], colon [47], and prostate; hypertension and osteoporosis[48]; multiple sclerosis; and other health problems.

If sunshine is the "medicine" in these diseases, then vitamin D and melatonin are the most likely by-products of sunlight exposure. Vitamin D has demonstrated the ability to enhance the immune system to fight off tuberculosis.[49] Our primitive ancestors consumed or produced about 5 times more vitamin D than we get, because they ate whole foods, ate lots of fish, and lived outside in the sun. Most Americans and nearly all women receive far below the RDA (400-800 iu) for vitamin D.[50] One international unit (1 iu) of vitamin D-3 (a measurement of biological activity) is equal to 0.025 micrograms in weight.

IS SUN EXPOSURE GOOD FOR US?

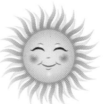

excess sun exposure (free radicals) on fair skin with excess PUFA diet (vulnerable to free radicals) with AOX deficient diet= cataracts, basal & squamous carcin, mac.deg.

Lowest incidence of melanoma found in outdoor constr.workers.
Sunnier climates have 50% reduction in risk for most other cancers.
Sun exposure lowers incidence of depression, auto-immune diseases.
Sunlight (UVB) generates 10,000 iu/day vit.D semi-naked adult.
RDA vit.D=400 iu
Most older Americans deficient in vitamin D
Vitamin D effective against infections, cancer, heart disease, osteoporosis, depression, auto-immune diseases.
40,000 iu (1000 mcg=1 mg) toxic
Vieth, R., Am.J.Clin.Nutr., vol.69, no.5, p.842,May 1999; Am.J.Clin.Nutr.,vol.77, p.204,Jan.2003

Ergosterol is a plant steroid that is converted commercially to vitamin D-2 and used to fortify milk, a move that has virtually eliminated the deficiency syndrome of rickets in cloudy regions of the world. Vitamin D-3, cholecalciferol, is the natural vitamin produced in the skin by the action of sunlight. Once activated in the kidneys and liver, the steroid version of vitamin D-3 is: 1 alpha 25 dihydroxy cholecalciferol (1,25 D-3), which works with the hormones of parathyroid and calcitonin to regulate calcium metabolism, absorption, transport, and regulate 20% of the human genome, and more.

So, how does all this information relate to the cancer process?-- probably by regulating calcium transport into and out of the cell, which has been shown to be crucial in the cell differentiation process.[51]

♦ In animals fed a high fat diet, which normally would produce a higher incidence of colon cancer, supplements of calcium and vitamin D blocked this carcinogenic effect of the diet.[52]

♦ Vitamin D inhibits the growth of breast cancer in culture, and also seems to subdue human breast cancer.[53]

♦ Cells from human prostate cancer were put into a "...permanent nonproliferative state.", or shut down the cancer process, by the addition of vitamin D.[54]

♦ Human cancer cells have been shown to have receptor sites, or stereo-specific "parking spaces" for vitamin D.[55]

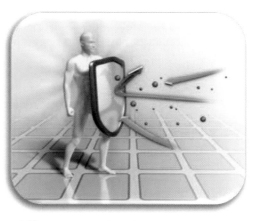

Vitamin D prevents the formation of gene fragments, or episomes, that may be the beginning of the cancer process. Bone cells that generate new blood and immune cells (hematopoietic cells) have receptors for 1,25 D-3, and activated macrophages from the immune system can synthesize 1,25 D-3.[56] Vitamin D induces differentiation to suppress cell growth in numerous tumor lines tested.[57] In tumor-bearing mice, vitamin D-3 supplements inhibited the immune suppression from the tumor secretion (granulocyte/macrophage colony stimulating factor, GM-CSF), while also reducing tumor growth and metastasis.[58] Due to the success of vitamin D at down-regulating various forms of cancer, many drug companies are researching patentable vitamin D analogs to treat cancer. But nothing works like Mother Nature's original.

SAFETY ISSUES

Nature has checkpoints in place to control the possibility of vitamin D toxicity in the body. People who are native to sunny climates have darker skin, which is full of melanin to reduce the production of vitamin D in the skin, while also protecting against the damaging effects of ultraviolet light. Dark-skinned people are also more vulnerable to rickets (vitamin D deficiency) when moving to cloudy climates. African-Americans have a much higher incidence of several cancers, diabetes, and obesity; probably from a vitamin D deficiency.[59]

In order for dietary intake of vitamin D to become toxic, there needs to be activation of vitamin D in the kidney and liver, which are other safeguards in the body. Nonetheless, young children are potentially vulnerable to vitamin D toxicity, which may begin as low as 1,800 iu/day for extended periods of time. [60]   Symptoms of toxicity include hypercalcemia, hypercalciuria, anorexia, nausea, vomiting, thirst, polyuria, muscular weakness, joint pains, and disorientation.[61]

On a summer's day, a sunbather at the beach will produce about 10,000 iu of vitamin D before the body says "that's enough" and shuts off the production mechanism for D.   Good research published in the *American Journal of Clinical Nutrition* shows that vitamin D toxicity for most adults may begin at 40,000 iu per day (100 x RDA).[62] Since there are 40 iu per microgram, this means that toxicity is at 1000 micrograms=1 milligram of D…a speck of dust.

E (succinate, and/or mixed natural tocopherols) 200-1,000 iu
Natural E stimulates immune functions and works as an antioxidant.
E succinate may be selectively toxic to tumor cells.

Since vitamin E is an antioxidant, and chemo and radiation work by generating pro-oxidants to kill cancer cells, it was assumed, therefore, that vitamin E would reduce the efficacy of medical therapy in cancer patients. Nothing could be further from the truth.   Vitamin E is a valuable ally for both the cancer patient and the oncologist.

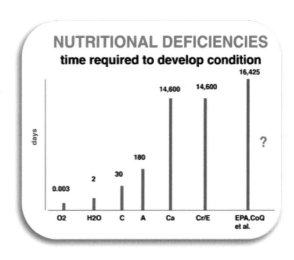

In the 1970s vitamin E was considered "a vitamin in search of a disease." In one study, healthy students were deprived of vitamin E in the diet for up to 2 years with no blatant vitamin deficiency syndrome, such as is found with vitamin C and scurvy, or vitamin D and rickets. Deficiencies of vitamin E cause an increase in lipid peroxidation (pro-oxidants) that decrease energy production (due to mitochondrial membrane damage), increase mutation of DNA, and alter the normal transport mechanisms in the cell membrane. [63]   Hemolytic anemia (premature bursting of red blood cells) has been found in infants who are fed a diet high in polyunsaturated fats (which generate lipid peroxides) and iron (which can be a pro-oxidant). Malabsorption syndromes, such as biliary cirrhosis (blockage of the liver duct to the gallbladder), can generate blatant vitamin E deficiency in humans.[64]

Actually, clinical deficiencies of vitamin E probably take decades to turn into full blown cataracts, Alzheimer's, heart disease, arthritis, or cancer. While 1 milligram of vitamin E (alpha tocopheryl acetate) equals 1 international unit (iu), other versions (racemates) of E are not as potent, and hence have less iu per mg.

Most substances in life are either fat soluble (can be dissolved in alcohol) or water soluble, with a few magical exceptions, like the phospholipid lecithin, able to work in either universe. Vitamin E is the most critical of all fat-soluble antioxidants. Imagine that little "fires", or pro-oxidants, break out all over the human body all of the time. The primary "fire extinguisher" that can put out fires in the fat-soluble portion of the body, including the vulnerable cell membrane, is vitamin E.[65] Because of this fundamental role in cell biology, vitamin E helps to:

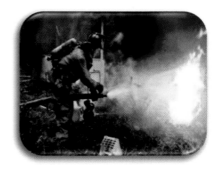

- ◆ protect the beneficial prostaglandins
- ◆ stimulate immune function
- ◆ protect healthy cells against toxins and radiation, while making cancer cells more vulnerable to medical therapy
- ◆ a special form of vitamin E (succinate) is selectively toxic to cancer cells.

Vitamin E actually refers to a family of 8 related compounds, the tocopherols and tocotrienols. Tocopherols got their name from "pherein", meaning to carry, and "tocos", meaning birth, because vitamin E from wheat germ was found to be essential for fertility. True natural vitamin E is a mixture of alpha, beta, delta, and gamma tocopherols plus some tocotrienols, which are more concentrated in rice bran and palm oil. Vitamin E may help the cancer patient in numerous ways:

NUTRITIONAL SYNERGISM. Zinc deficiency in animals further compounds a vitamin E deficiency, meaning that zinc must be present to properly utilize vitamin E.[66] Also, vitamin E protects the body against the potentially damaging effects of iron and rusting fish oil. Human volunteers given high doses of fish oil experienced an immune abnormality (mitogenic responsiveness of peripheral blood mononuclear cells to concanavalin A), which was reversed with supplements of vitamin E.[67]

IMMUNE REGULATOR. Vitamin E plays a powerful role as an immune regulator.[68] When 32 healthy elderly adults were given supplements of 800 iu daily of vitamin E, there were measurable improvements in immune functions.[69] Following 28 days of supplements of vitamins E, C, and A researchers found that 30 elderly institutionalized patients had substantial improvements in immune functions (absolute T-cells, T4 subsets, T4:T8 ratio, and lymphocyte proliferation).[70] E seems to work by protecting immune factors from immediate destruction in their suicidal plunge at cancer cells. E also works by bolstering the activity of the thymus and spleen organs to stimulate lymphocyte proliferation. In burned animals, vitamin E supplements offered substantial protection in the intestinal mucosa to prevent bacterial translocation (gut bacteria migrating into the blood to cause septicemia).[71]

PROTECTION FROM TOXINS. Vitamin E protected animals from the cancer-causing effects of alcohol on the esophagus[72] and a carcinogen on the colon.[73] Vitamin E and selenium protected animals against the potent carcinogenic effects of DMBA from tobacco.[74] Vitamin E protected the damaged liver of rats from developing fatty liver and collagen content.[75] Vitamin E protects us against the greatest toxin and essential nutrient of them all--oxygen, as shown in exercised animals.[76] By sparing fats in the blood from becoming lipid peroxides, vitamin E supplements were very effective at preventing heart disease.[77] Vitamin E prevents the formation of one of the more common carcinogenic agents in humans--nitrosamines--which are formed by the combination of nitrates in the diet and amino acids in the stomach. Vitamin E prevents damage to the skin from ultraviolet radiation.[78] According to researchers from Bulgaria, vitamin E protects us against the harmful effects of too many iron-generating free radicals and damage to our detoxification system, cytochrome P-450. Much of the damage caused by iron in the human body is due to:

1) wrong form of iron, we need chelated iron, not iron salts as we get in fortified white flour

2) not enough antioxidants to prevent this oxidizing metal from "rusting" in the cell and creating harm.

3) lowering of pH, or acidosis, which causes iron to become unbound from its protective shells of hemoglobin and transferrin

REVERSE PRE-CANCEROUS CONDITION. Vitamin E supplements (200-400 mg/d for 3 months) reversed fibrocystic breast disease (a major risk for breast cancer) in 22 out of 26 women.[79] Other women have found reversal of fibrocystic breast disease through elimination of caffeine, chocolate, and colas, which contain methylxanthines.

PROSTAGLANDINS. We can generate very healthy prostaglandins, if we have the right dietary precursors in our blood, which come from (for more on prostaglandins, see the chapter on Lipids):

♦ enough fish oil (EPA) or flax oil (ALA) and borage oil (GLA)
♦ healthy levels of blood sugar (60-100 mg%)
♦ optimal amounts of vitamin E[80]

Because of this beneficial impact on prostaglandins, vitamin E helps to inhibit platelet adhesion[81], which helps to slow down the spreading of cancer. Vitamin E does not influence blood clotting, or prothrombin time, which is good news for people worried about proper clotting during and after surgery.

SLOWS AND REVERSES CANCER. In human studies, low intake of vitamin E increases the risk for cancer of various body sites.[82] Patients with head and neck cancers are more likely to have a recurrence if they have low blood levels of vitamins E, A, and beta-carotene.[83] Vitamin E injected into animal mouth tumors was able to significantly reduce or completely eliminate tumors.[84] In patients with colorectal cancer, vitamin E, C, and A supplements were able to reduce the growth of abnormal cells in the colon, indicating a possible slowing of the cancer process.[85] In human epidemiology studies, people with the highest intake of E (still very low compared to ideal intake) had a 40% reduction in the risk for colon cancer.[86] In animals, vitamin E supplements prevent lung tumors from developing.[87]

VITAMIN E SUCCINATE AND CANCER. When vitamin E is esterified (combined) with succinic acid, a new molecule is formed (vitamin E succinate) with surprising ability to selectively shut down cancer growth, but not harm healthy tissue,[88] slowing the growth of brain (glioma and neuroblastoma) and melanoma cells in culture.[89] E succinate is able to reduce the genetic expression of c-myc oncogenes in cultured cancer cells.[90] E succinate inhibits virally-induced tumors in culture.[91] E succinate has been studied as a potent regulator of cell proliferation.[92]

IMPROVES MEDICAL THERAPY OF CANCER. Vitamin E helps generally toxic medical therapies to distinguish between healthy and cancerous cells. The best proposed mechanism for this action is the anaerobic state of many tumors. Vitamin E apparently is not well absorbed, or needed, by tumors, since they are anaerobic (without oxygen). An antioxidant is of little interest to an oxygen-independent cell. Because of this function of vitamin E, chemotherapy and radiation can be made much more selectively toxic to the cancer cells, while protecting the patient from host damage.

It has long been known that a vitamin E deficiency, common in cancer patients, will accentuate the cardiotoxic effects of adriamycin.[93] The worse the vitamin E deficiency in animals, the greater the heart damage from adriamycin.[94] Patients undergoing chemo, radiation, and bone marrow transplant for cancer treatment had markedly depressed levels of serum antioxidants, including vitamin E.[95] Given the fact that

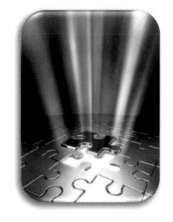

both chemo and radiation can induce cancer, which reduces the chances for survival, it is noteworthy that vitamin E protects animals against a potent carcinogen, DMBA.[96] Vitamin E supplements prevented the glucose-raising effects of a chemo drug, doxorubicin.[97] Since cancer is a sugar-feeder, preventing this glucose-raising effect may be another valuable contribution from vitamin E in patients receiving chemo. Meanwhile, vitamin E improves the tumor kill rate of doxorubicin.[98] Vitamin E modifies the carcinogenic effect of daunomycin (chemo drug) in animals.[99]

Human prostate cancer cells were killed at a higher rate when adriamycin (chemo drug) was combined with vitamin E at concentrations that can easily be obtained from supplementation.[100] Vitamin E supplements (1,600 iu/day) taken one week prior to adriamycin therapy protected 69% of patients from hair loss, which is nearly universal in adriamycin-treated patients.[101] Vitamin E helped to repair kidney damage caused by adriamycin in animals.[102] Vitamin E and selenium supplements in animals helped to reduce the heart toxicity from adriamycin.[103] Selenium and vitamin E supplements were given to 41 women undergoing cytotoxic therapy for ovarian and cervical cancers, with a resulting drop in the toxicity-related rise in creatine kinase.[104] Vitamin E, A, and prenylamine reduced the toxicity of adriamycin on the hearts of animals studied.[105]

In animals with implanted tumors, those pretreated with vitamin E had a much greater tumor kill from radiation therapy.[106] Radiation therapists know that the ability to kill cancer with radiation diminishes as the tumor becomes more anaerobic or hypoxic. Vitamin E seems to sensitize tumors, making them more vulnerable to radiation therapy. In cultured human cancer cells, vitamin E increased the damaging effects of radiation on tumor cells.[107] Brain cancer cells were easier to kill once pretreated with vitamin E succinate.[108] Tumor kill in animals receiving radiation therapy was greatly increased by pretreatment with vitamin E.[109] Vitamin E supplements reduced the breakage of red blood cells in animals given radiation therapy.[110] Vitamin E supplements improved the wound recovery in animals given preoperative radiation.[111]

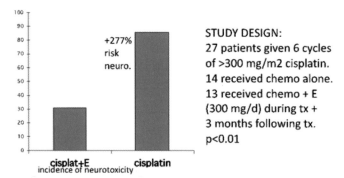

CAN VITAMIN E REDUCE NEUROTOXICITY FROM CISPLATIN?

+277% risk neuro.

STUDY DESIGN:
27 patients given 6 cycles of >300 mg/m2 cisplatin. 14 received chemo alone. 13 received chemo + E (300 mg/d) during tx + 3 months following tx. p<0.01

cisplat+E   cisplatin
incidence of neurotoxicity

Pace, A., J.Clin.Oncology, vol.21, no.5, p.927, Mar.2003

Vitamin E combined with vitamin K, leucovorin (anti-metabolite cancer drug), and 5FU (fluorouracil) significantly enhanced the cell growth inhibition curves for 5FU.[112] One of the more troublesome side effects of chemotherapy is peripheral neuropathy, or a tingling numbness in the extremities. Low vitamin E status is likely to blame for peripheral neuropathy.[113]

Oral mucositis, or sores in the mouth, is a common problem arising from the use of many chemotherapy drugs. These mouth sores are so painful that cancer patients stop eating, creating malnutrition, which really deteriorates the general health picture. Topical vitamin E healed 67% of cancer patients in a double-blind trial at M.D. Anderson Hospital in Houston.[114] To use this therapy, puncture the end of a soft gelatin vitamin E capsule and spread the vitamin E oil over the mouth sore. Do this several times each day.

Can't get enough in food

Vitamin E supplements have even been endorsed by the National Cancer Institute [115], American Heart Association, and the United States Department of Agriculture, because in order to consume 400 international units of vitamin E, you would have to eat either:

-2 quarts of corn oil, or

-5 pounds of wheat germ, or

-8 cups of almonds, or

-28 cups of peanuts

SAFETY ISSUES

Taking many times the RDA of vitamin E had some researchers worried about toxicity, so they fed 900 iu (90 times the RDA) daily to healthy college students for 12 weeks with no changes in liver, kidney, thyroid, **blood clotting,** or immunoglobulin levels.[116] These results are valuable, because vitamin E inhibits the platelet aggregation that can cause stroke, heart disease, or cancer metastasis; yet it does not alter blood clotting activity. Therefore, pre-surgical patients do not need to reduce vitamin E intake for fear of not clotting during and after surgery. According to a review of the world's literature on vitamin E toxicity, there are virtually no side effects at dosages under 3,200 iu/day.[117]

K2 and/or K3 50-200 mcg

Selectively toxic to tumor cells. In combination with vitamin C forms anti-cancer compound.

When vitamin K was first researched in 1929, it was labelled the "Klotting" factor by the Dutch scientist Henrik Dam. Since then, much has been learned about this fascinating molecule. There are three primary variations of vitamin K, all with certain levels of activity in the body.

♦ K-1, or phylloquinone, is produced in higher plants such as spinach, broccoli, Brussels sprouts, and kale.

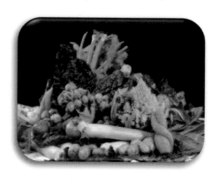

♦ K-2, or menaquinone, is produced by bacterial fermentation, which means that we manufacture varying amounts of vitamin K in a healthy human gut. Fermented foods such as cheeses and soy foods also carry some K.

♦ K-3, or menadione, is the synthetically-derived version of vitamin K, called Synkavite in drug form.

Although mother's milk will quickly begin generating vitamin K in the infant's gut, physicians have developed a standard hospital protocol of giving injections of Synkavite to all newborns. About 1/3 of all patients with chronic gastrointestinal problems have clinical vitamin K deficiency.[118]

There are several handsome lessons to be learned as we review vitamin K in :

♦ **Metavitamin functions**. Many nutrients develop unique functions when given at anything beyond survival doses. Niacin, vitamin A, vitamin C, fish oil, and others all reflect the fact that low dose of a nutrient will give you basic survival functions, while higher doses give us "above-vitamin" or meta-vitamin functions. In this case, vitamin K is basically a clotting factor that helps to activate prothrombin, so that we do not bleed to death when cutting open the skin envelope.[119] In higher doses, vitamin K becomes a potent anti-cancer agent that is non-toxic to healthy cells.[120]

♦ **Synergism yields two main benefits**: 1) significant increase in healing capacity; 2) the need for lower doses. Researchers found that combining vitamins C and K-3 against cultured human breast cancer cells allowed for inhibition of the cancer growth at doses 90-98% less than was required if only one of these vitamins was used against the cancer.[121]

♦ **Look beyond the obvious.** Coumarin (a.k.a. dicumarol, warfarin) is an anti-coagulant drug that holds promise in cancer treatment by shutting down cancer cell metabolism and helping to slow metastasis. Vitamin K has a primary function of inducing coagulation. The obvious deduction is that vitamin K (a coagulant) would neutralize the benefits of coumarin (anti-coagulant). In real life, Vitamin K-3 does not neutralize the effects of coumarin[122] but actually improves the anti-cancer effects of coumarin.[123] While K-1 reverses the effects of coumarin, K-3 does not reverse the effects of coumarin due to the slight difference in chemical structure in which K-3 cannot participate in the gamma carboxylation of prothrombin.

♦ **Similar is not the same as identical in chemical structures.** Oftentimes, drug companies find a substance that has therapeutic action, such as vitamin A or indole-3-carbinol from broccoli, and will try to create a slightly different molecule, so that it can be patented. These slight differences nearly always translate into high toxicity from these newly-formed molecules. For instance, the difference between a man and woman rests primarily in the difference between the hormones testosterone and estrogen, which are nearly identical molecules except for 3 OH group. Try slightly bending your house key and see how well it works in your home lock.

Over 40 years ago, Professor J.S. Mitchell of England showed that patients receiving K-3 had measurable shrinkage of tumors. Later, the drug doxorubicin was introduced as an anti-cancer drug. K-3, doxorubicin, and coumarin all share related chemical structures as "naphthoquinone" molecules. Yet, of all these compounds, K-3 has been shown by Chlebowski and colleagues at UCLA to have 70 times (7,000%!!!) more anti-cancer activity than coumarin and 25 times more cancer-killing capacity than vitamin K-1.

Vitamin K-3 works against cancer both by directly antagonizing cell replication in cancer cells[124] and also by inhibiting metastasis. K-3 also works as a potentiator of radiation therapy. In one study, patients with mouth cancer who were pre-treated with injections of K-3 prior to radiation therapy doubled their odds (20% vs. 39%) for 5-year survival and disease-free status.[125] Animals with implanted tumors had greatly improved anti-cancer effects from all chemotherapy drugs tested, when vitamins K and C were given in combination.[126] In cultured leukemia cells, vitamins K and E added to the chemotherapy drugs 5FU (fluorouracil) and leucovorin provided a 300% improvement in growth inhibition when compared to 5FU by itself.[127]

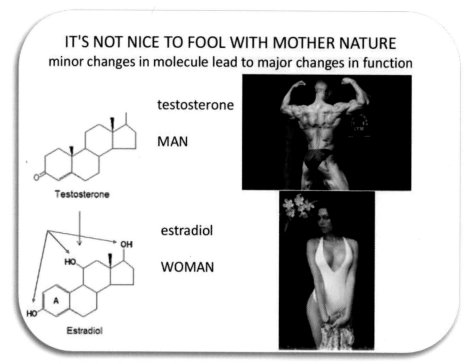

Animals given methotrexate and K-3 had improvements in cancer reversal, with no increase in toxicity to the host tissue.[128] In one case study, a patient with recurrent and drug-refractory bone cancer metastasized to the lungs was put on a regimen of hydrazine sulfate and vitamin K-3 injections, with a resulting weight gain and complete regression of her cancer.[129] In 13 cancer patients, some with demonstrated drug-resistant tumors, menadiol (vitamin K analog, a.k.a. K-4) was given at up to 3,200 mg per meter squared per week along with various chemo drugs, with no increase in host toxicity, but some improvements in tumor responses.[130]

Vitamin K2 has its own impressive resume of anti-cancer activity. K2 dramatically slowed the growth of lung cancer cells in test tubes.[131] And stomach cancer cells in vitro.[132] And liver cancer cells.[133] And hormone independent prostate cancer cells.[134] K2 induces apoptosis (suicide) in many cancer cell lines.[135] K2 shows extraordinary clinical promise in preventing and reversing bone loss, heart disease, cancer, etc.[136]

Therapeutic supplements of K2 as MK7 are taken at 150-180 micrograms daily, with K2 as MK4 at 150 mcg per day.

SAFETY ISSUES

There is no known toxicity associated with the plant-derived version, K-1.[137] The toxicity of menadione (K-3) is very low, with animals having no adverse side effects after being fed 1,000 times the daily requirement.[138] The typical dietary intake of K-1 in America is somewhere between 100-500 micrograms daily, with little understanding of the role played by the production of K-2 in the healthy human gut.

A special note on coumarin. Many cancer patients on coumarin are directed by their physician to avoid foods high in vitamin K-1, including kale, spinach, broccoli, and other anti-cancer greens. Actually, much more important is to have a PREDICTABLE intake of vitamin K-1. The doctor will take blood samples and conduct a Pro test (prothrombin test, time required for the blood to clot) and prescribe coumarin based on this test. It is much more essential to have a PREDICTABLE amount of vitamin K-1 in the diet than to avoid it, which will allow for the safest and most effective use of anti-coagulant drugs.

C 200-10,000 mg (from ascorbic acid and/or buffered sources like sodium ascorbate or calcium ascorbate)
Immune stimulant, antioxidant, helps envelop cancer, shuts down cancer growth, intravenously can selectively destroy cancer

---

If vitamin A is the mother of all anti-cancer vitamins, then vitamin C is the grandmother of all. The problem started millions of years ago, when primates lost the liver enzyme necessary to convert sugar into vitamin C.[139] Of the millions of animals, reptiles, amphibians, insects, and other things that walk, crawl, fly, and swim--humans are among the few creatures on earth that do not make our own vitamin C. Our primitive ancestors were able to consume 300-500 milligrams daily of vitamin C, which definitely prevents scurvy. Throughout the golden ages of world exploration by ship, thousands of people died--sometimes up to half of the crew--due to scurvy. Highly perishable fresh fruits and vegetables are the richest sources of vitamin C and were unavailable on ship voyages longer than a few weeks. Around 1750, the English physician, James Lind, found that limes could prevent and reverse scurvy. Does that make limes a prescription drug?

"Time lags" are a known phenomenon that separate a discovery from the actual implementation of a breakthrough. It was another 50 years after Dr. Lind's research before limes were required to be carried aboard ships, thus costing the world thousands of unnecessary deaths in this delay. Are we doing the same thing by delaying aggressive nutrition support for millions of cancer patients?

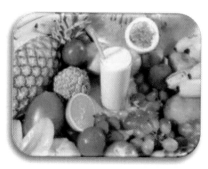

Vitamin C is one of the more versatile vitamins in human nutrition:

♦ protects against free radicals
♦ maintains tough connective tissue (collagen and elastin), which is the "glue" that keeps our body together
♦ produces adrenaline for energy
♦ produces serotonin for thought and calmness
♦ stimulates various immune components
♦ converts cholesterol into bile for its elimination in the bowels
♦ maintains fat stores in the adipose tissue to prevent heart disease
♦ regulates bone formation
♦ detoxifies pollutants
♦ reduces allergic reactions by preventing histamine release
♦ regulates insulin to better control blood sugar levels

HOW MUCH???

Part of the controversy surrounding vitamin C is the extreme range of dosages that can be consumed in humans or produced in animals:

- 10 milligrams daily will prevent blatant scurvy in most healthy adults
- 60 mg is the Recommended Dietary Allowance
- 200-300 mg would be consumed by people who are following the NCI suggestion of 5 servings of fruit and vegetables daily
- 300 mg of supplemental vitamin C was shown to increase quantity of life by 6 years in men
- 1,000 mg is required in many hospitalized patients, just to maintain adequate serum ascorbate levels

- 10,000 to 20,000 mg is often taken by many people using C to curtail some illness, such as cancer, AIDS, viral infections, and injury recovery
- 100,000 mg/day has been given intravenously with no side effects
- 20,000 mg is produced daily by many animals, such as goats and dogs, on a per weight basis using a 154 pound reference man; internal production goes up further when the animal is exposed to stress, infections, or toxins

Although Linus Pauling, PhD, was not the first scientist to suggest that vitamin C might help cancer patients, he was definitely the most vocal and decorated of the lot. With two unshared Nobel prizes and three Presidential citations, you would think that the scientific community would be more open to Dr. Pauling's comments. Though Pauling was considered to be one of the two greatest scientists of the 20th century, along with Albert Einstein, the 1970s found Pauling to be an academic nomad for his innovative views on vitamin C.

However, as time marched on, data continued to gather to support Pauling's viewpoint. By 1982, the National Academy of Sciences was willing to admit that vitamin C might prevent cancer.[140] And by 1990, the National Institutes of Health hosted a conference on "Vitamin C and Cancer", which showed that Pauling was truly on to something.[141] While Pauling's strident critics claimed that he was trying to cure cancer with vitamin C, in fact Pauling only suggested high doses of C in concert with medical therapies would augment cancer outcome.

Pauling later went on to explain the reasons that vitamin C may improve outcome in cancer treatment, including the increased need for C in cancer patients, the ability of C to prevent cancer breaking down connective tissue for metastasis, the ability of C to help "wall off" or encapsulate the tumor, the role of C in immune attack on cancer, and the role of C in hormonal balance.[142] One of the highlights of my career was having Dr. Pauling eat supper at my house in 1992, spry and alert at 91 years of age.

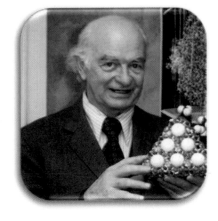

Vitamin C can help cancer patients in several ways:

1) Prevention. Cancer patients have already demonstrated a genetic vulnerability to cancer and toxins. Cancer patients will likely be exposed to even more potent carcinogens in medical therapy. Therefore, the need to prevent secondary and iatrogenic tumors is great. In a study encompassing 16 groups in 7 countries covering 25 years, higher vitamin C intake was strongly related to lowering cancer incidence.[143] Another study examined the cancer-protective effect of vitamin C and found that 33 of 46 epidemiological studies showed it helped, while none showed any increase in cancer with higher vitamin C intake.[144] Vitamin C protects humans against a whole assortment of toxic chemicals [145] while accelerating wound recovery[146] and stabilizing iron compounds (ferritin) in the blood.[147] Vitamin C reduced the incidence and severity of kidney tumors in animals exposed to the hormones estradiol or diethylstilbestrol.[148] Through a wide variety of mechanisms, vitamin C is a potent inhibitor of cancer.[149]

2) Augmenting medical therapy. C may be able to enhance the toxicity of chemo and radiation against the cancer cells, while protecting the patient from possible harm. C was able to enhance the effectiveness of a drug (misonidazole) that improves outcome in radiation treatment of cancer.[150] C improved the tumor-stopping abilities of a wide range of medical therapies against brain cancer (neuroblastoma) cells in culture.[151] Animals given the chemo drugs vincristine (from the periwinkle plant) and vinblastine were given supplements of vitamin C, with an increase in the excretion of these very toxic drugs.[152] Animals given adriamycin (a common chemotherapy drug) along with vitamin C had a significant prolongation of life and reduction in the expected heart damage (cardiotoxicity) from this drug.[153] Given the widespread use of adriamycin and its known lethal toxicity on the heart [154], it should be standard procedure to give high doses of antioxidants prior to administration of adriamycin.

Animals with implanted tumors were injected with high doses of C one hour prior to whole-body radiation therapy, all scaled to mimic the effects in a human cancer patient. Vitamin C did not affect the tumor-killing capacity of the radiation, but did provide substantial protection to the animals.[155] 50 previously untreated cancer patients were randomly divided into 2 groups, with group #1 receiving radiation therapy only and group #2 receiving radiation plus 5 grams daily of C. After 1 month, 87%

of the vitamin C group had achieved a complete response (disappearance of all tumors) compared to 55% in the control group.[156]

   3) **Slowing or reversing cancer.**   High doses of C are preferentially toxic to tumor cells, while not harming healthy tissue. One of the explanations why C kills cancer but not healthy cells lies in the fact that C generates large amounts of hydrogen peroxide, H_2O_2, a potent free radical, which is neutralized in healthy cells by catalase.[157] Cancer cells do not have catalase to protect them. Animals exposed to a carcinogen and then vitamin C had their basal cell cancers examined under electron microscope. The cancer cells exposed to C showed a disintegration of cell structure, cell membrane disruption, increased collagen synthesis, and general reduction in the number and size of tumors.[158] The researcher concluded: "...vitamin C exerts its antineoplastic effects by increasing cytolytic and autophagic activity, cell membrane disruption, and increased collagen synthesis, and thus, inhibits cancer cell metabolism and proliferation."

   C may be the ultimate selective toxin against cancer that researchers have been searching for.[159] Recent studies have found that vitamin C is absorbed well by tumor tissue. This study led to the "assumption" that cancer patients should not take vitamin C

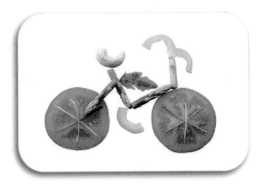

because it might reduce the effectiveness of chemo and radiation. Actually, no study has ever found that to be true. Vitamin C selectively kills cancer cells while protecting healthy tissue from the damaging effects of chemo and radiation. Vitamin C is absorbed by tumor cells because C is so similar in structure to glucose (sugar). Yet large amounts of a single antioxidant in an anaerobic environment, such as a tumor, have been shown to become a pro-oxidant, just like chemo, except the vitamin C only destroys cancer cells. Antioxidants in a team effort in an aerobic cell, such as healthy tissue, work in harmony to protect that cell against oxidation, like chemo and radiation.

   Vitamin C was toxic to melanoma cells but not to healthy cells in culture.[160] When researchers took leukemia cells from 28 patients and cultured them with vitamin C, 25% of the cultures were inhibited by at least 79%.[161] In animals with implanted tumors, vitamin C and B-12 together provided for significant tumor regression and 50% survival of the treated group, while all of the animals not receiving C and B-12 died by the 19th day.[162] C and B-12 seemed to form a cobalt-ascorbate compound that selectively shut down tumor growth. When vitamin C and K were combined with cancer cells in culture, the dosage required to slow and kill cancer cells dropped to only 2% compared to the dosage required by either of these vitamins alone.[163] Vitamin C or essential fatty acids were able to inhibit the growth of melanoma in culture, yet when combined, their anti-cancer activity was much stronger.[164]

In both case studies and clinical trials in the scientific literature, C helps many cancer patients and hurts no one. Show me a drug that has the same risk-to-benefit-to-cost ratio. There is compelling evidence that <u>high dose intravenous vitamin C</u> has a central role in cancer treatment.[165] High dose IVC as sole therapy has often been shown to be <u>effective in advanced cancer patients</u>.[166] Researchers from the NCI and other institutions have reported that in 2008 there were 172 doctors who <u>administered IVC to over 12,000</u> patients with remarkably few side effects and good clinical outcomes.[167] For more information on high dose intravenous vitamin C, see the chapter on Rational Cancer Treatment.

Pauling and Cameron found that 10,000 mg (10 grams) daily of vitamin C brought a 22% survival rate in end-stage untreatable cancer patients after 1 year on C, compared to a 0.4% survival in patients without C.[168] Charles Moertel, MD, of the Mayo Clinic allegedly followed the Pauling protocol and found no benefit with vitamin C.[169] Actually, even though Moertel did not follow Pauling's protocol, none of the untreatable, drug-refractory colon cancer patients in Moertel's study died while on vitamin C for 3 months.

4) Higher need. There is an elevated need for this nutrient during disease recovery. In one study, 15 patients with melanoma and colon cancer who were receiving immunotherapy (interleukin 2 and lymphokine-activated killer cells) showed blood levels of vitamin C indicative of scurvy.[170] In 20 adult hospitalized patients on Total Parenteral Nutrition (TPN), the mean daily vitamin C needs were 975 mg, which is over 16 times the RDA, with the range being 350-2,250 mg.[171] Of the 139 lung cancer patients studied, most tested deficient or scorbutic (clinical vitamin C deficiency).[172] Another study of cancer patients found that 46% tested scorbutic, while 76% were below acceptable levels for serum ascorbate.[173]

SAFETY ISSUES

Vitamin C is extremely safe, even in high doses. In one review of the literature regarding safety of vitamin C, 8 different double-blind placebo-controlled trials giving up to 10,000 mg daily of C for years produced no side effects.[174] In some sensitive individuals, doses of as little as 1,000 mg produce gastrointestinal upset, including diarrhea. Allegations that vitamin C mega-doses would produce oxalate kidney stones or cause B-12 deficiency have never been seen in millions of humans taking mega-doses of C for years. Up to 100,000 mg of C has been safely administered IV. As doses of oral C increase, the percentage that is absorbed goes down. Some experts claim that 1-2 grams of C per day is the upper threshold of what humans can tolerate and efficiently absorb. Use VitaChek C paper strips (316-682-3100) to monitor the vitamin C in urine. Maintaining maximum vitamin C in the urine can be helpful. Meanwhile, mineral-bound ascorbate provides a more prolonged and sustained blood level of serum ascorbate.

B-1 (thiamine mononitrate) 2-20 mg
Improves aerobic metabolism

When the British first learned to mill wheat and remove the outer bran and inner germ, they called the remaining cadaver of a food substance "the Queen's white flour". Bringing this technology around the world, the Dutch showed the South Pacific people of Java how to refine their rice, leaving only white rice behind and disposing of the bran and germ. Many of these people developed a condition of weakness and inability to function, called beri-beri, or literally translated: "I cannot. I cannot." Thiamin was one of the first vitamins to be studied and isolated in the early 20th century.

The importance of thiamin lies in its critical role in energy metabolism and the need for energy in every cell of the body. Thiamin becomes incorporated into a critical enzyme (thiamin pyrophosphate) for production of ATP energy. Low intake of thiamin was associated with an increase in the risk for prostate cancer.

"Better living through chemistry." DuPont Chemical 1935-82

Nutrition experiments:
1. milling of grain, white flour, 1000 AD Europe
2. beri-beri, 1897
3. saturated fat in butter to hydrogenated fats in margarine, trans vs cis fats
4. high fructose corn syrup
5. genetically modified organisms: GMO

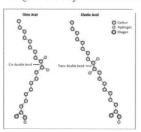

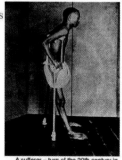

A sufferer – turn of the 20th century in

175

Although thiamin is added back to enriched white flour, it is not added back to pastry flour (as in doughnuts) and is often deficient in the elderly[176] and those who regularly consume alcohol.[177] Best food sources of thiamin include brewer's yeast, peas, wheat germ, peanuts, whole grains, beans, and liver.

B-2 (riboflavin) 2-20 mg
Improves aerobic metabolism

Again, like thiamin above, riboflavin is mainly concerned with generating ATP energy from foodstuffs through the enzyme FAD (flavin adenine dinucleotide).   However, riboflavin is also essential for the generation of a critical protective enzyme, glutathione peroxidase, which mops up free radicals. With optimal amounts of riboflavin in the body, there is less damage to cell membranes, DNA, and immune factors. Low intake of riboflavin is associated with an increased risk for cancer of prostate and esophagus. Although riboflavin is added back to enriched white flour, many elderly[178] and poor people are low in riboflavin intake.[179]   Alcohol interferes with the absorption and metabolism of riboflavin. Best food sources of riboflavin include brewer's yeast, kidney, liver, broccoli, wheat germ, milk, and almonds.

> **B-3 niacin (inositol hexanicotinate, or niacinamide) 100-1,500 mg**
> Improves aerobic metabolism and tumor-killing capacity of medical therapy, also may work like an enzyme to dissolve protective coating surrounding tumor.

Like the energy vitamins mentioned above, niacin generates ATP energy via the enzyme NAD (nicotinamide adenine dinucleotide) and also has other duties that impact the cancer patient. Niacin supplements in animals were able to reduce the cardiotoxicity of adriamycin, while not interfering with its tumor-killing capacity. [180] Niacin combined with aspirin in 106 bladder cancer patients receiving surgery and radiation therapy provided for a substantial improvement in 5-year survival (72% vs. 27%) over the control group. [181]

Tumors can hide from radiation therapy as hypoxic (low oxygen) lumps. Niacin seems to make radiation therapy more effective at killing these hypoxic cancer cells. [182] Loading radiation patients with 500 mg to 6,000 mg of niacin has been shown to be safe and is one of the most effective agents known to eliminate acute hypoxia in solid malignancies. [183] There is also intriguing evidence that high doses of niacin can act like enzymes, which means:

- ◆ changing the coating of the tumor to make it more vulnerable to the immune system and to medical intervention
- ◆ breaking up inefficient clumps of immune cells, or circulating immune complexes
- ◆ altering Tumor Necrosis Factor (TNF) that can lead to depression, weight loss, and pain.

> **B-5 (D-calcium pantothenate) 10-40 mg**
> Improves stress response

Pantothenic acid is named for "pantos", which is Greek for "found everywhere". Indeed, all plants and animals require or make pantothenic acid as part of a crucial energy enzyme, acetyl coenzyme A, which is vital for generating ATP energy and a chemical for stress response. Injections of pantothenic acid improved wound healing in rabbits. [184] Based on the fact that the average American diet provides about 6 mg of pantothenic acid daily, the recommended intake (no formal RDA) is 4-7 mg.

Deficiencies of pantothenic acid will generate symptoms of paresthesia (burning, prickling, tingling of extremities), headache, fatigue, insomnia, and GI distress. Pantothenic acid works closely with carnitine and CoQ to maximize the efficiency of burning dietary fats. Supplements of pantothenic acid can help in the stress response, proper balancing of adrenal hormones, energy production, and manufacturing of red blood cells. Best food sources of pantothenic acid are royal bee jelly, liver, kidney, egg yolk, and broccoli.

B-6 total of 50-100 mg; 2-15 mg from pyridoxal 5 pyrophosphate, and 10-40 mg from pyridoxine HCl
Improves immune functions and may reduce toxicity from radiation therapy

---

B-6 occurs in three natural forms: pyridoxine, pyridoxal, and pyridoxamine. B-6 works chiefly in an enzyme, pyridoxal-5-phosphate, which shifts amine groups from molecule to molecule in a process called transamination. At least 100 different enzyme systems in humans involving protein metabolism, catabolism, anabolism, or enzyme production all require B-6. B-6 is essential for:

♦ regulating proper blood glucose levels
♦ production of niacin from tryptophan
♦ lipid metabolism and carnitine synthesis
♦ making nucleic acids (RNA and DNA)
♦ immune cell production
♦ regulation of hormones.

Among its many functions, B-6 is required for producing thymidine, without which cells are more likely to develop cancerous mutations.[185] In a group of 12 non-medicated, newly diagnosed cancer patients who had been smokers, all showed indications (based on coenzyme stimulation) of B-6 deficiency.[186] A low intake of B-6 increases tumor susceptibility and tumor size.[187]

In huge surveys conducted by the United States Department of Agriculture, 80% of Americans did not consume the RDA of 2 mg daily of B-6. There are many aspects of the typical American lifestyle that will exacerbate a marginal deficiency of B-6: many drugs, common food dyes, alcohol, and a high protein intake. Deficiency symptoms will reflect the functions of B-6, which means that almost anything can go wrong.

In one study, 25 mg (1,250% of RDA) provided measurable improvements in immune functions in healthy adults. B-6 supplements (50-500 mg) have been shown to cure up to 97% of Carpal Tunnel Syndrome, a painful condition of the wrist and hands. B-6 is very helpful in preventing and reversing neuropathy, or a tingling numbness in the hands and feet, which is common in chemo patients and also preventing the "tanning" of blood proteins, a.k.a. glycosylation or glycation, which occurs when too much sugar is regularly found in the bloodstream.[188]

Above-normal intake of B-6 offers many possible benefits to the cancer patient, including immune stimulation[189], blood sugar control, protection from radiation damage, and inhibition of growth in melanoma.

Early studies in animals indicated that depriving them of B-6 might slow down tumor growth and increase survival time.[190] More recent studies find the opposite to be true. Animals supplemented with B-6 and then injected with a deadly strain of cancer, melanoma, showed an enhanced resistance to the disease.[191] B-6 inhibits melanoma in vivo.[192] B-6 supplements of 25 mg/day in 33 bladder cancer patients provided for marked reduction in tumor recurrence compared to the control group.[193]

CAN THERAPEUTIC NUTRITION LOWER TUMOR RECURRENCE?

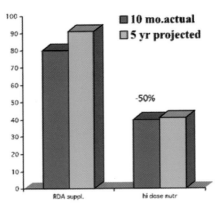

Study design: 65 patients w. transitional cell carcinoma of bladder, BCG immune tx, randomized to either RDA supplement 24 of 30 with tumor recurrence) or RDA + 40,000 iu A, 100 mg B-6, 2 gm C, 400 iu E, 90 mg Zn with 14 of 35 recurrence. Hi dose nutrients cut tumor recurrence in half.

% of bladder cancer patients with tumor recurrence
source: Lamm, DL, J.Urol.,151, 21, Jan.1994

More recently, oncologists randomized 65 patients with transitional cell carcinoma of the bladder into either the "one-per-day" vitamin supplement providing the RDA, or into a group which received the RDA supplement plus 40,000 iu of vitamin A, 100 mg of B-6, 2000 mg of vitamin C, 400 iu of vitamin E, and 90 mg of zinc. High-dose nutrients, including B-6, cut tumor recurrence in half.[194] B-6 supplements of 300 mg/day throughout 8 weeks of radiation therapy in patients with endometrial cancer provided a 15% improvement in survival at 5 years.[195]

SAFETY ISSUES

Less than 500 mg/day appears to be safe for most adults.[196] P-5-P appears to be the more readily available and active form of B-6, yet most people can convert pyridoxine into active P-5-P.

B-12 (cyanocobalamin) 500 mcg-3000 mcg
Assists in proper cell growth, i.e. making of new immune factors and proper division of other cells.   Combines with vitamin C to create selective anti-cancer compound

---

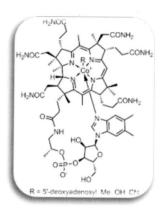

In 1926, Minot and Murphy were awarded the Nobel prize for showing that feeding large quantities of liver could cure the dreaded disease, pernicious anemia, or B-12 deficiency. As people mature beyond age 40, the likelihood of developing pernicious anemia goes up substantially as the gut loses its efficiency at binding with this gigantic molecule and escorting it across the intestinal mucosa. The RDA of 2 micrograms (mcg) can easily be obtained in a typical "meat and potatoes" diet in America, since the best sources are liver, meat, fish, chicken, clams, and egg yolk. Vegans must take B-12 supplements to prevent B-12 deficiency. However, absorbing the nutrient is another challenge. When this "intrinsic factor" in the gut is missing, large amounts in the diet can somewhat overwhelm the mucosal barrier in the gut and allow some absorption into the bloodstream, which is what happened when liver was used to cure pernicious anemia.

Since B-12 is a methyl donor, it is involved in all new cell growth, which makes it rather important in processes like red blood cell and immune cell formation, energy metabolism, and nerve function. There is a huge body of data now pointing to B-12 and folacin as primary nutrients that can interrupt the production of homocysteine, which is a major risk factor in heart disease.

For the cancer patient, B-12 supplements may bolster host defense mechanisms, plus it can combine with vitamin C to form a unique cobalt ascorbate complex that is selectively toxic to tumor cells. [197]

Folic acid 100-800 mcg as methyl folate
Assists in proper cell growth, is an immune stimulant, helps to check abnormal DNA production

---

Folic acid (a.k.a. methylfolate, folate, folacin) presents a unique challenge in cancer treatment. On one side of the fence stand the oncologists who have used the chemotherapy drug methotrexate for decades as an antagonist to the B vitamin, folic acid, to slow cancer growth, with leucovorin (folinic acid) as the rescue agent to summon the patient back from near death, or "the vital frontier". On the other side stand nutritionists who understand the pivotal role that folic acid plays in HEALTHY cell growth. The efficacy of methotrexate, now being used to treat some cases of rheumatoid arthritis, is not affected by patients taking supplements of folic acid.[198]

Without optimal amounts of folic acid in the cell, growth is erratic and prone to errors, such as birth defects and cancer. Low folate status during pregnancy will generate common birth defects, including spina bifida. Because of the irrefutable link between good nutrition in utero and healthy babies, groups like Vitamin Angels distribute vitamins to 70 million mothers annually in 70 different countries.[199] Humans with low B-12 and folate status present a clinical picture that looks like leukemia.[200] The importance of folate in new cell growth is highlighted in the fact that it is the only nutrient whose requirement doubles during pregnancy.

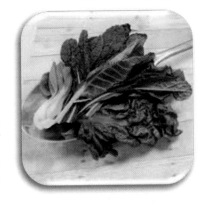

Folic acid is one of the common nutrient deficiencies in the world, since few people eat the plant foods rich in folacin. The name, folic acid, comes from the Latin term "folium", meaning foliage, since dark green leafy vegetables are a rich source of folic acid. Other good sources of folic acid include brewer's yeast, legumes, asparagus, oranges, cabbage, root vegetables, and whole grains. Since folic acid is essential for all new cell growth, disturbances in folic acid metabolism are far-reaching, including heart disease (due to more homocysteine in the blood), birth defects, immune suppression, cancer, premature senility, and a long list of other conditions. Without adequate folate in the diet, cell growth is like a drunk driver heading down the highway--more likely to do some harm than not.

Since folic acid and B-12 work together in methyl donor reactions, a deficiency of one can be masked by an excess of the other. Hence, the FDA has stipulated that non-prescription supplements cannot contain more than 800 micrograms of folic acid. Experts have estimated that up to 20% of all senility in older adults is merely a long-term deficiency of folic acid and vitamin B-12. The RDA of folate is 300 mcg for adults and 600 mcg for pregnant women, although the Center for Disease Control has recommended that 800 mcg of folic acid would prevent most cases of spina bifida. Without adequate folic acid in the body, there is a buildup of homocysteine in the blood, which probably generates 10% or more of the 1 million cases of heart disease each year in the U.S.

Cancer is not an "on-off" switch. There are varying shades of gray in between the black and white of normal cells and full-blown metastatic malignancies. In cervical cancer, there is a rating system where a stage I dysplasia shows abnormal cell growth, while stage IV is life-threatening cancer. In one study, 40% of women with stage I and II cervical dysplasia showed clear signs of folic acid deficiency.[201] In a double-blind placebo-controlled trial, 10 milligrams daily of folate (50 times the RDA) reversed cervical dysplasia in the majority of women tested.[202] Low folate intake increases the risk for colorectal cancer.[203] Human cells in a culture of low folate show immune suppression (impaired delayed hypersensitivity).[204] Folate deficiency is common throughout the world and America, especially among the elderly and adolescent females.[205] Alcohol and many drugs interfere with the absorption and metabolism of folate. Average intake of folate in the U.S. is about 240 mcg, which is one half to one fourth of what a good diet will contribute.

Biotin 10-50 mcg
Improves energy metabolism for glucose and fats, is involved in pH maintenance through carbon dioxide binding, and helps regulate cell growth.

Biotin is a B vitamin that is incorporated into 4 different carboxylase enzymes, which makes it essential for processing fats, sugar, and various amino acids. Biotin is also involved in the production of glucokinase, an enzyme in the liver that is essential for burning glucose. Biotin supplements have been helpful at improving glucose tolerance in insulin-dependent diabetics (Type 1, using 16 milligrams/day) and non-insulin-dependent diabetics (Type 2, using 9 mg/day). [206] Biotin supplements have been able to improve peripheral neuropathy (tingling numbness) in diabetics. Peripheral neuropathy is common in patients after extensive chemotherapy.

Richest food sources of biotin are brewer's yeast, liver, soy, rice, peanut butter, and oats. Biotin is also produced in the intestines through bacterial fermentation, which complicates the understanding of what an optimal intake might be. A healthy gut environment of adequate fiber, fluid, and probiotics probably improves the production of biotin in the gut. Recommended intake of biotin is 30-300 mcg per day.

For more information on how your body can fight cancer go to GettingHealthier.com.

PATIENT PROFILE: CONQUERED BREAST CANCER

D.S. was a 61-year old female diagnosed with Stage III breast cancer. Underwent radical mastectomy (1 breast) with 4 of 22 nodes found to have cancer. Two subsequent rounds of chemotherapy produced severe side effects--patient passed out within 5 minutes of beginning chemo. Told by oncologist that without chemo, D.S. had a 5% chance of survival. Discontinued chemotherapy anyway. Two years later went to different physician who detected possible disease in the remaining breast. Surgeon performed lumpectomy and there was no cancer in this tissue, as per the pathologist report. D.S. then began nutrition therapy as sole therapy. Three months later, she was found to have enlarged lymph nodes with possible recurrent breast cancer. Three months later these nodes disappeared. Last time I saw her was 3 years later and she was still in complete remission. She is very pleased with the healing power of nutrition.

ENDNOTES

[1]. Huang, ME, Am.J.Hematol., vol.28, p.124, 1988

[2] https://www.ncbi.nlm.nih.gov/pmc/articles/PMC4387950/

[3]. Watson, R., et al., Nutr.Res., vol.5, p.663, 1985

[4]. Zhang, XM, et al., Virchows Archiv.B Cell.Pathol., vol.61, p.375, 1992

[5]. Friedberg, EC, CANCER QUESTIONS, p.32, Freeman & Co, NY, 1992

[6] https://www.cambridge.org/core/journals/proceedings-of-the-nutrition-society/article/vitamin-a-and-immunity-to-viral-bacterial-and-protozoan-infections/8E1173F0F55C4FB4F4BE59436606D312

[7]. Semba, RD, Clin. Infect.Dis., vol.19, p.489, 1994

[8] https://search.proquest.com/openview/e2d8187c836887933c33a22fc0b71e65/1?pq-origsite=gscholar&cbl=42187

[9]. Pinnock, CB, et al., Aust.Paediatr.J., vol.22, p.95, 1986

[10]. Nutrition Reviews, vol.52, p.281, 1994

[11]. Micksche, M., et al., Onkologie, vol.1, p.57, 1978

[12]. Vagner, VP, et al., Klin.Med., vol.69, p.55, 1991

[13]. Michalek, AM, et al., Nutrition and Cancer, vol.9, p.143, 1987

[14]. Stich, HF, Am.J.Clin.Nutr., vol.53, p.298S, 1991

[15]. Lippman, SM, et al., J.Am.Coll.Nutr., vol.7, p.269, 1988

[16]. Pastorino, U., et al., J. Clin.Oncol., vol.11, p.1216, 1993

[17]. Hruban, Z, Am.J.Pathol., vol.76, p.451, 1974

[18]. Rothman, KJ, et al., N.Engl.J.Med., vol.333, p.1369, 1995

[19]. Hathcock, JN, et al., Am.J.Clin.Nutr., vol.52, p.183, 1990

[20]. Block, G., et al., Nutr.Cancer, vol.18, p.1, 1992

[21]. Mayne, ST, et al., J. Nat.Cancer Inst., vol.86, p.33, 1994

[22]. Krinsky, NI, Amer.J.Clin.Nutr., vol.53, p.238S, 1991

[23]. Zhang, L., et al., Carcinogenesis, vol.12, p.2109, 1991

[24]. Schwartz, JL, Biochem.Biophys Res.Comm., vol.169, p.941, 1990

[25]. Mathews-Roth, MM, et al., Photochem Photobiol., vol.42, p.35, 1985

[26]. Giovannucci, E., et al., J.Nat.Cancer Inst., vol.87, p.1767, 1995

[27]. Garewal, HS, et al., Archives Otolaryngol Head Neck Surg., vol.121, p.141, Feb.1995

[28]. Hazuka, MB, et al., J. Amer.Coll.Nutrition, vol.9, p.143, 1990

[29]. Burton, GW, J.Nutrition, vol.119, p.109, 1989

[30]. Tomita, Y., et al., J.Nat.Cancer Inst., vol.78, p.679, 1987

[31]. Santamaria, L., et al., Modulation and Mediation of Cancer by Vitamins, p.81, Karger, Basel, 1983

[32]. Bertram, JS, et al., Nutrients and Cancer Prevention, Prasad, KN (eds), p.99, Humana , 1990

[33]. Santamaria, L., et al., Nutrients and Cancer Prevention, p.299, Prasad, KN (eds), Humana , 1990

[34]. Seifter, E., et al., J.Nat.Cancer Inst., vol.71, p.409, 1983

[35]. Shklar, G., et al., Eur.J.Cancer Clin.Oncol., vol.24, p.839, 1988

[36]. Mills, EED, British J.Cancer, vol.57, p.416, 1988

[37]. Seifter, E., et al., J.Nat.Cancer Inst., vol.68, p.835, 1982

[38]. Nagasawa, H., et al., Anticancer Res., vol.9, p.71, 1989

[39]. Meyers, DG, et al., Archives Internal Med., vol.156, p.925, 1996

[40]. Alpha tocopherol beta-carotene cancer , New England J of Medicine, vol.330, p.1029, 1994

[41]. Schwartz, JL, Journal of Nutrition, vol.126, 4 suppl, p.1221S, 1996

[42] http://www.jnhrc.com.np/index.php/jnhrc/article/view/728

[43] https://www.mdpi.com/2072-6643/12/4/988

[44]. Norman, AW, in PRESENT KNOWLEDGE IN NUTRITION, p.120, Ziegler, EE (eds), ILSI, Washington 1996

[45]. Gorham, ED, et al., Intern.J.Epidemiol. vol.20, p.1145, Dec.1991

[46]. Lefkowitz, ES, et al., Intern.J.Epidemiol., vol.23, p.1133, Dec.1994

[47]. Garland, CF, et al., Lancet, p.1176, Nov.18, 1989

[48]. Barger-Lux, MJ, J. Nutr., vol.124, p.1406S, Aug.1994

[49]. Crowle, AJ, et al., Infection and Immunity, vol.55, p.2945, Dec.1987

[50]. Newmark, HL, Adv.Exp.Med.Biol., vol.364, p.109, 1994

[51] . Lancet, p.1122, May 16, 1987

[52] . Pence, B., et al., Proc Amer.Assoc. Cancer, vol.28, p.154, 1987

[53] . Colston, KW, et al., Lancet, p.188, Jan.28, 1989

[54] . Peehl, DM, et al., J. Endocrinol. Invest., vol.17, p.3,, 1994

[55] . Eisman, JA, et al., Modulation and Mediation of Cancer by Vitamins, p.282, Karger, Basel, 1983

[56] . Kizaki, M., et al., Vitamins and Cancer Prevention, p.91, Wiley-Liss, NY, 1991

[57] . DeLuca, HF, Nutrients and Cancer Prevention, p.271, Humana Press, NY, 1990

[58] . Rita, M., et al., Cancer Immunol. Immunother., vol.41, p.37, 1995

[59] https://academic.oup.com/ajcn/article/93/5/1175S/4597894

[60] . Food and Nutrition Board, National Research Council, Recommended Dietary Allowances, National Academy Press, p.97, Washington, DC, 1989

[61] . Buist, RA, Intern.Clin.Nutr.Rev., vol.4, p.159, 1984

[62] . Vieth, R., Am.J.Clin.Nutr., vol.69, no.5, p.842, May 1999; see also Vieth, R., Am.J.Clin.Nutr., vol.77, p.204, Jan.2003

[63] . Sokol, RJ, in PRESENT KNOWLEDGE IN NUTRITION, p, 132, Ziegler, ILSI, Wash DC, 1996

[64] . Munoz, SJ, et al., Hepatology, vol.9, p.525, 1989

[65] . Niki, E. et al., Amer.J.Clin.Nutr., vol.53, p.201S, 1991

[66] . Bunk, MJ, et al., Proc.Soc.Exp.Biol.Med., voo.190, p.379, 1989

[67] . Kramer, TR, et al., Am.J.Clin.Nutr., vol.54, p.896, 1991

[68] . Nutrition Reviews, vol.45, p.27, Jan.1987

[69] . Meydani, SN, et al., Am.J.Clin.Nutr., vol.52, p.557, 1990

[70] . Penn, ND, et al., Age Ageing, vol.20, p.169, 1991

[71] . Kuroiwa, K, et al., J.Parenteral Enteral Nutr., vol.15, p.22, 1991

[72] . Odeleye, OE, et al., Nutr.Cancer, vol.17, p.223, 1992

[73] . Cook, MG, et al., Cancer Research, vol.40, p.1329, 1980

[74] . Horvath, PM, et al., Anticancer Research, vol.43, p.5335, Nov.1983

[75] . Sclafani, L, et al., J.Parenteral Enteral Nutr., vol.10, p.184, 1986

[76] . Packer, L., Med.Biol., vol.62, p.105, 1984

[77] . Rimm, EB, et al., New Engl J.Med., vol.328, p.1450, 1993

[78] . Record, IR, et al., Nutr.Cancer, vol.16, p.219, 1991

[79] . J.Amer Med.Assoc, vol.244, p.1077, 1980

[80] . Panganamala, RV, et al., Annals NY Acad Sci, vol.393, p.376, 1982

[81] . Jandak, J., Blood, vol.73, p.141, Jan.1989

[82] . Knekt, P., et al., Am.J.Clin.Nutr., vol.53, p.283S, 1991

[83] . deVries, N., et al., Eur.Arch.Otorhinolaryngol, vol.247, p.368, 1990

[84] . Shklar, G., et al., J.Nat.Cancer Inst., vol.78, p.987, 1987

[85] . Paganelli, GM, et al., J.Nat.Cancer Inst., vol.84, p.47, 1992

[86] . Longnecker, MP, et al., J.Nat.Cancer Inst., vol.84, p.430, 1992

[87] . Yano., T., et al., Cancer Letters, vol.87, p.205, 1994

[88] . Prasad, KN, et al., J. Amer.Coll.Nutr., vol.11, p.487, 1992

[89] . Rama, BN, et al., Proc.Soc.Exper.Biol. Med., vol.174, p.302, 1983

[90] . Cohrs, RJ, et al., Int.J.Devl.Neuroscience., vol.9, p.187, 1991

[91] . Kline, K., et al., Nutr.Cancer, vol.14, p.27, 1990

[92] . Prasad, KN, et al., NUTRIENTS AND CANCER PREVENTION, Prasad, KN (eds), p.39, Humana Press, 1990

[93] . Singal, PK, et al., Mol.Cell.Biochem., vol.84, p.163, 1988

[94] . Singal, PK, et al., Molecular Cellular Biochem., vol.84, p.163, 1988

[95] . Clemens, MR, et al., Am.J.Clin.Nutr., vol.51, p.216, 1990

[96] . Shklar, G., et al., J.Oral Pathol.Med., vol.19, p.60, 1990

[97] . Geetha, A., et al., J.Biosci., vol.14, p.243, 1989

[98] . Geetha, A., et al., Current Science, vol.64, p.318, Mar.1993

[99] . Wang, YM, et al., Molecular Inter Nutr.Cancer, p.369, Arnott, MS, (eds), Raven Press, NY, 1982

[100] . Ripoll, EAP, et al., J.Urol., vol.136, p.529, 1986

[101] . Wood, L, N.Engl.J.Med., vol.312, p.1060, 1985

[102] . Washio, M., et al., Nephron, vol.68, p.347, 1994

[103] . VanVleet, JF, et al., Cancer Treat.Rep., vol.64, p.315, 1980

[104] . Sundstrom, H., et al., Carcinogenesis, vol.10, p.273, 1989

[105] . Milei, J., et al., Am.Heart J., vol.111, p.95, 1986
[106] . Kagerud, A., et al., vol.20, p.1, 1981
[107] . Prasad, KN, et al., Proc.Soc.Exper.Biol.Med., vol.161, p.570, 1979
[108] . Sarria, A., et al., Proc.Soc.Exper.Biol.Med., vol.175, p.88, 1984
[109] . Kagerud, A., et al., Anticancer Research, vol.1, p.35, 1981
[110] . Hoffer, A., et al., Radiation Research, vol.61, p.439, 1975
[111] . Taren, DL, et al., J.Vit.Nutr.Res., vol.57, p.133, 1987
[112] . Waxman, S., et al., Eur.J.Cancer Clin.Oncol., vol.18, p.685, 1982
[113] . Traber, MG, et al., N.Engl.J.Med., vol.317, p.262, 1987
[114] . Wadleigh, RG, et al., Amer.J.Med,vol.92, p.481, May 1992
[115] . J.Nat.Cancer Inst., vol.84, p.997, July 1992
[116] . Kitagawa, M., et al., J. Nutr.Sci. Vitaminology, vol.35, p.133, 1989
[117] . Hathcock, JN, NY Acad Sciences, vol.587, p.257, 1990
[118] . Nutrition Reviews, vol.44, p.10, Jan.1986
[119] . Suttie, JW, in PRESENT KNOWLEDGE IN NUTRITION, p.137, Ziegler, EE (eds), ILSI, Washington, 1996
[120] . Chlebowski, RT, et al., Cancer Treatment Reviews, vol.12, p.49, 1985
[121] . Noto, V., et al., Cancer, vol.63, p.901, 1989
[122] . Dam,H., in Harris, VITAMINS AND HORMONES, p.329, vol.18, Academic Press, NY, 1960
[123] . Chlebowski, RT, et al., Proc.Am.Assoc.Cancer Res., vol.24, p.653, 1983
[124] . Nutter, LM, et al., Biochem.Pharmacol., vol.41, p.1283, 1991
[125] . Krishanamurthi, S., et al., Radiology, vol.99, p.409, 1971
[126] . Taper, HS, et al., Int.J.Cancer, vol.40, p.575, 1987
[127] . Waxman, S., et al., Eur.J.Cancer Clin.Oncol., vol.18, p.685, 1982
[128] . Gold, J., Cancer Treatment Reports, vol.70, p.1433, Dec.1986
[129] . Gold, J., Proc.Amer Assoc Cancer Researchers, vol.28, p.230, Mar.1987
[130] . Nagourney, R., et al., Proc.Amer.Assoc.Clin.Oncol., vol.6, p.35, Mar.1987
[131] https://www.spandidos-publications.com/10.3892/ijo.23.3.627
[132] https://www.spandidos-publications.com/ijmm/17/2/235
[133] https://www.spandidos-publications.com/10.3892/ijo.29.6.1501
[134] https://www.sciencedirect.com/science/article/abs/pii/S0278691518300838
[135] https://www.sciencedirect.com/science/article/pii/S0083672907000106
[136] https://www.urologyofva.net/articles/category/longevity/59613/vitamin-k-protection-against-cancer-page-1-life-extension
[137] . National Research Council, VITAMIN TOLERANCE OF ANIMALS, National Academy Press, Washington, DC 1987
[138] . Suttie, IBID
[139] . Levine, M., et al., in PRESENT KNOWLEDGE IN NUTRITION, p.146, ILSI, Washington, 1996
[140] . National Academy of Sciences, DIET NUTRITION AND CANCER, National Academy Press, Washington, 1982
[141] . Block, G., Annals Intern.Med., vol.114, p.909, 1991
[142] . Cameron, E., Pauling, L., Cancer Research, vol. 39, p.663, Mar.1979
[143] . Ocke, MC, et al., Int.J.Cancer, vol.61, p.480, 1995
[144] . Block, G., Am.J.Clin.Nutr., vol.53, p.270S, 1991
[145] . Tannenbaum, SR, et al., Am.J.Clin.Nutr., vol.53, p.247S, 1991
[146] . Ringsdorf, WM, et al., Oral Surg, p.231, Mar.1982
[147] . Nutrition Reviews, vol.45, p.217, July 1987
[148] . Liehr, JG, Am.J.Clin.Nutr., vol.54, p.1256S, 1991
[149] . Bright-See, E., et al., Modulation and Meditation of Cancer by Vitamins, p.95, Karger, Basel., 1983
[150] . Josephy, PD, et al., Nature, vol.271, p.370, Jan.1978
[151] . Prasad, KN, et al., Proc.Natl.Acad.Sci., vol.76, p.829, Feb.1979
[152] . Sethi, VS, et al., in Modulation and Mediation of Cancer by Vitamins, p.270, Karger, Basel, 1983
[153] . Fujita, K., et al., Cancer Research, vol.42, p.309, Jan.1982
[154] . Minow, RA, et al., Cancer Chemother.Rep., vol.3, p.195, 1975
[155] . Okunieff, P., Am.J.Clin.Nutr., vol.54, p.1281S, 1991
[156] . Hanck, AB, Prog.Clin.Biol.Res., vol.259, p.307, 1988
[157] . Koch, CJ, et al., J.Cell.Physiol., vol.94, p.299, 1978

[158]. Lupulescu, A., Exp.Toxic.Pathol. vol.44, p.3, 1992

[159]. Riordan, NH, et al., Medical Hypotheses, vol.44, p.207, 1995

[160]. Bram, S., et al., Nature, vol.284, p.629, Apr.1980

[161]. Park, CH, et al., Cancer Research, vol.40, p.1062, Apr.1980

[162]. Poydock, ME, Am.J.Clin.Nutr., vol.54, p.1261S, 1991

[163]. Noto, V., et al., Cancer, vol.63, p.901, 1989

[164]. Gardiner, N, et al., Pros.Leuk., vol.34, p.119, 1988

[165] http://ar.iiarjournals.org/content/29/3/809.short

[166] https://www.cmaj.ca/content/174/7/937?sid=c4b05

[167] https://journals.plos.org/plosone/article/file?type=printable&id=10.1371/journal.pone.0011414

[168]. Cameron, E., Pauling, L., Proc.Natl.Acad.Sci., vol.75, p.4538, Sept.1978

[169]. Moertel, CG, et al., N.Engl.J.Med., vol.312, p.137, 1985

[170]. Marcus, SL, et al., Am.J.Clin.Nutr., vol.54, p.1292S., 1991

[171]. Abrahamian, V., et al., Ascorbic acid requirements in hospital patients, JPEN, 7, 5, 465-8, 1983

[172]. Anthony, HM, et al., Vitamin C status of lung cancer patients, Brit J Ca, 46, 354-9, 1982

[173]. Cheraskin, E., Scurvy in cancer patients?, J Altern Med, 18-23, Feb.1986

[174]. Bendich, A., in BEYOND DEFICIENCIES, NY Acad.Sci., vol.669, p.300, 1992

[175]. Kaul, L., et al., Nutr.Cancer, vol.9, p.123, 1987

[176]. Bowman, BB, et al., Am.J.Clin.Nutr., vol.35, p.1142, 1982

[177]. Rindi, G., in PRESENT KNOWLEDGE IN NUTRITION, p.163, ILSI, Washington, 1996

[178]. Elsborg, L., Int.J.Vitamin Res., vol.53, p.321, 1983

[179]. Lopez, R., et al., Am.J.Clin.Nutr., vol.33, p.1283, 1980

[180]. Schmitt-Graff, A., et al, Pathol.Res.Pract., vol.181, p.168, 1986

[181]. Popov, AI, Med.Radiol. Mosk., vol.32, p.42, 1987

[182]. Kjellen, E., et al., Radiother.Oncol., vol.22, p.81, 1991

[183]. Horsman, MR, Radiotherapy Oncology, vol.22, p.79, 1991

[184]. Aprahamian, M., et al., Am.J.Clin.Nutr., vol.41, p.578, 1985

[185]. Prior, F., Med.Hypotheses, vol.16, p.421, 1985

[186]. Chrisley, BM, et al., Nutr.Res., vol.6, p.1023, 1986

[187]. Ha, C., et al., J.Nutr., vol.114, p.938, 1984

[188]. Solomon, LR, et al., Diabetes, vol.38, p.881, 1989

[189]. Gridley, DS, et al., Nutrition Research, vol.8, p.201, 1988

[190]. Tryfiates, GP, et al., Anticancer Research, vol.1, p.263, 1981

[191]. DiSorbo, DM, et al., Nutrition and Cancer, vol.5, p.10, 1983

[192]. DiSorbo, DM, et al., Nutrition and Cancer, vol.7, p.43, 1985

[193]. Byar, D., et al., Urolog7, vol.10, p.556, Dec.1977

[194]. Lamm, DL, et al., Megadose vitamin in bladder cancer: a double-blind clinical trial, J Urol, 151:21-26, 1994

[195]. Ladner, HA, et al., Nutrition, Growth, & Cancer, p.273, Alan Liss, Inc., 1988

[196]. Cohen, M., et al., Toxicology Letters, vol.34, p.129, 1986

[197]. Poydock, ME, Am.J.Clin.Nutr., vol.54, p.1261S, 1991

[198]. Leeb, BF, et al., Clin.Exper.Rheumat., vol.13, p.459, 1995

[199] https://www.vitaminangels.org/

[200]. Dokal, IS, et all, Br.Med.J., vol.300, p.1263, 1990

[201]. Fekete, PS, et al., Acta. Cytologica, vol.31, p.697, 1987

[202]. Butterworth, CE, et al., Am.J.Clin.Nutr., vol.35, p.73, 1982

[203]. Freudenheim, J., Int.J.Epidemiol., vol.20, p.368, 1991

[204]. Levy, JA, BASIC AND CLINICAL IMMUNOLOGY, p.297, Lange, Los Altos, 1982

[205]. Werbach, M., NUTRITIONAL INFLUENCES ON ILLNESS, p.625, Third Line , Tarzana, 1996

[206]. Koutsikos, D., et al., Biomed.Pharmacother., vol.44, p.511, 1990

Chapter 21

FOOD EXTRACTS

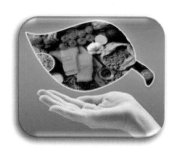

"If people let the government decide what foods they eat and what medicines they take, their bodies will soon be in as a sorry state as the souls who live under tyranny." - Thomas Jefferson

WHAT'S AHEAD

While whole foods are the foundation of this nutrition program, some ingredients in foods are so valuable as cancer fighters that they merit inclusion as concentrated supplements to:

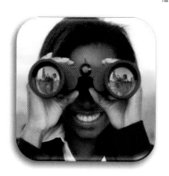

- ✓ Stimulate immune functions
- ✓ Regulate the body's cell division
- ✓ Escort any excess estrogen from the body
- ✓ Detoxify the body

> **Cruciferous (as diindolylmethane DIM) 50-300 mg**
> Detoxifying agent, helps to neutralize the damaging effects of estrogen, may selectively slow the cancer process

During the cold war era of 1950 researchers fed two different groups of animals either beets or cabbage and then exposed them to radiation, thinking nuclear war was imminent. The animals fed cabbage had much less hemorrhaging and death from radiation. But since no one in those days could conceive of a radio-protective effect of a food, the scientists concluded that "something in beets makes radioactive exposure more lethal." [1] Actually, "something" in cabbage makes radiation much less damaging to healthy tissue.

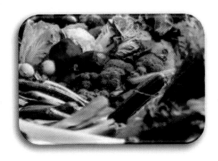

Cruciferous vegetables include cabbage, broccoli, Brussels sprouts, cauliflower, and others. Among the phytochemicals in cruciferous vegetables that have been researched, sulforaphane is one of the more promising as a cancer fighter. It was Professor Lee Wattenburg of Minnesota who found that cabbage extract has the ability to prevent the initiation and promotion of cancer cells. [2] The various fractions in cruciferous plants, including indole-3-carbinol, isothiocyanates, glucosinolates, dithiolethiones, and phenols, are able to:[3]

♦ Prevent chemicals from being converted into cancer-causing compounds
♦ Induce liver detoxification systems, such as glutathione S-transferase and P-450, to help rid the body of poisons
♦ Scavenge free radicals, thus working as an antioxidant
♦ Prevent tumor promoters from reaching their cell targets, such as blocking the binding of estrogen to estrogen-dependent tumors

> **Maitake D-fraction (10-60 mg)**
> Adaptogen, immune stimulant

Mushrooms, or fungi, have long been valued for their contributions as foods and medicines for humans. Penicillin was first discovered as bread mold, which is actually fungi generating a substance in its perimeter to inhibit bacterial growth. Mushrooms usually grow as mold on rotten tree stumps or in manure. Various mushrooms that have been tested for their medicinal value, including lentinan, AHCC, Shiitake, and PSK, Cordyceps, and Maitake (Grifola frondosa) with Maitake demonstrating consistent anti-cancer effects from oral intake.

Maitake literally means "dancing mushroom" since Japanese people who discovered these basketball-sized mushrooms growing on tree stumps would "dance with joy" at the prospects of the taste and health-giving properties. In the 1980s, Japanese firms began cultivating Maitake mushrooms on sawdust and intensely investigating the therapeutic value of this mushroom. An isolated fraction, D-fraction with active constituents of 1,6 and 1,3 beta-glucans, has been found to be the most potent and best-absorbed from the diet.

Maitake may help cancer patients via:

- Immune stimulation, capable of doubling the activity of Natural Killer cells in animals. D-fraction was able to increase interleukin-1 production from macrophages and potentiate delayed type hypersensitivity response, which is indicative of tumor growth suppression[4]
- Adaptogen that lowers hypertension,[5] lowers excess blood sugar levels, protects the liver, and has anti-viral activity[6]
- Inhibition of metastasis of cancer by 81% in one animal study[7]
- Augmenting the anti-cancer activity of drugs like Mitomycin. In a comparison study between Maitake D-fraction and Mitomycin C, Maitake provided superior tumor growth inhibition of 80% vs. 45% for the drug. Yet when both were given together, but at half the dosage for each, tumor inhibition was 98%
- Reducing toxic side effects from chemotherapy while augmenting tumor kill of the drug. There was a 90% drop in the incidence of appetite loss, vomiting, nausea, hair loss, and leukopenia (deficiency of immune cells) in human cancer patients treated with Maitake D-fraction while undergoing chemotherapy.

Garlic

Immune stimulant[8], detoxifying agent, antioxidant[9], powerful anti-fungal compound[10], protects[11] and rebuilds the liver[12], controls blood sugar levels, reduces the toxic effect of chemotherapy and radiation[13] on healthy cells, increases energy.

First mentioned as a medicine about 6,000 years ago, garlic has been a major player in human medicines throughout the world. In the tomb of the Egyptian king, Tutankhamen, were found gold ornaments and garlic bulbs. Slaves who built the Great Pyramids relied heavily on the energizing power of garlic for their work. Hippocrates, father of modern medicine, used garlic to heal infections and to reduce pain. Although garlic has been a medical staple of many societies for over 4,000 years, only in the past few decades when over 2,000 scientific studies have proven its healing value, has garlic received the respect and attention that it deserves.

Garlic grown on selenium-rich soil, such as found in Kyolic, may be directly toxic to tumor cells.[14] Garlic may be able to impact the cancer process[15] by inhibiting:

♦ carcinogen formation in the body (i.e. nitrosamines)
♦ the transformation of normal cells to pre-cancerous cells[16]
♦ the promotion of pre-cancerous cells to cancer[17]
♦ spreading (metastasis) of cancer cells to the surface of blood vessels
♦ formation of blood vessels in tumor mass, i.e. anti-angiogenesis

The debate continues regarding the active ingredients in garlic, but they may include amino acids (like the branched chain amino acids of leucine and isoleucine), S-allyl cysteine, allicin, and organically-bound selenium. In a double-blind trial in humans with high serum cholesterol, aged deodorized garlic with no allicin content was able to lower serum cholesterol by 7%.[18] While garlic in general, as either aged, fresh, cooked, or in supplement form, is a healthy addition to anyone's nutrition program, aged garlic extracts were effective at protecting animals from liver damage.[19] An extensive review of the literature on

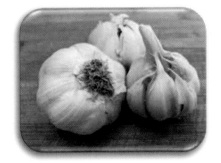

garlic and its influence on the cancer process shows the impressive and multiple ways that garlic can help the cancer patient.[20] In a Chinese study, people who ate more garlic had a 60% reduction in the risk for stomach cancer.[21]

Aged garlic was effective at preventing the initiation and promotion phase of esophageal cancer in animals.[22] In one animal study, garlic was more effective against bladder cancer than the drug of choice in human bladder cancer, BCG (bacillus Calmette-Guerin).[23] Garlic grown on selenium-rich soil was more effective than selenium supplements at inhibiting carcinogen-induced tumors in animals.[24] A study published in the *Journal of the National Medical Association* referred to garlic as "...a potent, non-specific biologic response modifier."[25] Garlic protects against the DNA-damaging potential of DMBA[26] and the liver carcinogen, aflatoxin.[27] It stimulates immune functions by activating macrophages and spleen cells[28] as well as enhancing Natural Killer cell activity.[29]

Lycopene 3-20 mg
Potent antioxidant and immune stimulant

Lycopene is one of the most potent antioxidants yet tested, having double the protective capacity of beta-carotene.[30] Lycopene is the reddish pigment from the carotenoid family. Tomatoes are the richest source of lycopenes, with watermelon and red grapefruit containing appreciable amounts of lycopenes.[31] 100 grams of raw tomatoes, or about 1 cup, contains about 3 milligrams of lycopene. Lycopene has made headlines around the world, and cheers in many college dorms, in December of 1995 when a scientific study 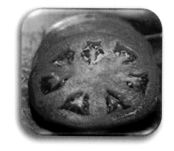 published in the *Journal of the National Cancer Institute* found that men who ate more PIZZA experienced less prostate cancer.[32] Pizza is obviously not a "nutrient dense" healthy food with all the fat, difficult-to-digest cheese, and white flour. Yet lycopene from tomatoes is such a potent antioxidant, immune stimulant, and regulator of cancer gene expression that a little tomato sauce on the pizza could neutralize the otherwise unhealthy meal of pizza and offer significant protection against the second most common cancer in American men.

As little as one serving per week of tomatoes could reduce esophageal cancer risk by 40% and other sites by 50%.[33] In another study, blood samples from 25,000 people were frozen for 15 years. Of the people in this study who developed cancer, those with the highest levels of lycopenes had the lowest incidence of pancreatic cancer.[34]

Bovine cartilage 2-9 gm
Immune stimulant, anti-mitotic agent (shuts down cell division in abnormal cells), anti-angiogenesis (shuts down production of blood vessels from tumors), adaptogen.

Bovine tracheal cartilage (BTC) is one of the more crucial and fascinating of all nutrition factors to help the cancer patient, so we will spend more than a little time discussing this ingredient. Imagine these headlines: "Major drug company finds new treatment for cancer, arthritis, shingles, and many other infectious disorders." The story would be featured on TV and newspapers around the world. The stock value of that company would skyrocket. But what if that same substance was a humble little unpatentable food extract? Would the enthusiasm be as great? Bovine cartilage may be in that category.

Good luck never hurt anyone's career. In 1954, John Prudden, MD (Harvard), PhD (Columbia), noticed an article from the reknowned Columbia-Presbyterian researchers, Drs. Meyer, Regan, and Lattes, on how topical cartilage could neutralize the disastrous effect that cortisone had on inhibiting wound recovery. This tip on the therapeutic value of cartilage had come from a mysterious "Dr. Martin" from Montreal, who has never since been located.

The next lucky event for Prudden came when a 70-year-old woman came to him with advanced breast cancer that was literally eating away her chest cavity in stage IV fungating breast cancer. Prudden tried the topical bovine cartilage along with injecting bovine cartilage solutions into obvious tumor areas with the hopes that it might help to heal these awful, ulcerated wounds so that Prudden could operate. Surprisingly, the woman returned to Dr. Prudden with the wounds healed AND the cancer gone. It has been said that "chance favors the prepared mind".

Over the course of 40 years, Prudden has been involved in $7 million of research to better understand BTC. Prudden received a patent on cartilage in 1962 for its anti-inflammatory properties when topically applied to arthritic regions of the body. Prudden was an affable man and dog lover who saved one of his dogs from mastocytoma (a terminal cancer) using BTC, before passing away in 1998.

Prudden found that the wind pipe of cows was considered offal, among the waste products of the butchering process. Given the world's hunger for beef, this seemed to be a bountiful supply of inexpensive raw material. Prudden developed the complex process for removing the fat from the cartilage, then drying, and powdering it. He named his original product Catrix, short for Cicatrix, which means "healed wound".

Cartilage resembles fetal mesenchyme, which is the source for developing muscle, bones, tendons, ligaments, skin, fat, and bone marrow. It probably is this unique origin that gives rise to the many therapeutic benefits of cartilage.

Anti-angiogenesis? Lane's theory that shark cartilage may shut down the making of blood vessels from tumors (anti-angiogenesis) has some foundation. In 1976, Dr. Robert Langer of MIT and Dr. Judah Folkman of Harvard published work showing that something in cartilage can shut down angiogenesis in cultured tumors.[35] Later studies by this same group showed that rabbits with corneal cancers had measurable benefits from cartilage topically applied in slowing the growth of tumors.[36] In 1983, Langer and colleague Anne Lee found that something in shark cartilage could slow the growth of tumors through anti-angiogenesis.[37]

Langer pursued this line of research, finding that tumors could not grow larger than 1-2 centimeters (1/2 to 1 inch) without vascularization to support further growth.[38] Dr. Patricia D'Amore of Harvard endorsed the concept that if you shut down angiogenesis, then you shut down tumor growth.[39] Folkman's team then found that when a cell switches from normal growth (hyperplasia) to rapid and uncontrolled tumor growth (neoplasia), then the angiogenesis process gears up dramatically.[40] Other Harvard researchers found that something in cartilage definitely shuts down angiogenesis, which is essential for tumor growth.[41] Japanese researchers reported on this anti-angiogenic agent found in shark cartilage.[42] More Harvard researchers reported on the strong link between angiogenesis and tumor progression.[43] Folkman further explained the importance of anti-angiogenesis in cancer, yet added that perhaps genetic regulation is more important than some dietary protein.[44]

BOVINE CARTILAGE IN HUMAN CANCER

31 patients over 11 yrs with refractory end stage cancer treated with 9 gm/d BTC

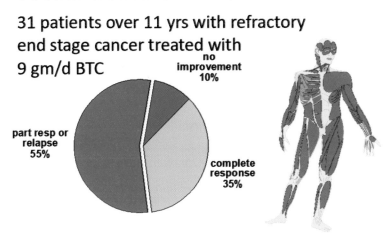

Prudden, J.Biol.Resp.Mod.,4,551,1985

In discussions with pathologists and Dr. Prudden, there seems to be a difference between the blood vessels that extend cork screw-like from a tumor and the blood vessels that extend "tree root-like" from healthy tissue. If there is an anti-angiogenesis factor in cartilage, then it cannot inhibit the making of normal healthy blood vessels. How does a baby shark grow into a large adult shark if shark cartilage shuts down the making of ALL blood vessels?

Prudden believed that BTC is effective because it is a biodirector, or "normalizer". There are parallels of these "homeostatic regulators" in the botanical medicine field called adaptogens, such as ginseng or astragalus, which will raise your blood pressure if it is too low or lower it if it is too high. Think about the enigma of cartilage:

♦ topically applied, it **accelerates** healthy growth for wounds, but **slows** abnormal cancer growth

♦ taken internally, it **increases** various immune factors, including B-cells (from the bone), macrophages (literally: "big eaters"), and cytotoxic T-cells (important in the "war on cancer"); YET it also **slows** down auto-immune attacks involved in allergies, arthritis, and lupus

◆ taken internally, it slows the wasting disease, cachexia, caused by cancer and AIDS
◆ taken internally, it **slows** the division in abnormal cells (anti-mitotic), but **allows** healthy cells to divide
◆ taken internally, it **reduces** inflammation, such as in arthritis.

Prudden pioneered the use of BTC for its:
◆ wound healing properties, which culminated in textbook acceptance[45]
◆ anti-inflammatory agent in arthritis[46]
◆ anti-cancer activity.[47]

Prudden's peer-reviewed article showed a 90% response rate in 31 human cancer patients followed for 15 years. Of the 31 total patients, 35%, or 11 of these terminal patients were **cured** using 9 grams daily of oral bovine tracheal cartilage as sole therapy, while 55% or 17 showed some benefit then relapsed, and 10% or 3 showed no improvement. Prudden used BTC in over 1,000 cancer patients, with good follow-up on 100 patients.

Dr. Brian Durie has found equally impressive results using BTC to halt cancer growth in vitro.[48] Prudden's other research shows that BTC probably works by turbo-charging the immune system.[49] For his noteworthy persistence and brilliance in spearheading BTC research, Prudden received the coveted "Linus Pauling Scientist of the Year" award at the Third International Symposium on Adjuvant Nutrition in Cancer Treatment in Tampa, in September of 1995.

Nucleic acids (nucleotides from brewer's yeast)
DNA 500-1500 mg and RNA 500-1500 mg
Immune stimulants, help to regulate genetic expression and discourage the excessive production of Tumor Necrosis Factor, which can lead to tissue wasting.

At the very core of our cells are the "blueprints" of DNA that allow that cell to make another exact copy. RNA has various forms that basically are the "servants" of DNA, clamping on the DNA to read the base pair sequence, then going out into the cell to construct proteins, enzymes, or whatever the cell needs based on the DNA blueprints. Obviously, this is a very crucial pathway for human health. When DNA goes awry, cancer can result. Somehow the DNA in the healthy host tissue can become corrupted and start creating cells that lack normal regulation properties, have no plan, and reproduce without any restraint.

We make our own DNA and RNA (also called nucleic acids) in our cells from amino acids in the purine and pyrimidine pathways. We also eat some DNA/RNA in metabolically active foods including brewer's yeast, liver, seeds (especially the germ), organ meats, and bee pollen. The debate has never been over the value of DNA/RNA, but rather "can we absorb these nutrients into the bloodstream intact?" To answer that question, we need to step back and look at other examples of:

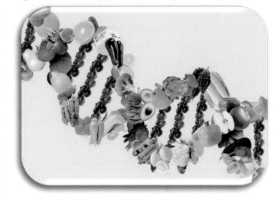

- ◆ fatty acids that are dissected with bile salts and enzymes in the GI tract and then reassembled in the bloodstream
- ◆ the known passage of large proteins through the intestinal wall to cause food allergies in the bloodstream
- ◆ the use of glandular therapy (such as natural desiccated thyroid) to treat the target gland with a large protein molecule that should be destroyed in the acid bath of the gut.
- ◆ how infants receive their immunity from the immunoglobulins in mother's milk.

Either these molecules have special "windows" in the gut or these molecules are torn apart in the gut and then reassembled on the other side of the intestinal mucosa in the bloodstream. Supplements of RNA/DNA have shown benefits in both immunity and wound recovery, when taken orally in both human and animal studies.

Animals fed a nucleotide-deficient diet had impaired immune functions which were corrected when fed uracil (a DNA precursor).[50] In protein depletion, RNA supplements may be essential in order to return immune functions to normal.[51] Several human trials have studied an enteral formula, Impact, which uses RNA, arginine, and fish oil to provide substantial improvement in immune factors.[52] RNA seems to improve wound recovery after surgery.[53] RNA supplements provide a boost to memory in the elderly.[54] RNA supplements were able to help regenerate the damaged livers of rats.[55] Early indications were that RNA may be able to help cancer patients.[56] Of course, a patentable drug (Poly A/Poly U) was developed to continue these studies, with very encouraging results.[57] RNA supplements seem to encourage Natural Killer cells to attack cancer and bacteria.[58]

Large amounts of RNA and DNA taken orally could shut down the tissue wasting process (cachexia) that is so common in cancer and AIDS. Precursors to make more nucleic acids seem to dampen down the cytokines (Tumor Necrosis Factor) that trigger the downward spiral of cancer cachexia.

Probiotics
Reduced production of carcinogens in the gut, maintenance of gut integrity and immune functions.

We have the seeds of our demise within our gut. Those same "seeds" are 100 trillion microorganisms which will become part of 21st century medicine. Throughout history, "gut shot or stabbed" meant an awful death, because the bacteria from the colon will invade the bloodstream and cause septicemia, a nasty way to go. However, if kept in their " dormitory" of the gut, these critters become an important part of healing from cancer.

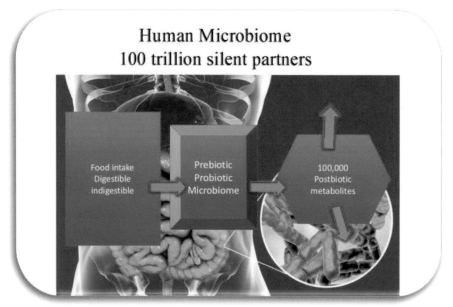

Scientists involved in the Human Microbiome Project (2007-2016) were dazzled at the elegant and complex ways in which the 100 trillion organisms in our gut interact with our body. There is cross talk, or chemical messengers between the post biotics (by products of metabolism from the microbes) and the intestinal lumen. Gut Associated Lymphoid Tissue (GALT) and mucosal associated lymphoid tissue (MALT) showed scientists that up to 70% of the human immune system surrounds the gut, making gut health crucial for immune support. Then there is "quorum sensing" in which the balance of microbes swings the health of the gut in favor of illness or disease, not unlike an election in a democratic country. More bad guys than good guys spells trouble.

We take in food, preferably with some fiber (resistant starches or prebiotics) and our critters in the microbiome (probiotics) eat this fiber, stay healthy, and give off an amazing array of by-products, called postbiotics.

It was the Nobel Laureate from Russia, Dr. Eli Metchnikoff, who told us at the turn of the century: "Death begins in the colon." Metchnikoff isolated the bacteria in yogurt, Lactobacillus, that ferments milk sugar, and he spent much of his illustrious career shedding light on the function of bacteria in the gut.

In order to better appreciate the importance of probiotics for cancer patients, we need to rewind the video cassette recorder to Louis Pasteur's deathbed confession in 1895: "I have been wrong. The germ is nothing. The terrain is everything." Pasteur was the famous French chemist who developed pasteurization, or the killing of bacteria with heat. Pasteur spent much of his life trying to figure out how to kill all the bacteria in the universe. Didn't work. By "terrain", Pasteur was referring to the land that bacteria grow in--your body.

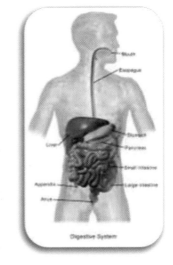

We now find that some bacteria are helpful, such as those that manufacture biotin and vitamin K in the gut. Many bacteria are relatively harmless, unless we have compromised immune functions. Many bacterial infections are called "opportunistic" because they only happen when the bacteria seize the opportunity while the host is weakened. Many bacteria in the gut can produce carcinogens and estrogens, to further a cancer process.[59] Oncologists have toiled for decades trying to isolate cancer patients from all external bacteria, since death from infections is so common in cancer patients, especially those treated with chemotherapy.

Oncologists working in bone marrow transplant (BMT) units will isolate cancer patients from family members and tell the patient to avoid fruits and vegetables, hoping to prevent an infection in the immune-compromised patient. Some BMT units even autoclave the food to try to reduce exposure to bacteria. Meanwhile, we have more bacteria in our gut than all the cells in our body. There is an ongoing struggle in your gut between bifidobacteria (good guys) and putrefactive bacteria (bad guys). The typical American diet (too much fat, sugar, and beef and not enough whole grains, fruits, and vegetables) will often create a very lethal mixture of bacteria in the gut. Add in the 30 millions pounds of antibiotics that we eat indirectly via meat and dairy products, since animals are fed antibiotics to allow them to stay alive under unhealthy conditions and abnormal diet.

What happens in too many cancer patients is that the infection comes from the inside, called bacterial translocation, not from the outside.[60] Only one of three factors needs to be present for disease-causing bacteria from the intestines to slide through the intestinal wall and create a life-threatening infection in the blood (sepsis):
- Disruption of the ecological balance of the normal intestinal microflora, resulting in overgrowth of certain harmful bacteria
- Impairment of host immune functions
- Physical disruption of the gut mucosal barrier.

Probiotics include a wide assortment of favorable bacteria, including Lactobacillus acidophilus from yogurt. Our ancestors did not have refrigeration to preserve food. Fermenting food became an essential art in creating lactic acid to preserve the food and the trillions of friendly bacteria in fermented food that supports our gut health. There are between 500 and 1,000 different species of microbes that inhabit the human gut. There is a bewildering array of probiotics available for human consumption OTC, with my favorite being Three Lac Probiotic.

When comparing the dietary habits of 1,000 women with and 1,000 women without breast cancer, yogurt was found to be the most protective of all foods analyzed.[61] Yogurt also helped to prevent the normal intestinal side effects caused by radiation therapy in women undergoing radiation for ovarian and cervical cancer.[62] There are soil-based organisms found in dirt and the gut that are equally intriguing as means of rectifying an imbalanced collection of bacteria in the human gut. Since dairy products are the most allergy-producing food in the world and can produce mucus in many individuals, it is unwise to recommend widespread use of yogurt for all cancer patients, though probiotic supplements can be of benefit.

Think of probiotics as "biological controls" within the gut. We have a septic tank inside of us. Our colon holds more than enough bacteria and fungi to kill us, yet when the gut flora is in balance, these deadly bacteria pass through us without doing any harm. Compare the balance of organisms in our gut with a healthy balanced organic garden. The birds and frogs (probiotics) eat the insects (unfriendly bacteria) and leave the vegetables (food in our gut) for us to digest and absorb.

Researchers in Russia gave gunshot-wounded animals either antibiotics, or probiotics, or no treatment (control) and found that probiotics were more effective than antibiotics at preventing surgical infection.[63] Bacterial translocation was dramatically reduced in animals who were given surgery on the gut, then probiotics.[64] Antibiotics can kill off the friendly bacteria in the gut, leaving the distinct possibility of bacterial translocation of the nasty bacteria into the bloodstream.

In an animal study, the probiotic Saccharomyces boulardii was able to reduce the incidence of bacterial translocation from antibiotics.[65] Bone marrow transplantation operations often trigger a "graft versus host" disease, which means the patient who received the new immune cells is having an allergic response because this is not the patient's own DNA. German oncologists found that giving yogurt to patients undergoing allogeneic bone marrow transplantation (getting immune cells from someone else versus getting your own—autologous) dramatically reduced the bacterial translocation of enteric bacteria.[66]

Use fermented foods, like yogurt, kimchi, sauerkraut, and supplements with probiotics and prebiotics (fiber).

Bee pollen
Rich in amino acids, B-vitamins, and bioflavonoids; historically used as an energizer, blood builder, and immune stimulant

---

Bee pollen is a rich and well-balanced collection of B-vitamins, vitamin C, RNA and DNA, amino acids, polyunsaturated fats, enzymes, trace minerals, bioflavonoids, and an assortment of other unidentified nutrition factors.

Bee pollen has been used throughout history as a superfood to restore energy and recuperative powers to the ailing individual.[67] Bee pollen improves allergies in many individuals, and hence may have a regulating effect on the immune system by helping to dampen unnecessary autoimmune attacks, which saves immune warriors for the real cancer battle. There is no toxicity to bee pollen. Other bee products with extraordinary healing properties include royal bee jelly and propolis, which is the antibiotic compound used by bees to disinfect their hives before occupation. Some people use propolis as a substitute for antibiotics in non-life-threatening infections.

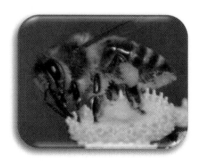

Lecithin (phosphatidylcholine)
Helps to detoxify the liver, regulates cell growth, contributes choline for many other functions in the body, becomes part of healthy cell membranes for proper nutrient intake and toxin removal

---

Most substances in life are either fat soluble, such as butter, or water soluble, such as vitamin C. Lecithin is on a very short list of substances (phospholipids) that can dissolve both fat and water soluble substances at the same time, also known as an emulsifier. Lecithin is used widely in the food industry to prevent separation of ingredients in cookies, etc. The richest sources of lecithin are soybeans and egg yolks.

Lecithin is a molecule that is similar in structure to triglycerides found in soy oil and beef, except that one of the fatty acids has been replaced by phosphatidylcholine. This simple exchange gives lecithin unique properties, including:

♦ lowering of serum cholesterol and reduction of platelet aggregation in humans[68]
♦ reversing the skin disease psoriasis[69]
♦ improving the course of Alzheimer's disease[70]
♦ reducing the tremors in tardive dyskinesia[71]

Lecithin seems to work in the cell membrane to enhance "cell membrane dynamics", works in the nervous tissue (sphingomyelin), and contributes a key B-vitamin, choline. Choline works with folate, methionine, and B-12 as methyl donors, which are responsible for all new cell growth.

Choline is one of the few nutrients tested in which merely a deficiency (without any other compounding factor, such as toxins or aging) is enough to spontaneously generate liver cancer in animals.[72] In animal and human studies, choline deficiency leads to fatty liver and compromised liver functions.[73] Lecithin is a major protective nutrient for the liver, helping to regenerate healthy liver tissue and excrete toxins. Protecting the liver, with substances like lecithin and milk thistle, is crucial for cancer patients.

Genistein (from non-genetically modified organism soy) 6 mg
Helps to selectively slow down cancer growth

When scientists reviewed the world's cancer incidences, they found some strange disparities. Japanese men had 1/5 the incidence of prostate cancer and Japanese women had 1/5 the incidence of breast cancer when compared to Americans. The reasons could be many, including a lower fat diet, more exercise, less beef, less obesity, and more vegetables and seaweed. But researchers settled in on soybean products, including tofu and tempeh, as the primary protector against cancer. It has now been well established that regular consumption of soy products may lower the incidence of many forms of cancer.[74] While there is a rich collection of isoflavones, protease inhibitors, and lectins in soybeans, researchers have focused on genistein as perhaps the cancer-protective bioflavonoid in soy.

Genistein may be able to:
- selectively kill cancer cells
- reduce the tumor growth capacity of sex hormones in both men and women
- induce programmed cell death (apoptosis) in cancer
- inhibit metastasis
- inhibit angiogenesis[75] (making of blood vessels from tumors)
- induce differentiation, to help regulate proper cell growth.[76]

Genistein is one of the few agents on planet earth that may be able to revert a cancer cell back to a normal healthy cell, in a process called prodifferentiation. [77]   Scientists have worked diligently to better understand the anti-cancer effects of protease inhibitors in soy.[78] Dr. Ann Kennedy spent 20 years at Harvard, and is now working at the University of Pennsylvania, researching the extraordinary ability of the Bowman Birk Inhibitor (a protease inhibitor found in soy) to prevent and reverse cancer while also reducing the toxic effects of chemo and radiation on animals.[79]

Soy and breast cancer. Based on the fact that soy contains weak phytoestrogens that can induce infertility in zoo animals kept on a high soy diet, some experts have cautioned against the use of soy in estrogen/progesterone-positive breast cancer. Tamoxifen is an estrogen binder drug that is given to women with estrogen-positive breast cancer. Tamoxifen has a similar chemical structure to genistein, yet genistein does not have any of the toxic side effects of Tamoxifen. <u>Phytoestrogens</u> 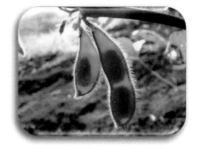 <u>have been</u> shown to lower the risk of breast cancer.[80] <u>Phytoestrogens have</u> <u>1,000 to 10,000</u> times lower estrogenic activity compared to estradiol, made in a woman's body.[81] Genistein inhibits both breast and prostate cancer.[82]   Genistein actually slows the growth of breast cancer cells in culture.[83] The macrobiotic diet uses large amounts of soy to help slow the growth of many cancers, including breast cancer.

Male vs female foods.   There are thousands of identified substances in plants. There are probably hundreds of thousands more substances yet to be isolated and studied. Mother nature has a palette that is awesome. Many chemicals in plants provide protection against fungus, bacteria, virus, or varmints. Many of those same noxious chemicals have been demonstrated to provide antioxidant, anti-inflammatory, anti-cancer, anti-aging effects in humans who consume these phytochemicals. Phytoestrogens are a unique study.

All studies point to the beneficial effects of men having ideal levels of testosterone in the body, including protective against heart disease, osteoporosis, obesity, depression, aging, and more. Phytoestrogens are probably beneficial for women, but may be detrimental to testosterone levels in men. Flax and soy are the blatant leaders in this area.

For more information on how your body can fight cancer go to <u>GettingHealthier.com.</u>

PATIENT PROFILE: REVERSING STAGE 4 STOMACH CANCER

B.C. was a 46 year old male diagnosed with stage 4 stomach cancer that had spread to 40% of his liver. His doctor gave him 6 months to 2 years to live. B.C.'s wife put him on the nutrition program in this book for a month at which point he then took chemo. He tolerated the chemo much better than the doctors had anticipated, probably because B.C. was taking many nutrition supplements which the doctor told him not to do. Three months later, the stomach cancer was gone and liver showed 3 remaining spots. Added herbal teas to their regimen which reduced the abdominal bloating. CAT scans 5 months later showed only 1 small spot remaining on the liver. Doctor was ecstatic. B.C. credits his wife's nutrition research with saving his life.

ENDNOTES

[1]. Lourau, G., et al., Experientia, vol.6, p.25, 1950

[2]. Wattenburg, LW, Cancer Res. (suppl), vol.52, p. 2085S, 1992

[3]. Kensler, TW, et al., p.154-196, in FOOD CHEMICALS AND CANCER PREVENTION, vol.1, American Chemical Society, Wash DC, 1994

[4]. Hishida, I., et al., Chem.Pharm.Bull., vol.36, p.1819, 1988

[5]. Adachi, K., et al., Chem.Pharm.Bull., vol.36, p.1000, 1988

[6]. Nanba, H., J. Orthomolecular Med., vol.12, p.43, 1997

[7]. Nanba, H., Cancer Prevention, NYAS, p.243, Sept.1995

[8]. Lau, BHS, et al., Molecular Biotherapeutics, vol.3, p.103, June 1991

[9]. Imai, J., et al., Planta Medica, p.417, 1994

[10]. Tadi, PP, et al., International Clinical Nutrition Reviews, vol.10, p.423, 1990

[11]. Nakagawa, S., et al., Phytotherapy, Research, vol.1, p.1, 1988

[12]. Horie, T., et al., Planta Medica, vol.55, p.506, 1989

[13]. Lau, BHS, International Clinical Nutrition Reviews, vol.9, p.27, 1989

[14]. Ip, C., et al., Nutr.Cancer, vol.17, p.279, 1992

[15]. Dausch, JG, et al., Preventive Medicine, vol.19, p.346, 1990

[16]. Wargovich, MJ, et al., Cancer Letters, vol.64, p.39, 1992

[17]. Belman, S, Carcinogenesis, vol.4, p.1063, 1983

[18]. Steiner, M., et al., Amer.J.Clin.Nutr., vol.64, p.866, 1996

[19]. Nakagawa, S., et al., Phytotherapy Res., vol.1, p.1, 1988

[20]. Dausch, JG, et al., Preventive Med., vol.19, p.346, 1990

[21]. You, WC, et al., J. Nat.Cancer Inst., vol.81, p.162, 1989

[22]. Wargovich, MJ, et al., Cancer Letters, vol.64, p.39, 1992

[23]. Marsh, CL, et al., J. Urology, vol.137, p.359, Feb.1987

[24]. Ip, C., et al., Nutrition and Cancer, vol.17, no.3, p.279, 1992

[25]. Abdullah, TH, et al., J.Nat.Med.Assoc., vol.80, p.439, 1988

[26]. Amagase, H., et al., Carcinogenesis, vol.14, p.1627, 1993

[27]. Yamasaki, T., et al., Cancer Letters, vol.59, p.89, 1991

[28]. Hirao, Y., et al., Phytotherapy Research, vol.1, p.161, 1987

[29]. Abdullah, TH et al., Onkologie, vol.21, p.53, 1989

[30]. DiMascio, P., et al., Arch.Biochem.Biophysics, vol.274, p.532, 1989

[31]. Mangels, AR, et al., J.Am.Diet.Assoc., vol.93, p.284, 1993

[32]. Giovannucci, E., et al., J.Nat.Can.Inst., vol.87, p.1767, 1995

[33]. Franceschi, S., et al., Int.J.Cancer, vol.59, p.181, 1994

[34]. Comstock, GW, et al., Amer.J.Clin.Nutr., vol.53, p.260S, 1991

[35]. Langer, R. et al., Science, p.70, July 1976

[36]. Langer, R. et al., Proceedings National Academy of Sciences, vol.77, no.7, p.4331, July 1980

[37]. Lee, A., et al., Science, vol.221, p.1185, Sept.1983

[38]. Folkman, J, et al., Science, vol.235, p.442, Jan.1987

[39]. D'Amore, PA, Seminars in Thrombosis & Hemostasis, vol.14, p.73, 1988

[40]. Folkman, J., et al., Nature, vol.339, p.58, May 1989

[41]. Moses, MA, et al., Science, vol.248, p.1408, June 1990

[42]. Oikawa, T., et al., Cancer Letters, vol.51, p.181, 1990

[43]. Weidner, N., et al., New England Journal of Medicine, vol.324, p.1, Jan.1991

[44]. Folkman, J., Journal Clinical Oncology, vol.12, p.441, Mar.1994

[45]. Madden, JW, in SABISTON'S TEXTBOOK OF SURGERY, p.268, WB Saunders, Philadelphia, 1972

[46]. Prudden, JF, et al., Seminars in Arthritis and Rheumatism, vol.3, p.287, Summer 1974

[47]. Prudden, JF, Journal of Biological Response Modifiers, vol.4, p.551, 1985

[48]. Durie, BGM, et al., Journal of Biological Response Modifiers, vol.4, p.590, 1985

[49]. Rosen, J, et al., Journal of Biological Response Modifiers, vol.7, p.498, 1988

[50]. Kinsella, J., et al., Crit.Care Med., vol.18, p.S94, 1990

[51]. Pizzini, RP, et al., Surgical Infection Society abstract, p.50, 1989

[52]. Cerra, FB, Am.J.Surg., vol.161, p.230, 1991; see also Cerra, FB, et al., Nutrition, vol.6, p.88, 1990; see also Lieberman, M., et al., Nutrition, vol.6, p.88, 1990

[53]. Aarons, S., et al., J.Surg.Onc., vol.23, p.21, 1983

[54]. Cameron, DE, et al., Am.J.Psychiatry, vol.120, p.320, 1963

[55]. Newman, EA, et al., Amer.J.Physiol., vol.164, p.251, 1951

[56]. Pilch, YH, Am.J.Surg., vol.132, p.631, 1976

[57]. Michelson, AM, et al., Proc.Soc.Exper.Biol. Med., vol.179, p.1, 1985

[58]. Wiltrout, RH, et al., J.Biol.Resp.Mod., vol.4, p.512, 1985

[59]. Tomomatsu, H., Food Technology, p.61, Oct.1994

[60]. Deitch, EA, Archives Surgery, vol.125, p.403, Mar.1990

[61]. Le, MG, et al., J.Nat.Cancer Inst., vol.77, p.633, Sept.1986

[62]. Salminen, E., et al., Clin.Radiol., vol.39, p.435, 1988

[63]. Nikitenko, VI, J.Wound Care, vol.13, no.9, p.363, Oct. 2004

[64]. Seehofer, D., J.Surg.Res., vol.117, no.2, p.262, Apr.2004

[65]. Herek, O, Surg. Today, vol.34, no.3, p.256, 2004

[66]. Gerbitz, A, Blood, vol.103, no.11, p.4365, Jun 1, 2004

[67]. Page, LR, HEALTHY HEALING, p.76, Healthy Healing Publ, 1996

[68]. Brook, JG, et al., Biochem.Med.Metab.Biol.,vol. 35, p.31, 1986

[69]. Gross, P, et al., NY State J.Med., vol.50, p.2683, 1950

[70]. Little, A., et al., J.Neurology, Neurosurgery & Psychiatry, vol.48, p.736, 1985

[71]. Jackson, IV, et al., Am.J.Psychiatry, vol.136, p.11, Nov.1979

[72]. Yokoyama, S, et al., Cancer Res., vol.45, p.2834, 1985

[73]. Zeisel, SH, et al., Fed Amer Soc Exper Biol., vol.5, p.2093, 1991

[74]. Messina, M., et al., J.Nat.Cancer Inst., vol.83, p.541, 1991

[75]. Fostis, T., et al., Proc. Natl. Acad.Sci., vol.90, p.2690, 1993

[76]. Boik, J., CANCER & NATURAL MEDICINE, p.184, Oregon Medical, Princeton, MN 1995

[77]. Watanabe, T., et al., Exp.Cell Res., vol.183, p.335, 1989

[78]. Hocman, G., Int.J.Biochem., vol.24, p.1365, 1992

[79]. Kennedy, AR, in ADJUVANT NUTRITION IN CANCER TREATMENT, p.129, Quillin, P. (eds), Cancer Treatment Research Foundation, Arlington Heights, IL 1994

[80] https://acsjournals.onlinelibrary.wiley.com/doi/full/10.3322/CA.57.5.260

[81] https://erc.bioscientifica.com/view/journals/erc/13/4/0130995.xml

[82]. Adlercreutz, H., et al., Lancet, vol.342, p.1209, Nov.1993

[83]. Peterson, G., et al., Biochem.Biophy.Res.Commun., vol.179, p.661, 1991

Chapter 22

MINOR DIETARY CONSTITUENTS

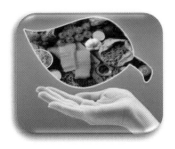

"The bad news is that half of what we have taught you is wrong. The worse news is that we can't tell you which half is wrong."
spoken at any graduation ceremony

WHAT'S AHEAD

MDCs are nutritional compounds that are not yet considered essential, yet may hold the key to optimal health by:
- ✓ Improving energy metabolism
- ✓ Providing full-spectrum antioxidant protection
- ✓ Bolstering detoxification pathways.

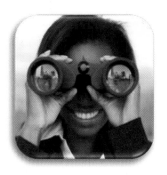

While there are around 50 nutrients that are considered essential in the diet of humans, there are literally thousands of other "accessory factors" found in various foods. There is increasing evidence that we may need these substances in our diet in order to maintain optimal health. These accessory factors or minor dietary constituents may someday be considered "conditionally essential" nutrients, which means that during some phases of life (i.e. very young, older, sick), these nutrients would become essential in the diet. For example, arginine is an amino acid (protein) that is not considered essential for most healthy adults, but is essential in the very young, old, and sick; hence arginine is a recognized conditionally essential nutrient. EPA and DHA from fish oil fit into a similar category.

Cancer patients often have a compromised system that is unable to manufacture optimal amounts of these nutrients in the body. The difference between "surviving" and "thriving to beat cancer" may rest in the intake of these accessory factors.

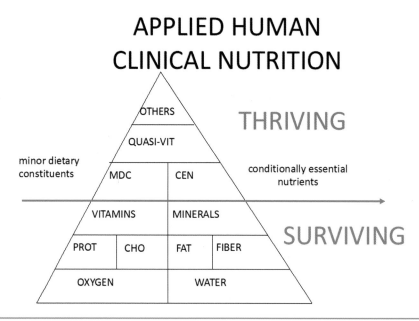

Coenzyme Q-10, 100-800 mg
Improves aerobic metabolism, immune stimulant, membrane stabilizer, improves prostaglandin metabolism.

CoQ is found in the energy transport system of mammals, specifically the mitochondrial membrane. Dr. Peter Mitchell was awarded the Nobel Prize for his work in 1975 on CoQ. CoQ is nearly a wonder drug in reversing cardiomyopathy.[1] CoQ is either manufactured in the human body from the amino acid tyrosine and mevalonate or consumed in the diet, with heart and liver tissue being particularly rich in CoQ-10 for humans. Hence, CoQ, along with carnitine, EPA, and other nutrition factors, are considered "conditionally essential nutrients", since we may not be able to manufacture enough of these nutrients at certain phases of the life cycle. Niacin is an essential vitamin that also is produced within the body from the amino acid tryptophan (endogenous source) and consumed in the diet (exogenous sources). CoQ is also called ubiquinone, since various forms of this molecule are found everywhere (as in ubiquitous). CoQ may help cancer patients by:

- correcting CoQ deficiency states[2], since we don't eat liver or heart and lose the capacity to make CoQ within as we age
- radical scavenger (antioxidant) that works with vitamin E in the fat-soluble portions of the body and cells[3]
- stabilizing cell membranes through interaction with phospholipids[4]
- correction of mitochondrial "leak" of electrons during oxidative respiration, which improves aerobic production of ATP[5]
- improving prostaglandin metabolism[6]
- stabilizing calcium-dependent channels on cell membrane receptor sites[7]

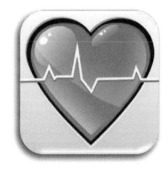

CoQ may enhance immune functions.[8] CoQ reduces the damage to the heart (probably by sparing mitochondrial membranes) from the chemotherapy drug adriamycin.[9] Long-term users of adriamycin risk cardiac arrest, unless given adequate CoQ, vitamin E, niacin, and other nutrients to reduce the damage to the heart. Using 300 mg daily of CoQ as sole therapy, 6 of 32 breast cancer patients (19%) experienced partial tumor regression, while one woman took 390 mg daily and gained complete remission.[10] 35 million Americans are taking the prescription drug category of statins to lower serum cholesterol. CoQ is best absorbed in the presence of fats in your digestive tract, especially lecithin, fish, shark, and borage oils. Statins lower CoQ production in the body which probably requires CoQ supplements during statin treatment.[11]

Lipoic acid 100-800 mg
Alpha lipoic acid (a.k.a. thioctic acid) is involved in energy metabolism, but also works as a potent antioxidant, regulator of blood sugar metabolism, chelator (remover) of heavy metals, improves memory, discourages the growth of cancer, and prevents glycation (sugar binding to cell membranes) that can change the flexibility of cell membranes and blood vessels.

Lipoic acid has so much potential to prevent and reverse common ailments, that drug companies salivate over a patentable look alike. Lipoic acid has been used <u>clinically for decades with extraordinary results</u>, including rescuing people from liver transplant procedures by rejuvenating the liver through IV lipoic acid.[12]

Lipoic acid works with pyruvate and acetyl CoA in a critical point in energy metabolism.[13] Partly because of this pivotal job in generating ATP, lipoic acid becomes an incredibly multi-talented nutrient. Though lipoic acid is not considered an essential nutrient yet, as humans age we produce less and less of lipoic acid 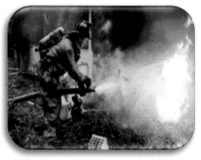 internally.[14] Because of its unique size and chemical structure, lipoic acid works as an antioxidant that can penetrate both fat-soluble (like vitamin E) and water-soluble (like vitamin C) portions of the body.[15] This gives lipoic acid access to virtually the entire body, whereas most antioxidants only protect isolated areas of the body. If we could see free radicals as the "fires" that destroy body tissue, then lipoic acid is a multi-talented fire extinguisher.

Lipoic acid prevents "glycation" or glycosylation, which means the binding of sugar molecules to important proteins in the bloodstream, cell membrane, nerve tissue, etc. Glycation is a disastrous "tanning" that occurs, not unlike turning soft cow skin into hard leather in the tanning process. These new proteins that are bound to sugars do not have the same abilities as before the glycation process.

Supplements of lipoic acid have been found to reverse the peripheral neuropathy from diabetes in as little as 3 weeks.[16] Lipoic acid improves blood flow to the nerves, which then improves nerve conduction.[17] Many cancer patients suffer peripheral neuropathy as a by-product of the damaging effects of chemotherapy. Lipoic acid may prevent and reverse this destruction of nerve tissue.

Because of its role in aerobic metabolism, lipoic acid supplements in animals provided an increase in the amount of oxygen reaching the heart by 72% and the liver by 128%. Since cancer is an anaerobic growth, enhancing aerobic metabolism in a cancer patient is like shining daylight on a vampire.

Lipoic acid increases the available levels of other antioxidants in the body, like vitamin E[18] and glutathione.[19] While there are many antioxidants found in a healthy diet and produced in the body (like uric acid), lipoic acid is the only antioxidant that meets the "wish list" for a "perfect" antioxidant:

- neutralize free radicals
- be rapidly absorbed and quickly utilized by the body cells
- be able to enhance the action of other antioxidants
- be concentrated both inside and outside cells and cell membranes
- promote normal gene expression
- chelate metal ions, or drag toxic minerals out of the body.[20]

Because of its role as an antioxidant and the critical need for immune cells to be protected from their own cellular poisons, lipoic acid has been shown to improve antibody response in immuno-suppressed animals.[21]

Lipoic acid also works to improve the efficiency of insulin by allowing blood glucose into the cells. Animal studies showed that supplements of lipoic acid increased insulin sensitivity by 30-50% and reduced plasma insulin and free fatty acids by 15-17%.[22]

S acetyl-glutathione 100-1,000 mg
Stimulator of immune system, detoxification, regulator of cell division and prostaglandin metabolism.

Glutathione is one of the most widely distributed and important antioxidants in all of nature, yet there has been some confusion regarding its use in cancer patients and its absorption. So keep your thinking cap on as we review this nutrient.

Glutathione is a tripeptide, meaning a molecule formed from three amino acids: glutamine, cysteine, and glycine. Some clinicians have chosen to use N-acetyl-cysteine as a means of augmenting the production of glutathione in the body. Glutathione, also abbreviated GSH, is one of the most widely-distributed antioxidants in plants and animals, and is the chief thiol (sulfur-bearing) molecule in most cells. Glutathione plays a central role in the enzyme system glutathione peroxidase, which is crucial for cell metabolism, cell regulation, detoxification, DNA synthesis and repair, immune function, prostaglandin metabolism, and regulation of cell proliferation through apoptosis (programmed cell death). [23] GSH is particularly helpful in protecting the liver from damage upon exposure to toxins. [24] GSH levels are decreased in most disease states, infertility, aging, toxic burden, and other unfavorable health conditions. [25] Lower levels of blood GSH are associated with more illness, higher blood pressure, higher percent body fat, and reduced general health status. [26] Cancer patients have less GSH in their blood than healthy people. [27] So far, no controversy.

glutamine+cysteine+glycine=glutathione

Help cancer patients? Some oncologists have reasoned that GSH provides one of the main protective mechanisms [28] for cancer cells to develop resistance to chemotherapy. [29] Thus, efforts have been made to develop drugs that deplete the cancer patient of GSH. However, supplements of glutathione in patients being treated for ovarian cancer with the drug cisplatin had an improvement in outcome and reduced kidney toxicity from the cisplatin. [30] In another study of 55 patients with stomach cancer, GSH prevented the neurotoxicity usually associated with cisplatin and did not reduce the anti-neoplastic activity of the drug. [31] In animals exposed to a potent carcinogen (DMBA), GSH provided significant reduction in the size and incidence of tumors. [32] Animals exposed to DMBA and given GSH, vitamin C, E, and beta-carotene had substantial reduction in the number and size of cancers. [33]

In animals with chemically-induced (aflatoxin) liver cancer (an extremely poor prognosis cancer), 100% died within 20 months, while 81% of the animals with liver cancer that were treated with GSH were disease-free 4 months later. [34] Eight patients with advanced refractory (resistant to medical therapy) liver cancer were given 5 grams daily of oral GSH, with most surviving longer than expected and one being cured. [35] Glutathione in the diet has been shown to protect the intestinal wall of animals from the insult of chemical carcinogens. [36] In cultured cancer cells, GSH was able to induce apoptosis (programmed cell death), which may be one of the ways that GSH can assist cancer patients.[37] Platin chemo drugs are notoriously destructive to nerve tissue, leaving the patient with neuropathy (pain, tingling) which often causes the cancer patient to withdraw from chemo treatment. Oncologists gave GSH intravenously just prior to oxaliplatin to cancer patients in a blinded controlled trial with GSH cutting <u>neuropathy in half in the treated group and no reduction</u> in the cancer killing effects of the oxaliplatin.[38]

S <u>Acetyl glutathione</u> is a relatively new form of nutrition supplement that has excellent bioavailability.[39] Best sources of GSH are dark green leafy vegetables, fresh fruit, and lightly cooked fish, poultry, and beef. Processing reduces the GSH levels of foods.

Trimethylglycine 10-500 mg (aka betaine)
Detoxifier, protects liver, lowers homocysteine, and energizer.

Trimethylglycine, or TMG, is the oxidative product of choline. If the body is made up of "bricks", then methylation is the laying of each individual bricks. TMG is heavily involved in methylation throughout the body, which means that TMG:
- lowers the cardiotoxic levels of homocysteine[40]
- protects the liver from alcohol ingestion[41]
- in animal studies, protects the liver from carcinogens[42]
- reverses non-alcoholic steatosis (fatty infiltration and deterioration of the liver)[43]

L-carnitine 100-800 mg
Involved in energy metabolism of fats, thus preventing fatty buildup in heart and liver and encouraging the complete combustion of fats for energy. Cancer cells prefer glucose for energy, not fat.

Think of carnitine as the "shoveler throwing fresh coals into the furnace" of the cell's mitochondria. Carnitine was first isolated from meat extracts in 1905, hence the "carnitine", refers to animal sources. Indeed, there is virtually no carnitine in plant foods, with red meats having the highest carnitine content.[44] The typical American diet provides from 5-100 mg/day of carnitine. Humans can manufacture carnitine in the liver and kidney from the precursors (raw materials to make) of lysine and methionine, and the cofactors of vitamin C, niacin, B-6, and iron. A deficiency of any of these precursors may lead to a carnitine deficiency, which involves buildup of fats in the blood, liver, and muscles and may lead to symptoms of weakness.

Vegans are completely dependent on their own internal ability to generate carnitine. Since infants require carnitine in their diet and other individuals have been found to have clinical carnitine deficiencies, some nutritionists have lobbied to have carnitine included as an essential nutrient, not unlike niacin.[45] Many chemo drugs inhibit the internal production of carnitine with the resulting symptoms causing multiple organ failure. <u>Carnitine supplements can prevent and reverse</u> this chemo-induced damage.[46]

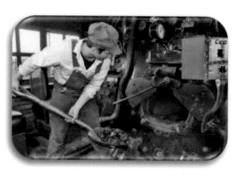

Carnitine may help the cancer patient by:
- protecting the liver from fatty buildup[47]
- improving energy and endurance[48]
- protecting the heart against the damaging effects of adriamycin.[49]
- In cultured cells, carnitine supplements provided for bolstering of immune functions (polymorphonuclear chemotaxis) and reduced the ability of fats to lower immune functions.[50]

Carnitine is probably essential in the diet for people who are very young, or sick, stressed, older, burdened with toxins, etc. Carnitine is one of the many reasons why I do not endorse a vegan diet.

Tocotrienols 20-40 mg
Antioxidant, immune stimulant, regulates fatty acid metabolism.

On a hike to the top of Mount San Gorgonio in southern California, I found the view was spectacular. However, when I pulled out my binoculars, I could see much more detail. And when I borrowed a pair of high-powered binoculars from a friend, the details of the surrounding landscape became even more defined and clear. The same thing is happening in the field of nutrition. As our analytical equipment becomes more sophisticated, our ability to see subsets of molecules that work together becomes more impressive. The star nutrient of today may become a supporting actress tomorrow. Such may be the case for vitamin E (tocopherols) and its kissing cousin, tocotrienols.

What started off as one vitamin, E, now appears to be at least 4 related forms of vitamin E plus slightly different cousins of vitamin E, of which there are 4 tocotrienols. While some nutritionists campaign against the use of palm oil, since it has a higher content of saturated fats than soy or corn oil, the data actually show that palm oil may LOWER the risk for heart disease, since it is rich in tocotrienols, which are potent antioxidants that protect the blood vessel walls.[51] Palm oil is the second largest volume of vegetable oil produced in the world.

α-Tocopherol $R_1=R_2=R_3=CH_3$
β-Tocopherol $R_1=R_3=Ch_3, R_2=H$
γ-Tocopherol $R_2=R_3=CH_3, R_1=H$
δ-Tocopherol $R_3=CH_3, R_1=R_2=H$

α-Tocotrienol $R_1=R_2=R_3=CH_3$
β-Tocotrienol $R_1=R_3=Ch_3, R_2=H$
γ-Tocotrienol $R_2=R_3=CH_3, R_1=H$
δ-Tocotrienol $R_3=CH_3, R_1=R_2=H$

Tocotrienols are very similar in structure to tocopherols, which is vitamin E. Palm oil and rice bran are the richest sources of tocotrienols. Tocotrienols have only 30% the vitamin E activity when compared to D-alpha-tocopherol, the "gold standard" of vitamin E.[52] Yet tocotrienols have demonstrated a greater anti-cancer activity than vitamin E.[53] Tocotrienols were able to delay onset of cancer in animals, while mixed carotenes from palm oil were able to regress these same cancers.[54] In vitro and in vivo, dietary palm oil (richest source of tocotrienols) was able to exhibit a "dose dependent" anti-tumor activity against several carcinogenic compounds.[55] Tocotrienols target several signaling pathways to inhibit cancer growth.[56]

Quercetin 100-1000 mg
Bioflavonoid with unique immune stimulating and anti-neoplastic activity.

"...quercetin may have a key role in anticancer treatment."

Quercetin is a bioflavonoid with extraordinary capacity to prevent and reverse cancer, as shown in several reviews of the scientific literature.[57] While a review paper from 1983 estimated that about 500 varieties of bioflavonoids existed in nature[58], more current estimates go as high as 8,000 different bioflavonoid compounds.   Bioflavonoids are basically accessory factors used by plants to assist in photosynthesis and reduce the damaging effects from the sun while also serving as naturally-occurring pesticides. Best sources of bioflavonoids are citrus, berries, onions, parsley, legumes, green tea, and bee pollen. The average Western 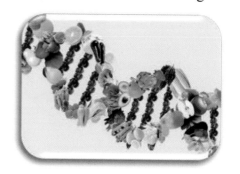 diet contains somewhere between 150 mg/day[59] and 1,000 mg/day[60] of bioflavonoids, with about 25 mg/day of quercetin. Quercetin is only found in plant food, with apples, berries, red wine, onions, and other fresh fruits and vegetables as ideal sources.   Of all the nutrition factors discussed in this book, only a few, including quercetin, have shown the potential to revert a cancerous cell back to a normal healthy cell, called prodifferentiation.[61]

Quercetin has many talents that may help the cancer patient:[62]

♦ Induces apoptosis, or programmed cell death in otherwise "immortal" cancer cells[63]
♦ Inhibits inflammation, by reducing histamine release
♦ Inhibits tumor cell proliferation
♦ Competes with estrogen for binding sites, thus defusing the damaging effects of estrogen
♦ Helps to inhibit drug resistance in tumor cells[64]
♦ Potent antioxidant
♦ May inhibit angiogenesis (making of blood vessels from the tumor)
♦ Inhibits capillary fragility, which protects connective tissue against breakdown by tumors

- Has anti-viral activity
- Reduces the "stickiness" of cells, or aggregation, thus slowing cancer metastasis
- Reduces the toxicity and carcinogenic capacity of substances in the body[65] YET at the same time may enhance the tumor-killing capacity of cisplatin[66]
- Helps to eliminate toxic metals through chelation[67]
- Increases the anti-neoplastic activity of hyperthermia (heat therapy) on cancer cells
- May revert cancer cells back to normal cells (prodifferentiation), possibly by repairing the defective energy mechanism in the cancer cells. [68]

In animals fed 5% of their diet as quercetin, there was a 50% reduction in the incidence of tumors after exposure to carcinogens, while animals fed 2% quercetin had a 25% reduction in tumor incidence.[69] Quercetin has been shown to inhibit estrogen-dependent tumors by occupying the critical 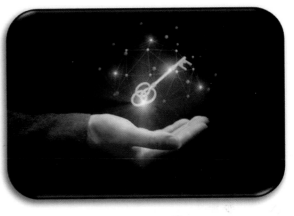 estrogen receptor sites on the tumor cell membranes.[70] Quercetin, at relatively low concentration, has been shown to inhibit the proliferation of squamous cancer cells.[71] Quercetin and other bioflavonoids have shown the ability to inhibit metastasis in cultured cells.[72] Quercetin significantly increased the tumor kill rate of hyperthermia (heat therapy) in cultured cancer cells.[73] Head and neck squamous cancers in humans are resistant to most medical therapies and have a high rate of tumor recurrence. Quercetin was selectively toxic in both in vitro and in vivo head and neck cancers in a dose-dependent fashion.[74]

One problem for cancer patients can be inflammation, or swelling of tissue. This is a crucial "tightrope walk", in which you want a certain amount of alarm in the immune system, which creates dumping of free radicals and swelling; yet you don't want too much of this, or it creates weakness, pain, discomfort, and tissue wasting. Quercetin can help reduce swelling by helping to produce anti-inflammatory prostaglandins. [75]

Quercetin inhibits the release of histamine from mast cells, thus reducing allergic reactions.[76] Quercetin also helps to stabilize cell membranes, decrease lipid peroxidation, and inhibit the breakdown of connective tissue (collagen) by hyaluronidase (one of the ways that cancer spreads).[77]

Medium chain triglycerides (MCT) 1-10 gm
Slows down lean tissue wasting, enhances thermogenesis (making of heat), and augments burning of fat

---

Fatty acids can have a length of anywhere from 2 carbons to 24 carbons. The long chain fats (or triglycerides, called LCT) include most dietary fats of soy oil and beef fat. LCT is difficult to absorb and requires special bile acids and absorption pathways in the lymphatic ducts.[78] Medium chain triglycerides (MCT) are much easier to absorb and are quickly burned in the human system. MCTs are primarily found in coconut oil and smaller amounts in other nuts. Almost like adding kindling (MCT) to a group of logs (LCT), medium chain triglycerides actually promote the burning of the body's fat stores, which helps to encourage thermogenesis (making of heat) in humans.[79] Cancer cells can be selectively destroyed by elevating the body temperature. In animals with implanted tumors, a ketogenic diet (high in fat and protein, low in carbs) coupled with fish oil and MCT was able to <u>dramatically slow the growth of tumors</u>.[80] MCT has been shown to be a useful tool:
- in the control of obesity
- lowering serum cholesterol
- as a concentrated and readily available source of energy
- helps to prevent immune suppression in critically ill people[81]
- maintains body (visceral) protein stores during wound recovery.[82]

MCT is extremely safe, provides quick energy for the person, does not feed the cancer, protects protein reserves in the body, and helps to slowly melt away unwanted fat stores in the adipose tissue.

L-glycine 1 gm
Energizer, calming agent, detoxifier, controls fat levels in the blood, builds energy stores (glycogen) in the liver, helps in wound recovery and collagen synthesis.

Glycine's name reflects its sweet flavor. It is considered a non-essential amino acid, since it can be formed from the amino acids threonine and serine. <u>Serine seems to augment cancer growth</u>, while glycine does not.[83] Glycine may help the cancer patient in several ways:

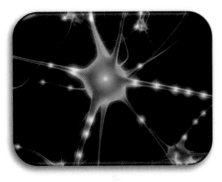

- ◆ Acts as a preservative in foods
- ◆ Sweetening agent, tastes much like sugar, does not alter glycemic index
- ◆ May be converted into glutathione (see that section) for antioxidant and detoxification benefits
- ◆ May be converted in the body into dimethylglycine (DMG)
- ◆ Works as a calming agent in the nervous system and also helps to improve spastic conditions[84] and muscular weakness[85]
- ◆ Promotes collagen formation, thus possibly helping the body to encapsulate tumors.

Glucaric acid (cal D glucarate) 500-1,000 mg
Improves detoxification in the gut and liver, escorts estrogen out of the system, may have anti-proliferative activity.

D-glucaric acid is a substance found in certain fruits (oranges) and vegetables (broccoli, potatoes). CDG has been shown to encourage critical phase II detoxification pathway. <u>D-glucaric acid has shown</u> promise as a powerful anti-cancer and detoxifying agent.[86]

For more information on how your body can fight cancer go to <u>GettingHealthier.com.</u>

PATIENT PROFILE: REVERSING INCURABLE CYTOMA

S.M. was a 44-year old male diagnosed with a rare form of cancer (hemangiopericytoma) that had caused pain and numbness in his back and legs. Began 13 rounds of radiation therapy to spinal region, which produced considerable relief from pain and weakness. One month later, CAT scans and liver biopsy found metastatic disease throughout pancreas, liver, kidneys, lungs, and pressing on spinal cord. Physicians agreed in medical staff meeting that this condition is "refractory to all medical therapy and invariably fatal." Patient began aggressive nutrition program of diet and supplements, along with detoxification (coffee enemas), 3 months chemotherapy (FUDR), and extensive prayer. CAT scans showed 50% shrinkage in tumors on pancreas, lungs and kidneys with elimination of tumors on liver. S.M.'s bloodwork was constantly normal, whereas one would expect declines in white cell count (leukopenia) and red blood cell count (anemia). When last in contact, three years later, S.M. still had some tumor burden, but had good quality of life and is well beyond the most optimistic predictions of his original oncologist.

ENDNOTES

[1] . Langsjoen, PH, et al., Int. J. Tiss Reac, vol.12, p.163, 1990

[2] . Folkers, K, et al., International Journal of Vitamin and Nutrition Research, vol.40,p.380, 1970

[3] . Sugiyama, S, Experientia, vol.36, p.1002, 1980

[4] . Gwak, S. et al., Biochem et Biophys Acta, vol.809, p.187, 1985

[5] . Turrens, JF, Biochem J., vol.191, p.421, 1980

[6] . Ham, EA, et al., J. Biol Chem, vol.254, p.2191, 1979

[7] . Nakamura, Y, et al., Cardiovasc Res, vol.16, p.132, 1982

[8] . Folkers, K., Med Chem Res, vol.2, p.48, 1992

[9] . Folkers, K., Biomedical and Clinical Aspects of Coenzyme Q, vol.3,p.399, Elsevier Press, 1981

[10] . Lockwood, K., et al., Biochem and Biophys Res Comm, vol.199, p.1504, Mar.1994

[11] https://www.sciencedirect.com/science/article/abs/pii/S1567724907000591

[12] https://www.amazon.com/Alpha-Lipoic-Acid-Breakthrough-Antioxidant-ebook/dp/B003L1ZVMC/ref=sr_1_1?dchild=1&keywords=burt+berkson&qid=1589208886&sr=8-1

[13] . Budavari, S. (eds), THE MERCK INDEX, p.1591, Merck & Co., Whitehouse Station, NJ 1996

[14] . Packer, L., et al., Free Radical Biol. Med., vol.19, p.227, 1995

[15] . Stoll, S., et al., Ann.NY Acad.Sci., vol.717, p.122, 1994

[16] . Passwater, R., LIPOIC ACID, Keats, New Canaan, CT, 1996

[17] . Nagamatsu, M., et al., Diabetes Care, vol.18, p.1160, Aug.1995

[18] . Podda, M., et al., Biochem.Biophys., Res.Commun., vol.204, p.98, 1994

[19] . Han, D., et al., Biochem.Biophys.,Res.Commun., vol.207, p.258, 1995

[20] . Ou, P., et al., Biochem.Pharmacol., vol.50, p.123, 1995

[21] . Ohmori, H., et al., Jpn.J.Pharmacol., vol.42, p.275, 1986

[22] . Jacob, S., et al., Diabetes, vol.45, p.1024, 1996

[23] . Bray, TM, et al., Biochem.Pharmacol., vol.47, p.2113, 1994

[24] . DeLeve, LD, et al., Pharmac.Ther., vol.52, p.287, 1991

[25] . Bray, TM, et al., Biochem.Pharmacol., vol.47, p.2113, 1994

[26] . Julius, M., et al., J.Clin.Epidemiol., vol.47, p.1021, 1994

[27] . Beutler, E., et al., J.Lab.Clin.Ned., vol.105, p.581, 1985

[28] https://onlinelibrary.wiley.com/doi/abs/10.1002/cbf.1149

[29] . Hercbergs, A., et al., Lancet, vol.339, p.1074, May 1992

[30] . DiRe, F., et al., Cancer Chemother.Pharmacol., vol.25, p.355, 1990

[31] . Cascinu, S., et al., J.Clin.Oncol., vol.13, p.26, 1995

[32] . Trickler, D., et al., Nutr.Cancer, vol.20, p.139, 1993

[33] . Shklar, G., et al., Nutr.Cancer, vol.20, p.145, 1993

[34] . Science, vol.212, p.541, May 1981

[35] . Ranek, DK, et al., Liver, vol.12, p.341, 1992

[36] . Lash, LH, et al., Proc.Natl.Acad.Sci., vol.83, p.4641, July 1986

[37] . Donnerstag, B., et al., Int.J.Oncol., vol.7, p.949, Oct.1995

[38] http://www.richmondhillnaturopath.com/uploads/1/3/3/5/13351706/glutathione__oxaliplatin.pdf

[39] https://www.clinicaleducation.org/resources/reviews/oral-glutathione-equivalent-to-iv-therapy/

[40] . Steenge, GR, J.Nutr., vol.133, no.5, p.1291, May 2003

[41] . Barak, AJ, Alcohol, vol.13, no.5, p.483, Sep.1996

[42] . junnila, M., Vet.Pathol., vol.37, no.3, p.231, May 2000

[43] . Abdelmalek, MF, Am.J.Gastroenterol., vol.96, no.9, p.2711, Sep.2001

[44] . Bremer, J., Physiol.Rev., vol.63, p.1420, 1983

[45] . Borum, PR, et al., J.Am.Coll.Nutr., vol.5, p.177, 1986

[46] https://www.sciencedirect.com/science/article/pii/S131901641000071X

[47] . Sachan, DS, et al., Am.J.Clin.Nutr., vol.39, p.738, 1984

[48] . Dragan, GI, et al., Physiologie, vol.25, p.231, 1987

[49] . Furitano, G, et al., Drugs Exp.Clin.Res., vol.10, p.107, 1984

[50] . DeSimone, C., et al, Acta Vitaminol. Enzymol., vol.4, p.135, 1982

[51] . Qureshi, AA, et al., Am.J.Clin.Nutr., vol.53, p.1042S, 1991

[52] . Farrell, PM, et al., in MODERN NUTRITION, Shils, ME (eds), Lea & Febiger, Philadelphia, 1994

[53] . Komiyama, K., et al., Chem.Pharm.Bull., vol.37, p.1369, 1989

[54] . Tan, B., Nutrition Research, vol.12, p.S163, 1992

[55] . Azuine, MA, et al., Nutr. Cancer, vol.17, p.287, 1992

[56] https://link.springer.com/content/pdf/10.1007/s12263-011-0220-3.pdf

[57] https://www.ingentaconnect.com/content/ben/cmc/2015/00000022/00000026/art00003

[58] . Havsteen, B., Biochem.Pharmacol., vo.32, p.1141, 1983

[59] . Murray, MT, ENCYCLOPEDIA OF NUTRITIONAL SUPPLEMENTS, p.321, Prima, Rocklin, 1996

[60] . Middleton, E., et al., in ADJUVANT NUTRITION IN CANCER TREATMENT, Quillin, P. (eds), p.319, Cancer Treatment Research Foundation, Arlington Heights, IL 1994

[61] . Middleton, E., et al., in ADJUVANT NUTRITION IN CANCER TREATMENT, Quillin, P. (eds), p.325, Cancer Treatment Research Foundation, Arlington Heights, IL 1994

[62] . Boik, J., CANCER & NATURAL MEDICINE, p.181, Oregon Medical Press, Princeton, MN 1995

[63] https://link.springer.com/article/10.1007/s13277-016-5184-x

[64] . Scambia, G., et al., Cancer Chemother. Pharmacol., vol.28, p.255, 1991

[65] . Wood, AW, et al., in PLANT FLAVONOIDS IN BIOLOG, p.197, Cody, V. (eds), Liss, NY, 1986

[66] . Scambia, G., et al., Anticancer Drugs, vol.1, p.45, 1990

[67] . Afanasev, IB, et al., Biochem.Pharmacol., vol.38, p.1763, 1989

[68] . Suolinna, E., et al., J.Nat.Cancer Inst., vol.53, p.1515, 1974

[69] . Berma, AK, et al., Cancer Res., vol.48, p.5754, 1988

[70] . Ranelletti, FO, et al., Int.J.Cancer, vol.50, p.486, 1992

[71] . Kandaswami, C., et al., Anti-Cancer Drugs, vol.4, p.91, 1993

[72] . Bracke, ME, et al., in PLANET FLAVONOIDS, p.219, Cody, E. (eds), Liss, NY, 1988

[73] . Kim, JH, et al., Cancer Research, vol.44, p.102, Jan.1984

[74] . Castillo, MH, et al., Amer.J.Surgery, vol.158, p.351, Oct.1989

[75] . Bauman, J., et al., Prostaglandins, vol.20, p.627, 1980

[76] . Middleton, E, et al., Arch.Allergy Appl.Immunol., vol.77, p.155, 1985

[77] . Busse, WW, et al., J.Allergy Clin.Immunol., vol.73, p.801, 1984

[78] . Bach, AC, et al., Am.J.Clin.Nutr., vol.36, p.950, 1982

[79] . Mascioli, EA, et al., J.Parenteral Enteral Nutr., vol.15, p.27, 1991

[80] https://bmccancer.biomedcentral.com/articles/10.1186/1471-2407-8-122

[81] . Jensen, GL, et al., J.Parenteral Enteral Nutr., vol.14, p.467, 1990

[82] . Maiz, A., et al., Metabolism, vol.33, p.901, Oct.1984

[83] https://www.sciencedirect.com/science/article/pii/S2211124714003477

[84] . Davidoff, RA, Annals Neurology, vol.17, p.107, 1985

[85] . Braverman, ER, et al., HEALING NUTRIENTS WITHIN, p.238, Keats, New Canaan, CT 1987

[86] https://journals.sagepub.com/doi/abs/10.1177/1534735403002002005

Chapter 23

CHANGING THE UNDERLYING
CAUSES OF CANCER

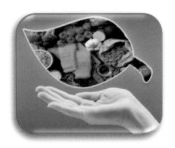

Sooner or later, we all sit down to a banquet of consequences.
Robert Louis Stephenson, author of Treasure Island, 1850-1894

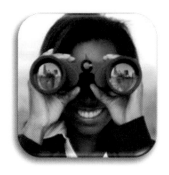

WHAT'S AHEAD
No one with a headache is suffering from a deficiency of aspirin. In order to achieve maximum results in cancer treatment, the underlying causes must be addressed. This process is easier said than done, but is essential.

No one with elevated serum cholesterol is suffering from a deficiency of clofibrate. Arthritis sufferers are not suffering due to lack of cortisone, and cancer patients are not lacking chemotherapy. All of these therapies are short term, symptom-fixing drugs that provide immediate relief, but do nothing to change the underlying causes of a disease.

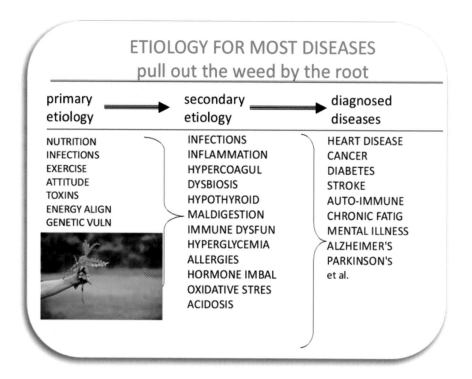

ETIOLOGY FOR MOST DISEASES
pull out the weed by the root

primary etiology	secondary etiology	diagnosed diseases
NUTRITION	INFECTIONS	HEART DISEASE
INFECTIONS	INFLAMMATION	CANCER
EXERCISE	HYPERCOAGUL	DIABETES
ATTITUDE	DYSBIOSIS	STROKE
TOXINS	HYPOTHYROID	AUTO-IMMUNE
ENERGY ALIGN	MALDIGESTION	CHRONIC FATIG
GENETIC VULN	IMMUNE DYSFUN	MENTAL ILLNESS
	HYPERGLYCEMIA	ALZHEIMER'S
	ALLERGIES	PARKINSON'S
	HORMONE IMBAL	et al.
	OXIDATIVE STRES	
	ACIDOSIS	

Doctors trained in detecting the underlying causes of your cancer can be found at:

♦ The Institute for Functional Medicine has a website that helps you to locate a health care professional who can help you solve the mystery of etiology of disease.[1]

♦ The American Association of Naturopathic Physicians also has a website to help you find a local talented doctor.[2]

♦ Life Extension Foundation also has a listing of innovative practitioners.[3]

Studies have proven that patients who undergo coronary bypass surgery have no extension in lifespan, because no one has changed the cause of the disease by replacing 4 inches of plugged up "plumbing" or arteries near the heart. Same goes for other drugs and conditions. Beta-blockers and diuretics for the 60 million Americans with high blood pressure make no change in longevity since they cause a loss of the crucial cardio-protective minerals of potassium and magnesium.[4]

This chapter is excerpted from <u>12 KEYS TO A HEALTHIER CANCER PATIENT</u>.[5] For more information, see that book. The ideal combination therapy for any disease would include short-term relief with minimal drugs, coupled with the long-term goal of changing the underlying causes of the disease. For more information, consult with your health care professional.

FIX WHAT'S BROKE

If you have a zinc deficiency, then a truckload of vitamin C will not be nearly as valuable as giving the body what it needs to end the zinc deficiency. If an accumulation of lead and mercury has crimped the immune system, then removing the toxic metals is more important than psychotherapy. If a low output of hydrochloric acid in the stomach creates poor digestion and malabsorption, then hydrochloric acid supplements are the answer. If a broken spirit brought on the cancer, then spiritual healing is necessary to eliminate the cancer.

This issue complicates cancer treatment tremendously and makes "cookbook" cancer treatment an exercise in futility. Our progress against cancer has been crippled not only by the complexity of cancer, but also by the need for Western science to isolate one variable. While it is easier to conduct and interpret research with one or two variables, cancer and the human body are far more complex than that. We will eventually help most cancer patients by fixing whatever bodily function needs repair.

1) PSYCHO-SPIRITUAL

Grief, loss of loved one, lack of purpose, depression, low self-esteem, hypochondriasis as means of getting attention, need love for self and others, touching, be here now, sense of accomplishment, happiness, music, beauty, sexual satisfaction, forgiveness, etc.

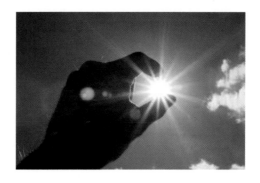

SOLUTION: Create a new way of thinking (crisis=opportunity or danger)

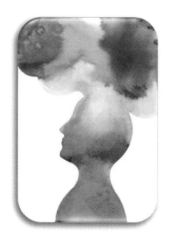

It was Hans Selye, MD, who first scientifically showed that animals subjected to stress undergo thymic atrophy (immune suppression), elevations in blood pressure and serum lipids, and erosion of the stomach lining (ulcers).[6] Since then, literally thousands of human studies have demonstrated that an angry, stressed, or depressed mind can lead to a suppressed immune system, which allows cancer and infections to take over. Drs. Locke and Horning-Rohan have published a textbook consisting of over 1,300 scientific articles written since 1976 that prove the link between the mind and the immune system.

We are finally beginning to accept what philosophers and spiritual leaders have been telling us for thousands of years: the mind has a major impact on the body and health. Proverbs 17:22 tells us "A joyful heart is good medicine, but a broken spirit dries up the bones." Over 100 years ago, observant physicians claimed that significant life events might increase the risk for developing cancer.[7] In the 1800s, emotional factors were related to breast cancer, and cervical cancer was related to sensitive and frustrated women. Loss of a loved one has long been known to increase the risk for breast and cervical cancer. When 2,000 men were assessed and then followed for 17 years, it was found that depression doubled the risk for cancer.

Researchers at the National Institute of Health, spearheaded by Candice Pert, PhD, have investigated the link between catecholamines, endorphins, and other chemicals from the brain as they influence cancer. A reknowned researcher, Jean Achterberg, PhD, has demonstrated a clear link between the attitude of the cancer patient and their quality and quantity of life.[8] This is especially true of breast cancer patients. There is even a medical textbook on the subject of "STRESS AND BREAST CANCER."[9]

Not only can mental depression lead to immune suppression and then cancer, but there may be a metaphorical significance to the location of the cancer. Divorced women may lose a breast as they feel a loss of their femininity. One of my patients developed cancer of the larynx a year after his wife left him. He tried to get her to talk about it, but she said there was "nothing left to say". And he developed cancer of the "say" box. Is it merely a coincidence that the great comedians, like Bob Hope (1903-2003), George Burns (1896-1996), and Milton Berle (1908-2002) lived decades longer than the average American male?

The good news is that the mind can be a powerful instrument at eliminating cancer. This is an empowering concept. Helplessness and hopelessness are just as lethal as cigarettes and bullets. Keep your eyes on the "prize" of a healing from your cancer.

Norman Cousins cured himself of a painful collagen disease by using laughter and attitude adjustment, along with high doses of vitamin C. Bernie Siegel, MD, a Yale surgeon, noticed that certain mental characteristics in his cancer patients were indicators of someone who would beat the odds: live each moment, express yourself, value your dreams, and maintain an assertive fighting spirit against the disease.

Carl Simonton, MD, a radiation oncologist, found that mental imagery and other mind techniques vastly improved the results in his cancer patients. In a National Cancer Institute study conducted at the University of Texas, researchers were able to predict with 100% accuracy which cancer patients would die or deteriorate within a two month period--strictly based upon the patient's attitude.[10]

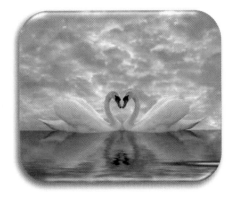

Enkephalins and endorphins, also called "the mind's rivers of pleasure", are brain chemicals that are secreted when the mind is happy. Endorphins improve the production of T cells, which improves the effectiveness of the immune system against cancer and infections. Enkephalins increase the vigor of T-cells attacking cancer cells as well as increasing the percentage of active T-cells. Essentially, your immune system is a well-orchestrated army within to protect you against cancer and infections, and your mind is the four-star general directing the battle. Depending on your attitude, your mind either encourages or discourages disease in your body.

The take-home lesson here is: you can take a soup bowl full of potent nutrients to fight cancer while you are being treated by the world's best oncologist, but if your mind is not happy and focused on the immune battle that must occur, then the following program of nutrition will not be nearly as effective as it should be.

We all have to drive over the "bumps in the highway of life". Your "shock absorber system"; like "lean on a higher Power", humor, prayer, meditation, music, friends, nature, gardening, sense of purpose, fun, etc; is your coping ability that makes stressful events less damaging to your well-being. Depending on whether you perceive cancer as an "opportunity for personal growth" or a "death sentence" may become self-fulfilling.

2) TOXIC BURDEN

Of the 10 million tons [11] of toxic substances released annually by industry around the world, 2 million tons are probable carcinogens. Of the 80,000 chemicals [12] in use in the USA, 60,000 were released without any data on safety in humans. The burden of proof rests on society to prove something is hazardous. Not easy to do when you realize that asbestos was approved by the Environmental Protection Agency, because they could not prove that asbestos was toxic. Asbestos has been banned in most developed countries, but still used in many developing countries and now kills at least 255,000 people [13] each year around the world.

43% of Americans breathe air that is unsafe, according to the American lung association. We add 1 billion pounds of pesticides to our food crops annually. Of the 3000 food additives in the American food supply, FDA has no knowledge of at least 1,000 of these, due to loopholes in the law via "generally regarded as safe" or GRAS status. 70% of Americans drink tap water that, by law, must contain fluoride, a known poison. [14] 91 contaminants are regulated by the Safe Water Drinking Act.

In 2020 the Covid virus swept the world killing over 1 million as of this writing. The disease had a 99% cure rate in younger healthier people, but was far more lethal in elderly patients who have immune senescence. Toxins, plus age, plus diseases, plus multiple nutrient deficiencies (D, C, iodine, selenium, etc.) plus prescription drugs, plus vaccinations (the flu vaccine increased risk for covid by 36%) increased risk of death from Covid by 100 fold. [15]

In 1996, hundreds of dead seals washed up on the beaches of Denmark and Germany. Scientists determined that a virus had killed these seals. However, the same virus exists in all healthy seals without creating any infection. Actually, it was pollution from the Rhine River that caused the immune systems of the seals to succumb to these normally-non-toxic viruses. At the same time in a forest just east of Los Angeles, California, a normal strain of beetles was decimating a huge stand of virgin pine trees. While these beetles normally live among these pine trees, it was the air pollution from Los Angeles that lowered the immune functions of the pine trees and allowed these innocuous beetles to devastate the forest.

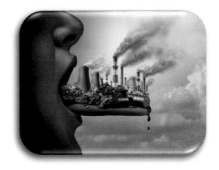

Meanwhile, thousands of bass fish are washing up on the shores of lakes in the southern plains of the US. Cause of death? A virus that normally inhabits the fish, but becomes lethal when the fish are exposed to pollutants, which lower immune defenses. Pollutants lower our defenses to everything from the common cold to cancer, while also jamming the body's many intricate biochemical reactions.

INTAKE from:
Toxins could be categorized as:
- ✓ Volatile organic chemicals, from industry and agriculture
- ✓ Tobacco
- ✓ Drugs, prescription and recreation
- ✓ Fungal by products, e.g. aflatoxin
- ✓ Heavy metals, including mercury, lead, cadmium, arsenic, aluminum and other metals
- ✓ Auto-intoxication, as by products from our gut, especially for those with an imbalance in gut microbiome
- ✓ Electromagnetic fields, cell phone towers, WiFi, high voltage power lines, radar, etc.
- ✓ Radiation, X-rays, radioactive fallout, sunlight, etc.

SOLUTION: DETOXIFICATION (EXCRETION) VIA:

◆ Urine. Increase intake of clean water, vitamin C, beans (sulfur amino acids are chelators), garlic, chelation EDTA therapy.

- Feces. 100 trillion microbes in the human gut. 40% of lymphoid tissue is surrounding the GI tract. Common constipation leads to toxic buildup, dysbiosis. Increase fluid, fiber, psyllium seed husk, senna, cascara sagrada, buckthorn, fructo-oligosaccharides, probiotics (lactobacillus, yogurt). Appropriate use of enemas, coffee enemas (every other day during intensive detox).
- Sweat. Skin is the largest organ of body, 2000 pores/square inch skin. Increase sweating through exercise, hot tubs, jacuzzi, sauna. Hyperthermia via far infrared saunas (SmartyHealth.com, Saunas.com, SunlightSaunas.com) can be useful. Bring core body temperature up to 102 F for 10-30 minutes/day. Do not use anti-perspirants.
- Liver. Most significant detoxifying organ of body, using conjugase (put together), oxidase, reductase, and hydrolase enzymes to neutralize poisons. Increase intake of glutathione (dark green leafy veg), silymarin, garlic, vitamin E, selenium.
- Other. Some chose chelation therapy, mercury amalgam removal, or magnets to neutralize electro-magnetic field pollution.

GET RID OF THE GARBAGE

Everyone is detoxifying their bodies all day throughout their lives--or they would die. But some people don't detox fast enough, and the toxins build up to encumber their bodily processes. One of the favored theories of aging says that eventually the accumulation of these cellular waste products overwhelms the cells, and they begin to die. Similarly, fermenting yeast creates alcohol to a certain point and then dies in its own toxins. Cell cultures of living tissue that are kept in a fresh nutrient solution and changed daily to eliminate toxin buildup will experience slowed aging.

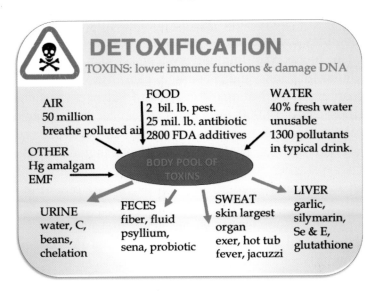

To summarize the essence of good health into one simple sentence: "supply your body with the physical and metaphysical needs while eliminating physical and metaphysical toxins." Each of the 37 trillion cells in your body is like a house in your neighborhood. Many cancer patients have erred at both ends of this equation: not enough essential nutrients, coupled with an accumulation of poisons.

A WORD ON COFFEE ENEMAS.

Enemas are one of the oldest healing modalities in human literature. Milk enemas are still used by noted surgeons and gastroenterologists to stem diarrhea that does not respond to medication. Coffee enemas were in the Merck Medical Manual for decades, until 1977, when editors of the manual claimed that this revered therapy was eliminated for "lack of space" in the new 3500 page manuscript. Actually, coffee enemas became the focal point in criticizing alternative cancer therapies. Coffee enemas help to purge the colon and liver of accumulated toxins and dead tissue. To prepare, brew regular organic coffee, let cool to body temperature, then use enema bag as per instructions with 4 to 8 ounces of the coffee.

After looking at the toxic burden carried by the average American adult, the question is not "why do 42% of us get cancer?", but a more appropriate question might be "why do only 42% of us get cancer?" Our cancer epidemic will not be abated until we get our environmental disaster cleaned up. By increasing the body's ability to purge poisons, detoxification may help the cancer recovery process for some individuals. Toxic burden blunts the immune system, erodes the delicate DNA, changes cellular functions, and encourages cancer growth.

According to the National Academy of Sciences, pesticide residues on food crops cause 14,000 new cases of cancer each year out of 1.6 million total cases, which means that about 1% of our cancer comes from pesticide use and abuse. That estimate did not include the more recent findings that pesticides amplify each other's toxicity by 500 to 1,000 fold!! That 1% is fairly insignificant, unless you are one of those 14,000 people.

Glyphosate (Roundup) is an herbicide first patented [16] in 1964 to clean boiler pipes. Glyphosate was patented again in 1974 as an herbicide, then again in 2003 as an antibiotic. The World Health Organization has listed glyphosate as a "probable carcinogen", which was instrumental in a jury awarding a patient with non-Hodgkins lymphoma $289 million verdict against Monsanto, the manufacturer. A couple was recently awarded $2 billion for the cancer they contracted from Roundup use. There are over 12,000 cases pending against Bayer/Monsanto for Roundup-induced cancer. 95 million pounds of glyphosate are used annually in the US.

TO CLEAN YOUR FRESH COMMERCIAL PRODUCE.
For those people who do not have easy access to organic produce, which is grown without pesticide use, peeling or washing produce is mandatory.
For produce that you consume entirely, like broccoli and apples, soak it in a solution of one gallon of warm water per 2 tablespoons of vinegar for 5 minutes, then rinse and brush.

From tainted water, food, and air; to exposure to carcinogens in the home and work place; to voluntary intake of poisons in drugs, alcohol, and tobacco; to showers of electromagnetic radiation falling on us--Americans are constantly pushing the outer envelope for toxin tolerance. Cancer patients need to do everything possible to eliminate accumulated wastes and minimize intake of new toxins.

Mercury. With more than 90% of the American population sporting at least a few mercury fillings in their teeth, the subject of mercury poisoning has become a hot topic. Lewis Carroll's classic book, ALICE IN WONDERLAND, showcased the "mad hatter" as representative of an industry that whimsically used mercury to give stiffness to formal felt hats. Mercury is a known carcinogen.[17] Mercury fillings arrive at the dentist office in a hazardous waste container, then are inserted in the mouths of 1 billion patients annually globally. Sweden, Norway, Germany, and other countries have banned mercury amalgams. Some

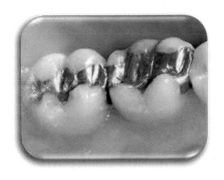

people have found relief from a wide assortment of diseases, including cancer, by having their mercury fillings replaced with non-toxic ceramic or gold material.[18] Mercury detox can be assisted with chelation therapy, both prescription and natural based: DMPS, EDTA, chlorella, kelp extracts, cilantro, and intravenous chelators from your doctor.

Half the weight of a "silver" filling is from mercury. According to Doctor's Data Lab, people with mercury fillings have 13 times more mercury in their stools than people without mercury fillings. With the assistance of common bacteria in the mouth, mercury in fillings becomes methylated and is then 100 times more toxic.[19] Roughly 78% of the 200 million adults in America have an average of 8 mercury fillings, which translates into 557 tons (1.1 million pounds) of mercury stored in the mouths of Americans today. For this reason, there are extraordinary levels of mercury gas emitted when cremating patients with the typical 8 mercury fillings. 90% of dentists still use mercury amalgams, adding another 100 million mercury fillings annually to the mouths of Americans alone.[20] Animal studies show that radioactively-labelled mercury from fillings quickly migrates to the kidneys, brain, and intestinal wall.[21] There are already class action law suits pending against the dental industry for mercury poisoning that will make any previous class action suits look like a socialite tea party.

In a famous case of blatant clinical mercury toxicity, the Chisso factory in Minamata, Japan dumped 100 tons (91,000 kilograms) of mercury wastes into the nearby bay in 1980, with the resulting fish being contaminated and the people eating the fish getting very sick. Nearly 500 people died, and thousands were declared severely brain damaged by acute mercury poisoning. But mercury rarely kills anyone outright. It slowly erodes all bodily functions until you wish you were dead. Multiple sclerosis (MS) patients have 800% the mercury levels in the cerebrospinal fluid around the brain and spinal cord as compared to healthy controls. Inorganic mercury is capable of producing symptoms that are identical to MS.[22] Mercury poisoning also can mimic Alzheimer's disease. Over 5 million Americans have Alzheimer's with a tripling (15 million) expected within a decade.

PATIENT PROFILE

GB was a bright, energetic, successful physician. He fancied himself a "health nut', running, working out with weights, fishing in nearby Lake Michigan, and eating the fresh fish. GB developed cardiomyopathy, or failure of the heart muscle, and was told by his fellow doctors that he needed a heart transplant. He questioned such invasive therapies and set out on a lengthy odyssey to find out why his heart was failing when he seemed to be doing all the healthy lifestyle things. He found he had mercury poisoning by eating fish from Lake Michigan. He commenced mercury detoxification in every conceivable way, including oral and intravenous chelating agents. Eventually, GB lowered his mercury load to a manageable level and used much of what he learned in this bizarre health odyssey to help his many patients. However, his heart gave out 13 years after he was told he needed a heart transplant operation. He added measurably to his life via mercury detox, but never would have had these problems if the fish in Lake Michigan had not been so criminally polluted with mercury.

If you overlay a map of mercury pollution in the US with elevated rates of cancer, they match. Mercury toxicity may be the initial insult which leads to depressed immunity, which leads to fungal and other infections, which leads to inflammation, hypercoagulability, and eventually some serious diagnosed disease like heart disease, stroke, cancer, diabetes, etc. If you want a truly terrifying piece of literature to read before bedtime, never mind the Steven King novels, download the "Mercury Study" from epa.gov on the Internet.

All this mercury has been cumulative. Mercury is immortal. There is no half-life. It never decomposes. Mercury in the air returns as mercury in the world's land and waterways, which enters the food chain through fish and seafoods. The World Health Organization (WHO) has conducted studies showing that the more fish you eat, the more mercury you have in your body. The higher the fish on the food chain (shark, tuna, swordfish are higher than salmon, cod, sole, and crab), the more the concentration of mercury in the flesh. States that have a higher mercury load have it in the water and soil, hence the food supply in general. WHO reports that the largest source of mercury in most people is from mercury dental fillings.

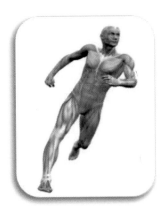

3) EXERCISE

Humans evolved as active creatures. Our biochemical processes depend on regular exercise to maintain homeostasis. A well-respected Stanford physician, Dr. William Bortz, published a review of the scientific literature on exercise and concluded: "our dis-eases may be from dis-use of the body."[23] Cancer patients who exercise have fewer side effects from oncology therapy. Exercise oxygenates the tissue, which slows the anaerobic cancer cell progress. Exercise stabilizes blood sugar levels, which selectively deprives cancer cells of their favorite fuel. Even if exercise is not a possibility for the cancer patient, deep breathing would be invaluable.

Exercise is an absolutely essential ingredient for health. It is a primary tool for detoxification, stabilizing blood glucose levels, improving digestion and regularity, proper oxygenation of tissue, stress tolerance, improving hormone output (i.e. growth hormone & DHEA), burning fatty tissue, and eliminating harmful by-products (i.e., estrogen, uric acid).

4) BLOOD GLUCOSE

Sugar in the blood can feed cancer growth. See the chapter on sugar and cancer for more information.

5) REDOX

Life is a continuous balancing act between oxidative forces (pro-oxidants) and protective forces (antioxidants). We want to fully oxygenate the tissue, which generates pro-oxidants, but we also want to protect healthy tissue from excess oxidative destruction, using anti-oxidants. Antioxidants are a sacrificial substance, to be destroyed in lieu of body tissue. Antioxidants include beta-carotene, C, E, selenium, zinc, riboflavin, manganese, cysteine, methionine, N-acetylcysteine, and many herbal extracts (i.e. green tea, pycnogenols, and curcumin).

> **SOLUTION:** Use an appropriate mix of antioxidants along with adequate breathing and oxygenation of cells for optimal redox levels to fight cancer.

6) IMMUNE DYSFUNCTIONS

We have an extensive network of protective factors that circulate throughout our bodies to kill any bacteria, virus, yeast, or cancer cells. Think of these 20 trillion immune cells as both your Department of Defense and your waste disposal company. The immune system of the average American is "running on empty". Causes for this problem include toxic burden, stress, no exercise, poor diet, unbridled use of antibiotics and vaccinations, and less breast feeding.

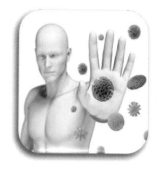

Most experts now agree to the "surveillance" theory of cancer. Cells in your body are duplicating all day every day at a blinding pace. This process of growth is fraught with peril. When cells are not copied exactly as they should be, then an emergency call goes out to the immune system to find and destroy this abnormal saboteur cell. It is the surveillance of an alert and capable immune system that defends most of us from cancer. See the chapter on immune functions.

Immunology: cops and army protecting body

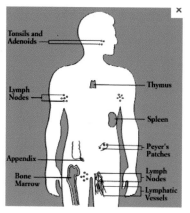

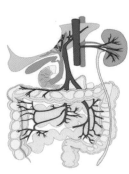

7) GLAND OR ORGAN INSUFFICIENCY

As we age, many glands and organs of the endocrine system produce less vital hormones and secretions.

- ✓ Stomach (hydrochloric acid)
- ✓ Pancreas (digestive enzymes)
- ✓ Thyroid (thyroxin)
- ✓ Adrenals (DHEA, cortisol)
- ✓ Thymus (thymic extract)
- ✓ Spleen (spleen concentrate)
- ✓ Joints (glucosamine sulfate)
- ✓ Pineal (melatonin)
- ✓ Pituitary (growth hormone)
- ✓ Replacing missing secretions often dramatically improves health.

After protein-calorie malnutrition, the second most common malnutrition condition in the <u>world is iodine deficiency</u>, with about 2 billion people suffering from this condition.[24] The mineral iodine feeds the thyroid gland, a small walnut-shaped gland in the throat region that produces a mere one teaspoon of thyroxin annually. But that thimble-full of thyroxin can make a huge difference in whether you will be bright or dull, fat or lean, healthy or sick, energetic or always tired. There are some regions of the world, particularly inland and mountainous areas, where iodine deficiency (goiter) is so common that the few people who do not have goiter are called "bottlenecks" for their abnormally slim necks. While the United States has made progress against goiter by adding iodine to salt, there are unsettling results from studies showing that about 33% of children with seemingly adequate iodine intake still have goiter.[25]

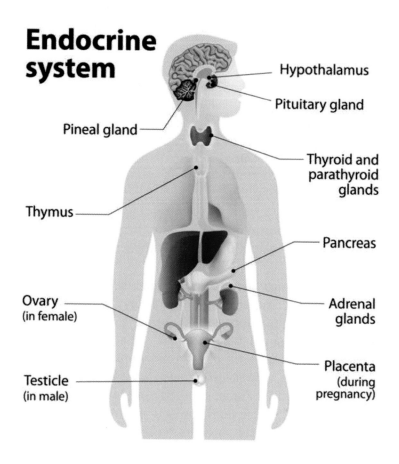

What does all this have to do with cancer? There is compelling evidence that low thyroid output substantially elevates the risk for cancer.[26] Based upon the groundbreaking work by Broda Barnes, MD, PhD, from 1930 through 1980, it is clear that about 40% of the population suffers from chronic hypothyroidism. Dr. Barnes earned his doctorate in physiology and medical degree from the University of Chicago. His primary interest was the thyroid gland. He found that people with a basal temperature of less than 97.8 F. were probably suffering from low thyroid. Symptoms include coldness; easy weight gain; constipation; sexual dysfunctions of infertility, frigidity, heavy periods, regular miscarriages, or impotence; elevated serum lipids to induce heart disease; mental confusion and depression; hypoglycemia and diabetes; and cancer. This may sound like an improbable grocery list of diseases that can all stem from one simple cause. But realize that the thyroid gland regulates energy metabolism throughout the body, which is the basis for all other functions.

Work with your physician on this issue. There is a strong link between iodine intake, thyroid function and breast health.[27] People who consume kelp, or sea vegetables, often have healthier thyroid functions and lower risk for breast cancer, which indicates that sea vegetables or kelp tablets should be consumed by cancer patients.[28] Here is another area of "simple solutions for major problems".

8) MALDIGESTION

After a lifetime of high fat, high sugar, overeating, too much alcohol, stress, drugs, indigestible foods (i.e., pizza), many Americans have poor peristalsis, insufficient stomach and intestinal secretions, damaged microvilli, and imbalances of friendly (probiotic) vs unfriendly (anaerobic, pathogenic) bacteria. One must remove, repair, replace, and re-inoculate. Food separation (combinations) may be of value for a brief time until the GI tract recuperates. Digestive enzymes and/or hydrochloric acid taken with meals may help.

Most of us have intestinal parasites. In some of us, these worms and bacteria are causing serious harm to the lining of the intestinal tract, such as a permeable gut, which allows allergies to form. Our ancestors developed many de-worming techniques that they used seasonally, such as fasting while consuming purgative herbs or regular flushing out with garlic. Work with your doctor on this issue.

9) pH (POTENTIAL HYDROGENS)

Acid alkaline balance (7.41 ideal in human veins) brought about by:
- ✓ proper breathing
- ✓ exercise (carbonic buffer from carbon dioxide in blood)
- ✓ diet (plant foods elevate pH, animal foods and sugar reduce pH)
- ✓ water (adequate hydration improves pH).
- ✓ other agents, such as cesium chloride, citric acid, sodium bicarbonate
- ✓ yeast infections that generate a collection of acids that lower pH

Cancer is acidic (low pH) tissue.[29] It is clear from all human physiology textbooks that pH in the blood, saliva, urine, and other areas is a critical factor for health. Blood pH is usually 7.35-7.45, with 7.41 thought to be ideal. Acceptable pH for saliva is 6.0-7.5, stomach 1.0-3.5, colon 5.0-8.4, and urine 4.5-8.4. pH is a logarithmic scale, meaning that moving from a healthy pH of 7.41 in the veins to 6.41 in the tumor tissue is a 10-fold (1,000 times) deterioration in the number of hydrogen ions influencing all chemical reactions. Most foods influence pH--pushing toward either acid or alkaline. Clinicians will spend much time adjusting parenteral feedings to achieve a proper pH in the blood. Diet can create a slightly <u>acidic environment in the blood</u> to encourage cancer.[30]

"diet-induced acidosis may influence molecular activities at the cellular level that promote carcinogenesis or tumor progression."

Just about everything that goes in your mouth can alter pH, including oxygen. The acidic pH of cancer cells also decreases the oxygen-carrying capacity of the surrounding blood so that tissue can become somewhat anaerobic--which are perfect conditions for cancer to thrive. Deep breathing has an alkalizing effect on the blood. An alkalizing diet of lots of plant food also helps to encourage removal of toxic heavy metals.

10) HYPOXIA

Humans are aerobic organisms. All cells thrive when there is proper oxygenation to the tissue. Red blood cell production is dependent on iron, copper, B-6, folate, B-12, protein, and zinc. Adequate exercise and proper breathing help. Cofactors, like CoQ, and B-vitamins improve aerobic energy metabolism in cell mitochondria. Fatty acids in diet dictate "membrane fluidity" of all cells and their ability to absorb oxygen.

Professor Otto Warburg received the Nobel prize in 1931 for his work on cell bioenergetics, or how the cell extracts energy from food. In 1966, Professor Warburg spoke to a group of Nobel laureates regarding his work on cancer cells:

"...the prime cause of cancer is the replacement of the respiration of oxygen in normal body cells by a fermentation of sugar."

Cancer cells are more like primitive yeast cells, extracting only a fraction of the potential energy from sugar by fermenting food substrates down to lactic acid.

Aerobic-enhancing nutrients. Yet, by oxygenating the tissue, you can exploit the "Achilles heel" of cancer. Cancer shrinks from oxygen like a vampire shrinking from daylight. Fuel is burned in the cellular furnaces, called mitochondria. As long as the mitochondrial membrane is fluid and permeable, oxygen flows in and carbon dioxide flows out and the cell stays aerobic. With a diet high in trans-fat, saturated fat, and deprived of essential fatty acid omega 3, the mitochondrial membrane becomes more rigid and less permeable to the flow of gases and electrons, which are essential to aerobic metabolism.

Nutrient factors that heavily influence aerobic metabolism include the B-vitamins, including biotin, B-1 thiamin, B-2 riboflavin, and B-3 niacin. Numerous herbal extracts, including ginseng and ginkgo biloba, can enhance the aerobic capacity of the cell. Coenzyme Q-10 is a nutrient that is the rate-limiting step in aerobic metabolism, not unlike the bridge that ties up traffic going into the city during rush hour. Most people are low in their levels of CoQ.Breathing is a lost art in our modern world. Proper breathing should include stomach and diaphragm deep breathing. Lay flat on your back on the floor. Place a book on your stomach. Begin inhaling through the nose and push out the stomach. Raise the book as high as you can, then complete inhalation by filling the chest with air. Exhale through the mouth slowly. This is diaphragm breathing, which more thoroughly oxygenates tissue and can be done by the most bed-ridden patient.

12) PHYSICAL ALIGNMENT

Spinal vertebrae must be in proper alignment. Chiropractic and osteopathic manipulations on spine, joints, and skull plates can be helpful. Accidents, poor muscle tone, and aging create alignment problems. Nerves and blood vessels radiate from the spinal column, which can become misaligned and cause compression on these vital channels of energy. Exercise, inversion, and physical manipulations from chiropractic or osteopathic physicians may solve these problems.

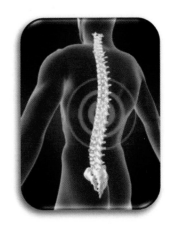

13) ENERGY ALIGNMENT

Meridians, chakras, and energy pathways were discovered by metaphysicians in ancient India. Use magnets, acupuncture, electro-acupuncture, and acupressure to correct these problems. Homeopathy probably works on this level.

PATIENT PROFILE

B.F was initially diagnosed with B-cell lymphoma. She was experienced problems with walking and visual disturbances. Initially B.F. was under the care of her oncologist and was doing chemotherapy per his recommendation. After her 6th chemotherapy session, and realizing the survival rate was limited, she began exploring other options. B.F. also underwent 2 Gamanite surgeries. Her oncologist told her the survival rate of those who have Gamanite surgery was 48%. At that time, she first met with her local naturopath who gave her hope. Then, in 2016 she watched The Truth About Cancer and saw Dr. Quillin's presentation, and shortly after scheduled a consultation. Following her consultation with Dr. Quillin B.F. bought the book Beating Cancer with Nutrition, which she still uses as a reference book. She has made many changes to her lifestyle including; improved diet - though she has always had a reasonably healthy diet, more sunshine (Vitamin D), exercising 5X week, enjoys Tai Chi, has a green smoothie 3X week, has removed stress from her life, says a gratitude prayer every morning, and has read many books on healing cancer naturally. Today B.F. is 69 feels great, has a grandchild on the way, and is looking forward to a long and healthy life.

For more information on the epigenetic (lifestyle controlled) factors that can help your body recognize and destroy cancer, read 12 KEYS TO A HEALTHIER CANCER PATIENT .[31]

ENDNOTES

[1] https://www.ifm.org/find-a-practitioner/
[2] https://www.naturopathic.org/AF_MemberDirectory.asp?version=2
[3] http://health.lifeextension.com/InnovativeDoctors/
[4] https://www.cochranelibrary.com/cdsr/doi/10.1002/14651858.CD002003.pub5/abstract
[5] https://www.amazon.com/Keys-Healthier-Cancer-Patient-Incredible/dp/0578564297
[6]. Selye, H, STRESS WITHOUT DISTRESS, JB Lippincott, NY, 1974
[7]. Newell, GR, Primary Care in Cancer, p.29, May 1991
[8]. Achterberg, J., IMAGERY IN HEALING, New Science, Boston, 1985
[9]. Cooper, CL (ed.), STRESS AND BREAST CANCER, John Wiley, NY, 1988
[10]. National Cancer Institute, NCI# NO1-CN-45133, National Institute of Health, Washington, DC 1977
[11] http://www.worldometers.info/view/toxchem/

[12] https://www.pbs.org/newshour/science/it-could-take-centuries-for-epa-to-test-all-the-unregulated-chemicals-under-a-new-landmark-bill

[13] https://en.wikipedia.org/wiki/Asbestos

[14] https://articles.mercola.com/sites/articles/archive/2012/05/21/fluoride-health-hazards.aspx

[15] https://www.ncbi.nlm.nih.gov/pubmed/31607599

[16] https://gmofreeusa.org/research/glyphosate/glyphosate-overview/

[17] https://www.sciencedirect.com/science/article/pii/S1383574216300266

[18]. Huggins, HA, IT'S ALL IN YOUR HEAD, Life Sciences Press, Colorado Springs, 1989

[19]. Heintze, G, et al., Scan.J.Dent.Res., vol.91, p.150, 1983

[20]. Berry, TC, et al., J.Am.Dent.Assn., vol.120, p.394, 1994

[21]. Zalups, RK, Pharmacol.Rev., vol.52, no.1, p.113, Mar.2000

[22]. Ahlrot, U., Nutrition Research, suppl. p.403, 1985, Second Nordic Symposium on Trace Elements in Human Health & Disease, Odense, Denmark, Aug.1987

[23]. Bortz, WM, Journal American Medical Association, vol.248, no.10, p.1203, Sept.10, 1982

[24] https://www.ncbi.nlm.nih.gov/pmc/articles/PMC6284174/#:~:text=At%20a%20global%20scale%2C%20aproximately,role%20when%20discussing%20treatment%20options.

[25]. Ziporyn, T., Journal American Medical Association, vol.253, p.1846, Apr.1985

[26]. Langer, SE, et al., SOLVED: THE RIDDLE OF ILLNESS, Keats, New Canaan, 1984

[27] https://breast-cancer-research.biomedcentral.com/articles/10.1186/bcr638

[28] https://breast-cancer-research.biomedcentral.com/articles/10.1186/bcr638

[29]. Newell, K, et al., Proceedings of National Academy of Sciences, vol.90, no.3, p.1127, Feb.1993

[30] https://www.ncbi.nlm.nih.gov/pmc/articles/PMC3571898/

[31] https://www.amazon.com/Keys-Healthier-Cancer-Patient-Incredible/dp/0578564297

Chapter 24

IS CANCER AN INFECTION?

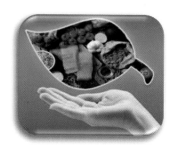

"I have been wrong.   The bacteria is nothing.   The terrain is everything."
Louis Pasteur 1822-1895

> ### WHAT'S AHEAD
> Cancer is a complicated disease, caused by many factors with no "magic bullet" cure anywhere on the horizon. Some cancers, and possibly many, are caused by chronic infections. This makes immune recognition critical:
> ✓ Nourish immune functions
> ✓ Use appropriate anti-microbial therapies.

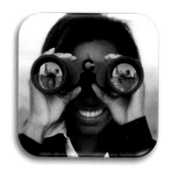

Ignaz Semmelweis (1818-1865) was an Austrian physician who found that washing hands with a dilute chlorine solution before delivering a baby would cut down the incidence of infections (puerperal fever) and mortality in the mother and newborn infant. His successes in his clinic in the 1840s were profoundly better than other physicians, who would go straight from the autopsy room then the stables without washing their hands to delivering an infant. Dr. Semmelweis had a logical, non-toxic, inexpensive, clinically-proven solution to a horrible problem of that era. His technique reduced mortality in mothers and newborns to 1.3% which was a 90% reduction from his colleagues' results of 11% mortality.

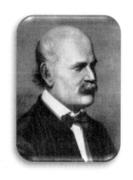

Unfortunately, his simple solution was rejected because his critics asked: "So, Dr. Semmelweis, what is causing these women to die?" "I don't know." replied Semmelweis. "And are we to suspect that 'spooks' are involved?" they laughingly chided. When Louis Pasteur peered into a microscope and cooked (pasteurized) bacteria to death, he presented his data to his colleagues: "I have found Dr. Semmelweis's spooks."

WHAT DO FUNGI AND CANCER CELLS HAVE IN COMMON?

"Differentiation of blastomycotic bone disease from tuberculosis, malignant disease or other fungal disease is difficult." p.53 Clinical Mycology, Kibbler, Wiley, 1996

FUNGUS	CANCER
Obligate glucose metabolizer	Obligate glucose metabolizer
Generates lactic & other acids	Generates lactic acid
Produce alpha-fetal proteins (second.metab.)	Produce alpha-fetal proteins (second.metab.) CEA, HCG
Produce proteolytic & other enzymes	Produce proteolytic enzymes, metastasis

Lung cancer often spreads to the brain.
Aspergillosis of the lungs (fungal) usually spreads to the brain.

Semmelweis died a broken man, yet many hospitals in Europe are named after this brilliant and courageous physician, now considered the "father of infection control". How many people died because critics of Semmelweis refused to accept his solution? How many cancer patients die because we are stuck in a half-century battle with cancer using outdated methods and theories? Many cancers are probably infections, with the infectious organism (fungi, virus, bacteria) becoming an intracellular pathogen, creating a hybrid DNA from the weaving of the pathogen with host human DNA. Bacteria are about 100 times larger than viruses and fungi are about 100 times larger than bacteria. Let's look at the facts.

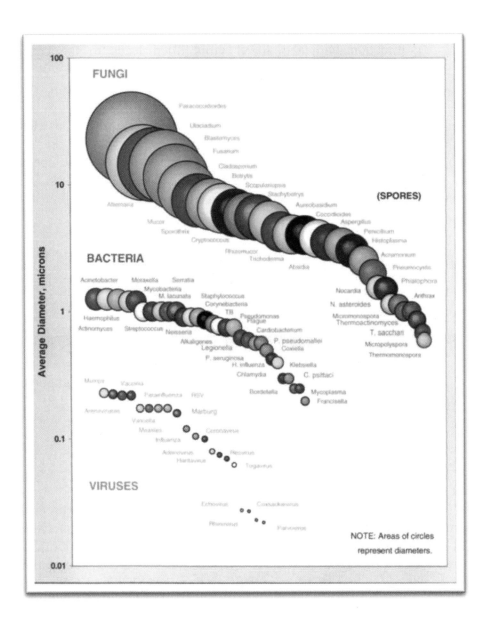

- The most conservative estimates show that 10% of all cancers are caused by infections.[1]
- Human papilloma virus (HPV) is associated with at least 80% of all cervical cancer. Virus is a piece of DNA or RNA that is wrapped in protein and invisible to standard microscopes.
- The bacteria Helicobacter pylori is a major risk factor for stomach cancer.[2]
- Infection with the AIDS virus often leads to the cancer lymphoma.
- Infection with Epstein-Barr virus often leads to Burkitt lymphoma.[3]
- Chronic infection with hepatitis B virus usually leads to liver cancer.[4]
- Any exposure to the fungal poison aflatoxin or extensive exposure to the fungal by-product alcohol will often cause liver cancer.[5]
- CRP is a valuable marker for the progression of cancer.[6] CRP measures inflammation as a by-product of infection.
- A National Science Foundation grant winner, Professor David Hess, has written a fascinating book linking infections as the underlying cause of many cancers.[7]
- Ketoconazole is an anti-fungal drug that is commonly used to treat prostate cancer.[8] It may work by killing fungal cells disguised as cancer cells.[9]
- Griseofulvin, an antifungal drug, killed human colon cancer cells in a culture dish by inducing apoptosis, or programmed cell death.[10]
- Milton White, MD found evidence that cancer is a blend (hybrid) of human DNA with spores of plant bacterial conidia.[11]

Mainstream physicians scoff at the notion of fungal infections in anyone but the most immune-compromised person. In the academic textbook on fungal infections in humans, PRINCIPLES AND PRACTICES OF CLINICAL MYCOLOGY, researchers note that in the majority of cases there are no good explanations for the immuno-compromised status in the patient with systemic fungal infection.[12] Lung cancer oftentimes spreads to the brain. So does the fungal infection Aspergillosis.[13]

PATIENT PROFILE: LUNG CANCER OR FUNGAL INFECTION?
D.M. came to me in 1998 in the end-stages of lung cancer. He was 75 years old and had failed the best chemo and immune protocols from his home town in Florida, the Harvard Deaconess Hospital and the National Cancer Institute. He had a sweet tooth, a history of toenail fungal infections, and the needle biopsy of his lung cancer was "indeterminate". I asked him to follow an anti-fungal diet, supplements, and for his physician to prescribe an antifungal medication (Diflucan) for his toenail fungal infection. Within 3 months, his lung cancer had shrunk by 40% based on CAT scans. Unfortunately, the congestive heart disease he had developed as a consequence of many cardiotoxic chemo agents caused his death. But the anti-fungal program was reversing his lung cancer.

PATIENT PROFILE: LUNG CANCER OR FUNGAL INFECTION?
C.T. was diagnosed with lung cancer and scheduled for a lobectomy, or surgical removal of a lobe of her lung. Another physician, who also held a doctorate in mycology (the study of fungi) examined the patient and found possibilities of a fungal infection in the lungs. The oncologist for C.T. was enraged that someone would have such a ludicrous idea that a board-certified oncologist did not know the difference between lung cancer and fungal infection in the lungs. The patient felt more comfortable with the possibility of fungal infection and went on anti-fungal medication rather than going in for surgery the next day. The patient recovered fully from her "lung cancer".

DIAGNOSIS: YOU CANNOT FIND WHAT YOU ARE NOT LOOKING FOR

In the definitive textbook on fungal infections, the experts tell us: "Despite uniformly negative blood cultures, necrotizing vasculitis and infarction are characteristic of zygomycosis." Meaning, you cannot pick up fungal infections from blood cultures, aka fungemia, until the patient is nearly dead. Fungi are fastidious microbes that do not culture well for visibility under the microscope. Fungi are masters of evasion, listed as dimorphic (two different shapes) in many textbooks, and pleomorphic (variable in size and shape) in some texts.

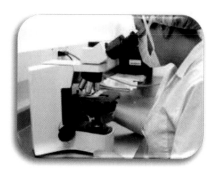

In 1999, doctors at the Mayo Clinic released a study showing that 96% of the chronic sinusitis patients they analyzed were suffering from a fungal infection. [14] Millions of American sinusitis patients have taken antibiotics over the past half century because doctors assumed the problem was due to a bacterial infection. These Mayo Clinic researchers used the sophisticated tool of PCR (polymerase chain reaction) to look for DNA fingerprints of fungi, which could not be found before without this valuable tool.

Realize that when doctors give the diagnosis of cancer, in many cases it is not as clear cut as it may sound. Pathologists, surgeons, radiologists, and other experts confer to assess this abnormal tissue. If, under a microscope or on a CAT scan, all the cancer cells were blue and all healthy cells were red, then diagnosis would be easy. But that is not the case. Cancer cells, infected cells, aging cells, and fungal colonies can become an indistinguishable blur. As Thomas Cox, MD wrote in *Journal of Family Practice*:

"Although artificial categories have been set up to divide a continuum of abnormal cells, nature's paintbrush is not as specific as we would like."

There is a great deal of subjectivity, discretion, judgment, and professional guessing that goes into the diagnosis of cancer. Cancer is sometimes misdiagnosed.

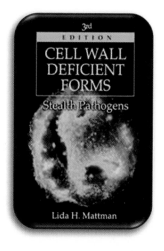

Enter the 2001 textbook CELL WALL DEFICIENT FORMS: STEALTH PATHOGENS, in which a Yale-trained microbiologist explains how microorganisms, including fungi, mutate throughout their life cycle into many different shapes (pleomorphism) and even shed their cell wall coating to become almost invisible under the microscope.

Pathologists routinely ignore a common staining technique when they are trying to assess tissue for a cancer diagnosis. Acridine Orange will find traces of nucleic acid from nearby cell wall deficient microorganisms. But it is not used. The only way you are going to see sparrows is to look up. If you don't look up, then you won't see any sparrows. Unless you stain the slide properly for microscopic evaluation, you won't find any pleomorphic cell wall deficient fungi in the cancer patient's tissue. Of all the agents that cause microorganisms to shed their cell wall and become "invisible", antibiotics are the most powerful. The scary part is that modern medicine disregards the importance of systemic fungal infections:

"Discovery of aspergillosis is often made at autopsy".[15]

ANTIBIOTICS: PROBLEM OR SOLUTION?

It was 1928 when Alexander Fleming noticed that a gray furry mold in his petri dish killed all the surrounding bacteria.[16] The chemical from the mold (Penicillium notatum) produced the first successful antibiotic (meaning "against life"), penicillin, for which Fleming was awarded the shared Nobel prize in medicine in 1945. Just ask any physician who remembers the 1950s, when medicine was shifting from sulfa drugs and colloidal silver to antibiotics. Doomed patients with bacterial infections were sometimes pulled from the brink of death by antibiotics. In ancient

SOMETHING CORRUPTS THE DNA
TO INDUCE CANCER

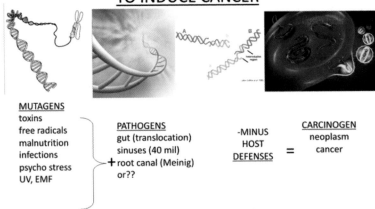

MUTAGENS
toxins
free radicals
malnutrition
infections
psycho stress
UV, EMF

PATHOGENS
gut (translocation)
sinuses (40 mil)
+ root canal (Meinig)
or??

-MINUS
HOST
DEFENSES

=

CARCINOGEN
neoplasm
cancer

Recombinant DNA, altered DNA resulting from the insertion into the chain by chemical, enzymatic, or biological means, of a sequence not originally present in that chain.

Ayurvedic medicine, the healer would apply a piece of moldy bread (rich in antibiotics) to a wound to prevent infection. Unfortunately, this warm and fuzzy story does not end here.

Antibiotics are chemical "no trespassing" borders that are excreted by fungi and some bacteria. Of the 100 different types of antibiotics available in modern healthcare, 10 are most commonly used. Most of the nearly one thousand antibiotics, or mycotoxins, that have been tested proved to be so toxic that they could not be used without killing the patient. One mycotoxin, aflatoxin B, is the most carcinogenic substance on the planet earth. Streptozotocin is an antibiotic that is too toxic for human use except as a chemotherapy drug for cancer patients. It is used in research to destroy the pancreas in experimental animals and generates insulin-dependent diabetes to do research on animals.[17] There are about a dozen different antibiotics used as chemo agents to treat cancer.

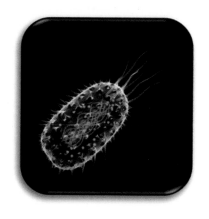

There is a thin line between killing the bacterial infection and killing the patient. After bee venom, the most hyper-allergenic substance in the world is penicillin. Today, Americans use about 60 million pounds (27 million kilograms) of antibiotics, half of which is used to make the 8 billion animals raised for human consumption grow faster.[18] The other half, 30 million pounds, is used to provide the 154 million annual prescriptions for antibiotics, which the Center for Disease Control estimates that at least 30% are inappropriate.

Most European countries do not allow antibiotics to be given at "sub-therapeutic" levels to make animals grow faster. In the 1950s, American farmers would add 5-10 parts per million of the antibiotic tetracycline to animal feed to accelerate the rate of growth by about 20%. Today, farmers need to use 50-200 ppm (10 to 40 times more than previous dosage) to get the same effect.

Bacteria carry within them little mysterious forms of life called plasmids. These "hitchhikers" get free room and board in exchange for their ability to "hack" the code on chemical poisons in the environment. Plasmids somehow figure out how to bypass the biochemical pathways of antibiotics, which makes the bacteria immune to the effects of this poison.[19] Bacteria exchange plasmids frequently, like a convention of hackers trying to beat the code. Antibiotics are extremely stable to heat, sun, and even passing through the digestive tract of an animal. Which means they remain active in the environment in raw sewage allowing the plasmids an opportunity at hacking the chemical combination that allows the bacteria to become drug resistant. We now have drug-resistant "bullet-proof" microbes (MRSA) that thrive in spite of our best drugs, including multiple antibiotic cocktails. Between 20-50% of patients now exhibit bacterial infections that are resistant to one or more formerly-effective antibiotics.

According to one study published in the *Journal of the American Medical Association*, 44% of children going to the doctor for a cold were given antibiotics, which is inappropriate therapy.[20] In a separate study, researchers observed 250 adults being treated for a fever that lasted less than a week. The physicians were wrong 50% of the time in assessing whether the patient had a viral or bacterial infection.[21] Intussusception is the leading cause of intestinal obstruction in young children in America. Antibiotic use triples the risk for intussusception in children. The antibiotic Cephalosporin increases the risk for intestinal obstruction by 20 fold.[22]

Antibiotics are useless against a virus, but may induce a fungal infection in the process. Antibiotics are given before, during and after nearly all medical and dental procedures; from a tooth cleaning to routine chemotherapy to bone marrow transplantation. Antibiotics are among the most toxic of all cancer therapy drugs, including adriamycin and bleomycin. Antibiotics kill most or all bacteria that they encounter, including the good bacteria (probiotics) in the digestive tract, which is where the real trouble begins.

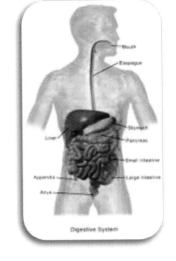

Digestive System

The average human has about 100 trillion microorganisms in the gut. Good bacteria in the gut help us to make vitamins (biotin, K, etc.), digest food, encourage regularity, and compete with or eat the unfriendly yeast that can overrun the gut. A healthy human gut is like a balanced ecosystem of a garden in which the birds eat the bugs, and the bugs do minimal damage to the vegetable garden. When we kill off the birds (friendly bacteria), the bugs (harmful yeast) have no predators and quickly overrun the garden. When we overuse antibiotics, we kill ALL the bacteria in the gut and commonly end up with a yeast infection that can become systemic.[23] All major clinical textbooks on fungal infections agree that antibiotic use is a leading cause of fungal infections in humans.[24] "Candida overgrowth and bloodborne dissemination are favored by...multiple antibiotics, catheters, and tubes."[25]

Antibiotics, if used appropriately, can save lives. Unfortunately, antibiotics are being wildly overused today. Antibiotic use increases the risk for breast cancer.[26]

PATIENT PROFILE

LC was a reasonably healthy 25-year old woman when she came down with a cold. After a few days of misery, she went to her doctor who gave her a prescription for antibiotics, having never taken a throat culture to see if the infection was bacterial. A week later, LC was still sick. More powerful broad-spectrum antibiotics were prescribed. Eventually, LC recovered from the cold. Three months later, LC began discharging blood in her stools. As the "solution" to this problem, her doctor performed an ileostomy, or removal of the colon and ileocecal valve and placed a plastic bag on her hip. No more normal toilet pooping. A few years later, LC developed vaginal bleeding. Her doctor surgically removed all of her female organs by hysterectomy and ovariectomy. She has since experienced hot flashes and chronic fatigue syndrome that would flatten anyone. It is quite possible that her nearly 30 years of health problems could have been avoided by not using antibiotics for a cold, or dealing with the inevitable yeast overgrowth from the antibiotics in ways other than removal of "elective" organs.

In 1908, the Nobel laureate, Elie Metchnikoff, PhD (1845-1916), who discovered the bacteria (Lactobacillus acidophilus) that makes yogurt, said "Death begins in the colon." Once the balance of power in the gut swings from healthy bacteria to unhealthy yeast overgrowth, illness in the body is inevitable and death is quite possible.

Orian Truss, MD wrote the seminal book on the subject of yeast infections, THE MISSING DIAGNOSIS. He describes a half century of his own medical practice and the bewildering collection of conditions produced in patients who had taken antibiotics.[27] Dr. Truss was working in the 1950s when antibiotics were being prescribed with great enthusiasm for many inappropriate conditions. Patients would return a few months later with rheumatoid arthritis, or Crohn's disease, or irritable bowel syndrome, or multiple sclerosis. Dr. Truss was the first one to link antibiotic side effects to yeast overgrowth and the limitless diseases that can be produced through fungal by-products, or secondary metabolites. Once you carpet bomb the gut with antibiotics, the delicate balance of 100 trillion microbes in the intestines has been disturbed.

The immune system is a collection of 20 trillion highly specialized warrior cells that patrol the human body looking for bad guys. You are either with us or against us. Recognize self from non-self. This is truly an amazing feat. When the immune system is suppressed, we get infections or cancer. When the immune system is overstimulated, we get auto-immune diseases as the immune system begins to attack our own tissues.

When antibiotics were first discovered in the 1930s, there were no auto-immune diseases known to modern medicine. Today there are 50 million Americans suffering from at least 80 different autoimmune diseases. Arthritis, juvenile diabetes, multiple sclerosis, scleroderma, ankylosing spondylitis, lupus erythematosus, Crohn's disease, and many others are growing exponentially in numbers. Overuse of antibiotics may generate systemic fungal infections. Fungi can either slow down the immune system to allow more infections and cancer,[28] or can upregulate the immune system to trigger an autoimmune attack.[29] Now the body is literally eating itself alive.

If antibiotics are not the answer to all infections, then what is? A healthy immune system. When our immune system is properly fortified with nutrients, and not impaired by toxins or stress, then our immune system can recognize and destroy the most evasive of microbes. Lymphocytes, Natural Killer cells, helper and suppressor cells, antibodies, and immunoglobulins constitute the world's most sophisticated army to repel invaders in our body.

The worst plague to hit the human race was the Black Plague of 1347, which started in Asia and arrived in Europe at the ports of Italy. Estimates vary widely, but somewhere between 25 and 75 million people,

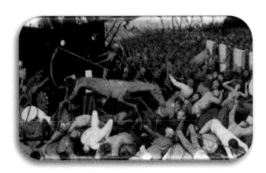

probably a third of Europe died from the plague.

Every year about 50,000 Americans die from pneumonia and another 36,000 from the flu, of which 90% are older people with compromised immune systems.[30] 2020 brought a pandemic plague which was no different. 90% of death from corona virus or Covid-19 were in older people with multiple co-morbidities (illnesses). As of this writing, 1 million people globally have died from Covid, out of the 7.8 billion earthlings. Covid has a 99.75% recovery rate in the population at large. Near zero risk for young people. Worst case scenario is 95% recovery among the elderly. Vitamin D, zinc, iodine, and a healthy immune system are critical to prevention and recovery from Covid and cancer. The authorities put schools, churches, travel industry, hotels, restaurants, conventions, and more on lockdown.

WHERE DO THE FUNGI COME FROM?

Doctors at Georgetown Medical Center in Washington, DC found that patients with unexplained chronic fatigue were nine times (900%) more likely to be suffering from sinusitis than the population at large. Patients with chronic pain were 6 times (600%) more likely to be suffering from sinusitis than the control group.[31] Maybe the fungi enters the body through the sinus cavities, creates an infection there, then spreads throughout the body to create pain, fatigue, and possibly eventually cancer.

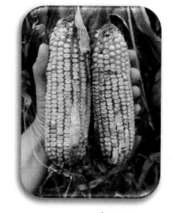

Fungi are so prolific and so fecund as to defy the imagination. A wood decay fungus (Ganoderma) sends out 5.4 trillion spores per season. Corn smut fungi produces 25 billion fungal spores per ear of corn. In one experiment, researchers on the first floor of a building took the lid off of a culture dish with fungi. Within 10 minutes, these unique fungi had traveled through the ventilation system, up to the 4th floor, and were measured in the thousands of fungi per cubic meter.[32]

The Government Accounting Office tells us that 20% of the 80,000 public schools in America have an air quality problem, usually including fungi, which cause breathing problems and more in school children. Close up a school for 3 months of a hot humid summer with plenty of food (books) for the fungi, and the possibility of mold-causing health problems in school children escalates. Americans have been to the moon, built the Panama Canal and the Internet, and have more Nobel laureates than any other country on earth, yet we are only beginning to look at one of the most powerful and potentially destructive creatures on the planet earth: fungi. Never mind Jaws or the Predator. Fungi can make these two horror films look like cartoons.

The definitive textbook on fungal infections in humans, PRINCIPLES AND PRACTICES OF CLINICAL MYCOLOGY, by world renowned physicians and researchers, says that fungal infections in the bone are virtually identical to bone cancer (i.e. leukemia, multiple myeloma) on an X-ray machine:

"Differentiation of blastomycotic bone disease from tuberculosis, malignant disease, or other fungal disease is difficult."

A.V. Costantini, MD, former professor at the University of California San Francisco Medical School and former head of the World Health Organization, has amassed an <u>impressive amount of data</u> showing that mycotoxins in our food supply can and do cause many forms of cancer, including breast and prostate.[33]

Where do the fungi come from? They come from the air around us and the fungi that live within our gut, mouth, sinuses, vaginal tract, and other body cavities.

THE ECOLOGIST AND UNDERTAKER

Early biologists noticed things that move and eat, aka animals and insects, and things that don't move and do conduct photosynthesis, aka plants. Then they noticed fungi, which does none of the above. Biologists consider there to be 6 main kingdoms of life, with fungi (mycota) as one.

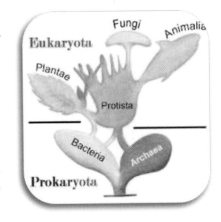

Fungi (also known as yeast, mold, rust, and mushrooms) are on top of the food chain on earth, because they degrade all organic matter once dead. Fungi turn us and everything else into dirt. There are an estimated 1.5 million different species on earth, of which 400 species can cause diseases in humans.

Candida is the species most often associated with human fungal infections, yet there are hundreds of other fungi that infect humans. The fungi, Aspergillus, "eat" damp grains and nuts in the field and give off aflatoxins, one of the most toxic and cancer-causing agents on the planet earth. Fungi are, basically, enzyme factories. They make enzymes to digest any organic matter on earth. When all the people, bugs, poop, and leaves have fallen, then fungi step in to degrade this organic matter back to the basic elements of carbon, hydrogen, nitrogen, oxygen, and minerals. Unfortunately, sometimes fungi are too eager to perform their duties. Fungi are at their best converting your back yard compost pile into rich soil. And at their worst in a dying patient.

WHAT IS YOUR VITALITY SCORE?

Why do we have so many Americans suffering from systemic fungal infections? Bacteria, yeast, virus, parasites are abundantly present all around us. What keeps you well is "your terrain", or your "non-specific host defense mechanisms". How does anyone recover from the flu, a laceration of the skin, or a broken bone? You recover through the miraculous healing properties within your body.

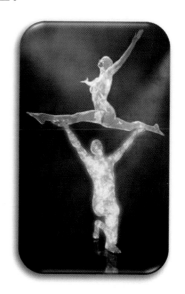

What is your "vitality score"? How healthy are you? If vitality exists as a continuum, with 0 meaning dead, 1 being very ill, and 10 being an Olympic athlete, then where are you on this scale? If we drop below 7 or so on the scale, fungi become eager to perform their duties in us.

This is where the bubble bursts on the American dream of a "magic bullet" drug to kill all disease-causing organisms in our body, while we consume 150 pounds per year of sugar, add 100 million mercury fillings to our mouths each year, lavishly overuse antibiotics, the only exercise that we get is coughing, and an endless stream of stress hormones from unhappy spirits. A malnourished, sugar-drenched, toxically-compromised, exhausted, and stressed-out person is an easy target for a fungal infection. When we are well, the fungi live as "commensal" organisms, creating small amounts of uric acid as an antioxidant to slow down the aging process.

As our vitality score drops, yeast switch into saprophytic mode, or begin to decay any available fuel in our body. When things really get ugly, the yeast becomes a parasite and can cause a slow torturous death with a bewildering assortment of medical labels, starting with autoimmune diseases and cancer. The typical American lifestyle generates a very low vitality score. Fungi are there to do their job. If you want to get well, then begin a healthy lifestyle that discourages the presence of fungal infections.

IF CANCER IS REALLY FUNGI, THEN..

In the hundreds of medical staff meetings and tumor boards that I have attended, brilliant physicians have presented their most puzzling cancer cases. How does a cancer cell secrete enzymes to break through the various epithelial barriers and eventually metastasize throughout the patient's body? Why does a cancer feed primarily on sugar (glucose), which is why we use a PET scan to find the cancer? How does a cancer cell generate a wide assortment of chemicals that mimic the human fetus, as if to create a regional immune suppression or "stealth coating"? How does cancer create substances (like lactic acid) that cause havoc with energy metabolism of the patient? How does cancer send out roots to burrow into the flesh of the host. Fungi can do all of this, and more.

Fungi is a formidable invader in the human body for many reasons. For instance, bacteria are prokaryotic cells that lack a membrane around the nucleus. It is easier for human immune cells to "smell" the difference between human and bacterial cells. Fungal cells mimic human cells as eukaryotic cells that do have a membrane around the nucleus, making it more difficult for the immune system to detect "good guys from bad guys".

GETTING WELL

Stop taking indiscriminate antibiotics. Regular use of antibiotics increases the risk for breast cancer. Cut back on sugar intake dramatically. Follow the dietary recommendations in this book and recipe chapter. Avoid processed foods. Detoxify the poisons from your body.

CONDITIONS THAT ENCOURAGE YEAST

- toxins (i.e. mercury, petrochemicals, pesticides, etc.)
- stress
- malnutrition (excess, deficiency, or imbalance or any nutrient)
- chronically-elevated blood glucose
- sedentary lifestyle
- mold overload (working around mold, animal dung, moldy attics)
- antibiotics
- constipation, dysbiosis

TO DETECT YEAST OVERGROWTH

organic acid urine analysis, Great Plains Labs, 913-341-8949

TO REVERSE YEAST OVERGROWTH

1) Starve it. Reduce fasting blood sugar to 60-90 mg% by incorporating intermittent fasting and a wholesome diet. Use a home blood glucose testing kit, available at your local drug store.

2) Kill it.
- Prescription anti-fungals and/or vitamins D and A at therapeutic levels as immune modulators.
- Garlic, oil of oregano, grapefruit seed extract, Essiac tea, castor oil, capryllic acid, medium chain triglycerides, olive oil
- Purge yeast sanctuaries. Maintain bowel regularity. Chronic constipation can create small intestine fungal overgrowth (SIFO) or SIBO (bacteria). Probiotics, like Three Lac, to establish healthy microbes in the gut.

3) Change the conditions that allow yeast to thrive. Add probiotics (yogurt, lactobacillus), detoxify heavy metals, endorphins (peace and happiness), exercise, immune stimulation, lots of greens (chlorella, spirulina, barley green), healthy prostaglandin mix through less omega 6 oils (corn, soy, safflower) and more omega 3 oils (fish), MSM (sulfur).

My sincere appreciation to Orian Truss, MD, Milton White, MD, A.V. Costantini, MD, William Crook, MD, "Doc" Pennington, and Doug Kaufmann for making the rest of the world more aware of an underdiagnosed problem: mycotoxins in our food supply and fungal infections in our bodies.

For more information on how your body can fight fungal infections go to GettingHealthier.com.

PATIENT PROFILE

"Doc" Pennington was an oil magnate who developed end-stage non-resectable (cannot be surgically removed) colon cancer with metastasis to the liver at the age of 70 in 1972. His doctors told him to "get his affairs in order". Pennington used no conventional cancer treatments, since they held little promise for him. He got his physician to write a prescription for Griseofulvin, an anti-fungal drug. Three months later, his oncologist found that Doc Pennington had no more colon cancer. Remember, Pennington had no medical therapy. Pennington died at age 97 in 1997, but not before spending $125 million of his own money to found the Pennington Biomedical Center to study the link between yeast, nutrition, and cancer. Researchers in Taiwan have found that Griseofulvin induced suicide, or apoptosis, in human colon cancer cells in a culture dish.[34]

WHAT DOES FUNGUS HAVE TO DO WITH CANCER?

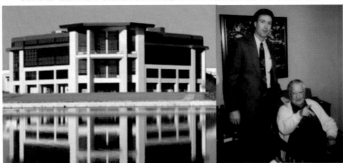

PENNINGTON BIOMEDICAL CENTER   Patrick Quillin
BATON ROUGE, LA   Doc Pennington

ENDNOTES

[1] . Dollinger, M., EVERYONE'S GUIDE TO CANCER THERAPY, p.8, Andrews McMeel, Kansas City, 2002

[2] . Sugiyama, T, Med.Electron.Microsc., vol.37, no.3, p.149, Sep.2004

[3] . Cheung, TW, Cancer Invest.vol.22no.5, p.787, 2004

[4] . Brechot,C., Gastroenterology, vol.127,5 suppl.1, p. S56

[5] . Williams, JH, Am.J.Clin.Nutr., vol.80, no.5, p.1106, Nov.2004

[6] . Mahmoud, FA, Curr.Oncol.Rep., vol.4, no.3, p.250, May 2002

[7] . Hess, DJ, CAN BACTERIA CAUSE CANCER?, New York Univ.Press, 1997

[8] . Peehl, DM, Urology, vol. 58, 2 suppl. 1, p.123, Aug.2001

[9] . Bok, RA, Drug Saf., vol.20, no.5, p.451, May 1999

[10] . Yuan-Soon, H., Int.J.Cancer, vol.91, p.383, 2001

[11] . White, MW, Medical Hypotheses, vol.55, no.4, p.302, 2000

[12] . Kemper, CA, PRINCIPLES AND PRACTICES CLINICAL MYCOLOGY, p.58, Wiley, NY, 1996

[13] . Graybill, JR, PRINCIPLES AND PRACTICES CLINICAL MYCOLOGY, p.96, Wiley, NY, 1996

[14] . Ponikau, JU, Mayo Clin.Proc., vol.74, p.877, 1999

[15] . Graybill, JR, ibid.

[16] . Mitchell, J. (ed.), RANDOM HOUSE ENCYCLOPEDIA, p.2191, Random House, NY, 1983

[17] . Mavrikakis, ME, et al., Exp.Clin.Endocrinol.Diabetes, vol.106, no.1, p.35, 1998

[18] . Levy, S., ANTIBIOTIC PARADOX,p. 149, Perseus Publ, Cambridge, MA, 2002

[19] . Levy, SB, THE ANTIBIOTIC PARADOX, Perseus Publ, Cambridge, MA, 2002

[20] . JAMA, vol.279, p.875, 1998

[21] . Brit.J.Gen.Practice, vol.51, p.998, 2001

[22] . Spiro, DM, et al., vol.157, no.1, p.54, Jan.2003

[23] . Verduyn, L, Diagn.Microbiol.Infect.Dis., vol.34, no.3, p.213, Jul 1999

[24] . Kibbler, CC, et al., PRINCIPLES AND PRACTICES OF CLINICAL MYCOLOGY, Wiley, NY, 1996; see also Calderone, RA, CANDIDA AND CANDIDIASIS, ASM Press, Washington, 2002

[25] . Graybill, JR, p.97, ibid.

[26] https://jamanetwork.com/journals/jama/article-abstract/198216

[27] . Truss, O., THE MISSING DIAGNOSIS, Missing Diagnosis, Inc., Birmingham, AL, 1985

[28] . Boutrif, E., et al., Global Significance of Mycotoxins, in MYCOTOXINS AND PHYCOTOXINS, p.3, deKoe, Netherlands, 2001

[29] . Norred, WP, et al., Toxicology and mechanisms of action of selected mycotoxins, in MYCOTOXINS AND PHYCOTOXINS, deKoe, Netherlands, 2001

[30] . US Mortality Public Use Data Tape, National Center for Health Statistics, Centers for Disease control and Prevention 2003

[31] . Chester, AC, Arch.Intern.Med., vol.163, no.15, p.1832, Aug11, 2003

[32] . Hudler, GW, MAGICAL MUSHROOMS, MISCHIEVOUS MOLDS, Princeton Press, 1998

[33] . Costantini, AV, PREVENTION OF BREAST CANCER, Oberlin Verlag, Germany, 1996

[34] . Yuan-Soon, H., Int.J.Cancer, vol.91, p.383, 2001

Chapter 25

RATIONAL CANCER TREATMENT

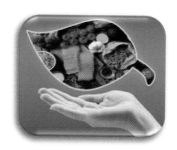

It was the best of times, it was the worst of times. It was the age of wisdom. It was the age of foolishness.
Charles Dickens, A Tale of Two Cities

WHAT'S AHEAD
Use an appropriate combination of:
✓ Cytotoxic therapies to reduce tumor burden
✓ An aggressive collection of naturopathic (cell-restorative) therapies to re-regulate the body and bolster host defense mechanisms.

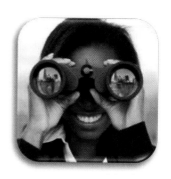

The purpose of this book is to provide detailed information on the role of nutrition as adjuvant (helpful) therapy in comprehensive cancer treatment. This book is not intended to be a compilation of all meaningful alternative cancer therapies. Among the very good books on this subject are <u>THE COMPLETE GUIDE TO ALTERNATIVE CANCER TREATMENT</u>[1] and <u>THE TRUTH ABOUT CANCER.</u>[2]

The combination of changing the underlying conditions that brought on the cancer (naturopathic) and attacking the cancer with therapies that kill cancer, but do not harm the host (cytotoxic), can be incredibly effective.

Chemotherapy, radiation, and surgery may be appropriate in certain cancers and for certain people. But make sure that the physician understands the concept of "restrained" medical therapies against cancer. I have worked with cancer patients who were devastated by unrestrained chemo, radiation, or surgery.

If you threw a hand grenade into your garage to get rid of the mice, then you may have accomplished the goal of killing the mice, but you don't have a garage anymore. Similarly, too many cancer patients are exposed to "maximum sub-lethal" therapies, which may provide an initial "response" or tumor shrinkage, but in the end may

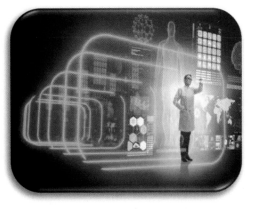

reduce the quality and quantity of life for the cancer patient by suppressing immune functions, damaging the heart and kidneys, and creating a tumor that is "drug resistant", or virtually bullet-proof.

There are other cancer therapies that may be more effective at killing cancer and less toxic to the cancer patients, such as hyperthermia, intravenous vitamin C, Burzynski's anti-neoplastons, PolyMVA, enzymes, Cell Specific Cancer Therapy, Ukrain, Govallo's vaccine, and others.

VITAMIN C. Vitamin C can become a targeted anti-cancer agent because it resembles the preferred fuel of cancer, glucose, and is absorbed by cancer cells in abundance. The ascorbic acid by itself in an anaerobic environment then becomes a powerful pro-oxidant and destroys the cancer cell--but only the cancer cells, since healthy cells have built-in mechanisms for absorbing the right amount of vitamin C along with the entire "symphony" of other antioxidants.

There is compelling evidence that high dose intravenous vitamin C has a central role in cancer treatment.[3] High dose IVC as sole therapy has often been shown to be <u>effective in advanced cancer patients.</u> [4] Researchers from the NCI and other institutions have reported that in 2008 there were 172 doctors who <u>administered IVC to over 12,000</u> patients with remarkably few side effects and good clinical outcomes.[5]

    A couple of hundred thousand years ago, humans lost the ability to convert blood sugar (glucose) into vitamin C (ascorbic acid). Some scientists have called this evolutionary shift a figurative "fall from the Garden of Eden". All but a few creatures on earth produce their own vitamin C in massive quantities, with higher internal production when the creature gets sick. For instance, a 150-pound goat makes about 10,000 milligrams daily of vitamin C. Meanwhile, the Recommended Dietary Allowance for a 156-pound reference human is 60 milligrams per day.

    Vitamin C is one of the more utilitarian nutrients in the human body, by assisting in the construction of connective tissue (the glue that keeps the body together), regulating the levels of fats in the blood, assisting in iron absorption, aiding in the synthesis of various brain chemicals for thought, and protecting against the damaging effects of free radicals. In a study done at the University of California at Los Angeles, men who took supplements of 300 mg daily of vitamin C (5 times the RDA) lived an average of 6 years longer than men who did not take supplements of vitamin C. Mark Levine, MD, researcher with the National Institutes of Health, finds evidence that 250 mg per day might be a more rational and healthy RDA for vitamin C.

    Meanwhile, oncologists worry about the possibility that vitamin C might inhibit the free radical activity of chemotherapy and radiation in destroying cancer cells. While it might seem logical that an antioxidant (like vitamin C) might reduce the effectiveness of a pro-oxidant (like chemo and radiation), the opposite has been found in animal and human studies: antioxidants protect the healthy tissue of the patient while allowing the cancer tissue to become more vulnerable to the damaging effects of chemo and radiation.

    Any antioxidant can become a pro-oxidant in a given chemical soup. That is why Nature always gives us droves of different antioxidants to play "hot potato" with unpaired electrons until their destructive energy is dissipated. No food has just one antioxidant. No human cell wants just one antioxidant. Antioxidants can become pro-oxidants when in isolation, which is exactly what happens to cancer cells when they selectively absorb only vitamin C, hoping to get some fuel for growth. The vitamin C is gulped by the cancer cells, then becomes toxic because <u>cancer cells</u>

cannot generate catalase to protect themselves against the hydrogen peroxide generated by vitamin C.[6]

Dozens of very well trained physicians have been giving high doses of intravenous vitamin C (10 to 100 grams daily) to thousands of cancer patients for decades with no side effects, and usually improved outcome.[7] Intravenous vitamin C seems to have selective anti-cancer activity, according to an article in the *Annals of Internal Medicine* (Apr.6, 2004, p.533), authored by several doctors including researchers at the National Institutes of Health. IV vitamin C supports cancer patients in many well documented pathways.[8] Dr. Hugh Riordan reported improved outcome in poor prognostic cancer patients who have been put in remission through use of high dose IV vitamin C.

COMPREHENSIVE CANCER TREATMENT INCLUDES:

1	2	3
change underlying cause(s) of disease	restrained tumor debulking	symptom management
NUTRITION	CHEMO?	PAIN**
DETOXIFICATION	RADIATION?	NAUSEA
DYSBIOSIS	SURGERY?	ANOREXIA
HORMONE BAL.	IV Vit C	ANEMIA
HYPERGLYCEMIA	CURCUMIN	LEUKOPENIA
INFECTIONS	Oxygen/OZONE	DEPRESSION
STRESS	BURZYNSKI	CACHEXIA
EXERCISE	HYPERTHERM	HAIR LOSS
ENERGY PATHWAYS	ALKALINIZE	
ETC.	PEMF	
	HERBALS	

Vitamin C supplements can be helpful in slowing cancer, while making medical therapy more of a selective toxin against the cancer and protecting healthy host tissue.

Don't take your vitamin C supplements--unless you want to live longer.

For more information on how your body can fight cancer go to GettingHealthier.com.

PATIENT PROFILE: SPIRIT OVER NUTRIENTS

H.G. was a fun-loving, guy who enjoyed cigarettes, wine, and a good laugh. He developed prostate cancer with bone metastasis while in his mid 50s. His doctor said: "Get your affairs in order." H.G. went to a psycho-neuroimmunology clinic to help him use his mind as a healing tool in his advanced untreatable cancer. He felt that he had been burdened with an endless procession of responsibilities, from high school to the Marines, to a profession, family, and more. He wanted to be free of all of this. He left his wife and his cancer went into remission. Meanwhile, his wife, B.G. was a non-smoker, drank very little, hiked, was in good shape, and ate a very good diet. One year after H.G. left her, B.G. developed advanced brain cancer and died within 6 weeks of diagnosis. Nutrition is an important factor in cancer outcome. But as a nutritionist, I must admit that what you are eating is not as important as what's eating you--as H.G. and his wife illustrated.

ENDNOTES

[1] https://www.amazon.com/Complete-Guide-Alternative-Cancer-Treatment/dp/1467515248/ref=sr_1_2?dchild=1&keywords=the+complete+guide+to+alternative+cancer+treatment&qid=1598897705&sr=8-2

[2] https://www.amazon.com/Truth-about-Cancer-Treatment-Prevention/dp/1401952259/ref=sr_1_3?dchild=1&keywords=ty+bollinger&qid=1598897858&sr=8-3

[3] http://ar.iiarjournals.org/content/29/3/809.short

[4] https://www.cmaj.ca/content/174/7/937?sid=c4b05

[5] https://journals.plos.org/plosone/article/file?type=printable&id=10.1371/journal.pone.0011414

[6] https://www.ncbi.nlm.nih.gov/pmc/articles/PMC5106370/

[7] https://www.ncbi.nlm.nih.gov/pubmed/15068981

[8] https://www.ncbi.nlm.nih.gov/pmc/articles/PMC5927785/

Chapter 26

BEATING CANCER SYMPTOMS

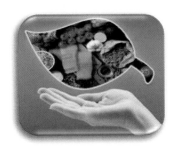

"What cancer cannot do: It cannot cripple love, or shatter hope, or corrode faith, or destroy peace, or kill friendship, or suppress memories, or silence courage, or invade the soul, or steal eternal life, or conquer the Spirit."
anonymous, from Ann Landers column

For many cancer patients, the side effects can be worse than facing a life-threatening disease. This concise guide may help to minimize many of the complications from cancer or the cytotoxic treatment.

At the very least, the cancer patient should have appropriate palliative care. No one should struggle with pain, depression, insomnia, and other common symptoms from cancer treatment. Seek help. Pain management doctors are trained to make your passage through cancer more tolerable.

BEATING CANCER SYMPTOMS

SYMPTOMS	ALLOPATHIC	NATUROPATHIC
NAUSEA	Zofran, Compazine	enzymes, ginger, acupressure wrist band, acupuncture
VOMITING	Phenergan, Tigan	suck on ice cubes, yogurt, ginger tea or caps, ginger ale, acupuncture
ANOREXIA	Megace, Marinol	enzymes, small meals, ginger, dining with others, zinc, B vitamins
MALNUTRITION	TPN, Advera, Impact	hydrazine sulfate, Dragon Slayer shake, enzymes, high protein meals
DIARRHEA	Lomotil, Imodium, Questran	yogurt, probiotics, SeaCure, glutamine, milk enemas, Pepto Bismol, acupuncture,blueberries
MALDIGESTION	enzymes, Hcl, Pancrease	SeaCure, enzymes, probiotics, betaine HCl, ginger, mustard, Zymarine
LYMPHEDEMA		lymph drainage therapy (iahe.com), rebounder (trampoline), massage, topical castor oil
CONSTIPATION	Senacote, Milk Magnesia, Mag Citrate, glycerin suppositories	probiotics,psyllium,Perfect7,sena, buckthorn,cascara sagrada, epsom salts,fiber, water, walking, aloe
GAS	Phyzeme, Propulsid, Reglan, Zantac	enzymes, probiotics, soil-based organisms, ginger, mustard, onions, walking; avoid beans, nuts, broccoli
ANEMIA	Epogen, Procrit (erythropoietin)	liquid liver extract, B-12, B-6, chelated iron supplements, folate, copper, beet juice, shark liver oil

LEUKOPENIA	Newpogen	ImmunoPower, PCM4, ImmKin, bovine cartilage, garlic, ginseng, propolis, olive leaf, shark liver oil, echinecea, vit. C, E, A, betacarotene, selenium, zinc, colloidal silver, astragalus, colostrum, golden seal, ginkgo
HAIR LOSS		1600 iu vit.E 1-2 weeks prior to beginning chemo, aloe, vit.D ointment
FATIGUE	Megace, antidepressants i.e. Prozac	B vit., B-12 sublingual, ginseng, mahuang , bee pollen, chromium, DHEA, caffeine from tea, high protein diet
ORAL MUCOSITIS	Mylanta, Maalox, Zylocaine Benadryl, Nystatin	vit.E oil from capsule topically applied 3x daily with cotton swab, prophylactic antioxidants
YEAST INFECTIONS	Diflucan, Ketoconazole, Sporonox, Amphotericin, Vitrex, Nystatin, DMSO with diflucan	grapefruit seed extract, topical Australian tea tree oil, garlic, undecenoic acid (castor), caprylic acid, MCT, probiotics, biotin, Essiac tea, vaginal suppository of gentian violet or boric acid capsules
DEPRESSION	Prozac, etc.	St. John's wort, SAMe, TMG, tryptophan, niacinamide sunlight, ginkgo, DHEA except for hormonal cancers
ANXIETY	Xanax, Ativan	hops, valerian, kava, homeopathic, 5HTP
INSOMNIA	Ambien, Xanax	melatonin, 5HTP, kava, hops, valerian
PAIN	Tylenol, morphine, colchicine	acupuncture, hypnosis, magnets, white willow, DL phenylalanine

Chapter 27

PARTING COMMENTS

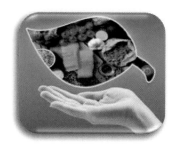

"Unless we put medical freedom into the Constitution, the time will come when medicine will organize itself into an undercover dictatorship."
Dr. Benjamin Rush, signer of the Declaration of Independence, 1776

From my cancer patients I have learned of the incredible tenacity of the human body and spirit. Of the immeasurable dignity and generosity that is waiting to be expressed by all of us. Of the undying passion and commitment shown by a dedicated mate when a loved one is failing. And above all-of the preciousness of life. In our increasingly callous world, it is easy to drift away from the true pleasures in life: love, family, friends, enthusiasm, laughter, freedom, meaningful work, skills developed, helping one another, and savoring the beauty in this emerald paradise planet. For many people, cancer has become the ultimate "truth serum" in helping them to establish real priorities.

While the scope of the book is to offer helpful advice on using nutrition to improve outcome in cancer treatment, there are some fundamental flaws in the structure of our health care system and governmental surveillance that impair our ability to investigate and use rational cancer treatments.

In many states, chemotherapy, radiation, and surgery are the only LEGAL options for cancer patients. Physicians have lost their licenses and even gone to jail for venturing outside the narrow confines of this allopathic model for cancer. There are 7 states in the U.S. that have passed an AMTA bill, or Access to Medical Treatment

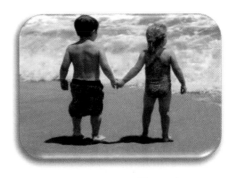

Act, meaning the licensed health care professional can offer whatever therapies the doctor and the patient agree to be appropriate. Such freedom is desperately needed if we are to truly win the war on cancer.

Strongly encourage all Americans to voice your opinion with your representative in state and federal legislatures regarding the need for more freedom and options in cancer treatment. Why do cancer patients have to leave the country or visit some "underground" clinic to seek alternative cancer treatment?

FIND A "CO-PATIENT" TO HELP YOU

Cancer is a difficult disease to treat. And it gets even more difficult to overcome when you are doing it all on your own. Find a "co-patient" to help. Someone who has faith, hope, and sense of humor, and encourages you. Spend as much time as you can with that person. It could be a spouse, family member, friend, neighbor, or member of your church or synagogue. Tell him or her that they will get as much out of this journey together as you, the patient, will receive. Bask in the glow of their enthusiasm and optimism. I find that cancer patients who have a "co-patient" are much more likely to beat the odds.

HARNESSING THE HEALING CAPACITY WITHIN YOU

Every day around the world there are about 8 million lightning strikes, each carrying about 1 billion volts of electrical energy. Your body consists of 37 trillion cells, each conducting about 100,000 chemical reactions per second. Nature is extraordinary in its power and orchestration. There are miracles happening in and around all of us. The quest of

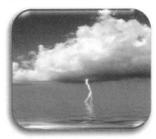

this book is to harness your internal healing capacity. The power of Nature to heal you from within.

A healthy human body is self-regulating and self-repairing. Embrace the lightning power of healing that is within you.

MAKING A DIAMOND OUT OF COAL

You are the pro-active and assertive cancer victor. You have been through some or all of the phases that come with the disease: anger, denial, rejection, isolation, fear, depression, withdrawal, and more. While the bulk of this book is spent providing nutritional facts to change the biochemistry of your body, my final parting comments are directed more at your soul, because cancer is a disease of the mind, body, and spirit.

Today, we wage full-scale chemical warfare on ourselves with potent agricultural and industrial carcinogens, while stripping our once-benevolent food supply of any vestige of nutritional value. We are subjected to intolerable stress from work and dissolving family structures, thousands of murders per year on TV and movies, and an endless procession of gut-wrenching stories on the nightly news.

Nourish your body, mind, and spirit. Take every opportunity to say: "I love you." Give away smiles with reckless abandon. Practice random acts of kindness and beauty. Savor each day as though it may be your last, because the same holds true for all of us. You have the opportunity to be born again with a renewed vigor and purpose in life.

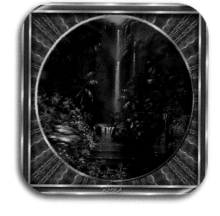

A diamond is nothing more than a piece of coal that was put under a lot of pressure. Make the cancer treatment process a transformation for you from a piece of coal to a diamond.

My prayer for you is the same thought that began this book--that you will soon be able to say: "Cancer is the best thing that ever happened to me." Make your life into a masterpiece painting.

PATIENT PROFILES: COMPARING 3 CASES OF MULTIPLE MYELOMA

Multiple myeloma: a relatively rare and poor prognostic cancer in which cancer cells crowd out the healthy cells in the bone marrow.

J.H. was a 41-year old white male diagnosed with multiple myeloma in 2001. JH had a consultation with PQ in which we discussed lifestyle changes, including diet and nutrition supplements. JH worked with his doctor on medical therapies for his condition. JH went into remission, was able to re-establish his pilot's license, continue to work as an attorney, and bestselling fiction author. JH had an excellent quality of life for the next 14 years, at which he went into a steep decline and died.

K.Q. was a 41-year old white male diagnosed with multiple myeloma in 1999. PQ worked with KQ to provide guidelines for lifestyle changes, including nutrition and supplements. KQ's oncologist said: "If you take any of these supplements, then I will not work with you." KQ died 18 months later with his wife pregnant with twins.

Michael Gearin-Tosh was a white male Oxford professor who was diagnosed with multiple myeloma in 1994 at the age of 54. He was told that he would die soon without conventional therapy. MGT took a different route for his therapies, including using Beating Cancer with Nutrition, intravenous vitamin C, high dose nutrition supplements, and more. MGT went into remission and lived another 11 years before passing away in 2005. Dr. Gearin-Tosh wrote a book, LIVING PROOF, A MEDICAL MUTINY to detail his journey toward wellness for longer than anyone expected.

For more information about
Beating Cancer with Nutrition
And
Patrick Quillin, PhD,RD,CNS

BCN   BeatingCancerwithNutrition.com

PQ   PatrickQuillin.com

Facebook: PatrickQuillinPhD

Linked In: Dr Patrick Quillin PhD RD CNS

Instagram: #drpatrickquillin

Twitter: @QuillinPatrick

YouTube: DrPatrickQuillinPhDRDCNS

Pinterest: PatrickQuillin PhD

Robert F. Miller - I read this book 18 years ago and still use it today!
In 1996 I was diagnosed with stage 3 pancreatic cancer. I was given the option of a Whipple (surgery), chemo and radiation. I did all three. After the surgery the "doctors" gave me no chance of survival as they discovered the cancer had migrated into my lymph system. During the chemo and radiation I was introduced to Patrick Quillin's book which became my food and nutrition bible then and as it is today. I followed everything in his book. Once it appeared that the cancer was gone I asked each doctor who had attended me if they would take credit for the fact I was still alive? Each one answered with an emphatic NO! To this day I still follow the nutrition protocols I learned from Patrick Quillin's book! Believe me it is never too late to change your lifestyle and diet.

Ronald Brown - My wife actually HAS beat cancer and she did it ...
My wife actually HAS beat cancer and she did it without Chemo or Radiation. She did it the Natural Way and this book is a wealth of information

Linda Thiessen - Restoration of life!!
This book is a true testimony of hope, incentive, and fact. I was diagnosed with uterine cancer that had metastasized. I went through the surgery to debulk the tumor and out-lying tissue. Through my protocol I'm doing much better and picking up strength and energy every day. Thank you so much for the enlightened encouragement and hope!!

Elizabeth – Excellent Book, A Must Read!!!
Words could not express the amount of gratitude I have for the author of this book. My mother was diagnosed with lung cancer three months ago. I started stuffing her with veggies and fruits, etc. as the book recommends (among other things). Upon her follow up appointment with the doctor her blood work was much better. I HIGHLY recommend this book to patients and loved ones facing cancer. Together, you CAN beat it.

Maureen Yorke – Excellent and Empowering
As an RD for 20 years, a former Oncology Nutritionist and a breast cancer survivor, I have bought so many copies of this book and given them away, I can't even count. Excellent resource, and empowering.... it is another tool that I use to stay healthy.